ACTION ON AIDS

Recent Titles in
Contributions in Medical Studies

"Hydropathic Highway to Health": Women and Water-Cure in Antebellum
America
Jane B. Donegan

The American Midwife Debate: A Sourcebook on Its Modern Origins
Judy Barrett Litoff

Planning for the Nation's Health: A Study of Twentieth-Century Developments in
the United States
Grace Budrys

Essays of Robert Koch
K. Codell Carter, translator

Photographing Medicine: Images and Power in Britain and America since 1840
Daniel M. Fox and Christopher Lawrence

The Tuberculosis Movement: A Public Health Campaign in the Progressive Era
Michael E. Teller

Families and the Gravely Ill: Roles, Rules, and Rights
Richard Sherlock and C. Mary Dingus

"Doctors Only": The Evolving Image of the American Physician
Richard Malmsheimer

Disease in the Popular American Press: The Case of Diphtheria, Typhoid Fever,
and Syphilis, 1870–1920
Terra Ziporyn

Biomedical Technology and Public Policy
Robert H. Blank and Miriam K. Mills, editors

Prescriptions: The Dissemination of Medical Authority
Gayle L. Ormiston and Raphael Sassower, editors

ACTION ON AIDS

National Policies in Comparative Perspective

Edited by
BARBARA A. MISZTAL
and
DAVID MOSS

Contributions in Medical Studies, Number 28

GREENWOOD PRESS
New York • Westport, Connecticut • London

Library of Congress Cataloging-in-Publication Data

Action on AIDS : national policies in comparative perspective / edited
by Barbara A. Misztal and David Moss.
    p. cm. — (Contributions in medical studies, ISSN 0886–8220 ;
no. 28)
    Includes bibliographical references.
    ISBN 0–313–26369–8 (lib. bdg. : alk. paper)
    1. AIDS (Disease)—Government policy—Comparative studies.
I. Misztal, Barbara A. II. Moss, David, 1946–   . III. Series.
RA644.A25A274   1990
362.1'9697'92—dc20   89–26034

British Library Cataloguing in Publication Data is available.

Library of Congress Catalog Card Number: 89–26034
ISBN: 0–313–26369–8
ISSN: 0886–8220

First published in 1990

Greenwood Press, 88 Post Road West, Westport, CT   06881
An imprint of Greenwood Publishing Group, Inc.

Printed in the United States of America

The paper used in this book complies with the
Permanent Paper Standard issued by the National
Information Standards Organization (Z39.48–1984).

10 9 8 7 6 5 4 3 2 1

Contents

Illustrations

ACTION ON AIDS

1   David Moss and Barbara A. Misztal

Introduction

Emergencies commonly reveal the disorder from which routine order is painfully extracted. They dramatize social fissures, inconsistencies, and ignorance that ordinarily remain hidden or can be ignored without damage or controversy. They transform the taken for granted into the up for discussion, compel the formation of decisions and accompanying justifications, and demand action of a special and urgent kind. To a world hardly short of such emergencies has recently been added "AIDS," an acronym formally designating the most developed stage of HIV infection but misleadingly used in our lexicon of public concern to stand for the disease as a whole. The scale and likely duration of the emergency are not yet even approximately clear. If the gloomiest predictions on the spread of the virus, the progression from asymptomatic infection to early death, and the difficulty of producing an effective vaccine turn out to be accurate, the past decade will turn out merely to be the first of many. If, instead, the most optimistic assertions about the scale and efficiency of scientific, educational, and behavioral responses are accurate, then the acquired immune deficiency syndrome will sooner rather than later join cholera, smallpox, and leprosy as an endemic disease, devastating to some individuals in some places but no longer a social, political, and medical drama. Although the unexpected collapse of one regime has already been attributed to AIDS, the political, social, and economic consequences of the epidemic are yet to be revealed.[1]

Because it is now commonplace to define the spread and consequences of AIDS as a *global* emergency, the light thrown by the disease onto the fragmented, incoherent, and unknown aspects of our social order takes on an international dimension. The senses in which AIDS has become a global phenomenon are straightforward and need no laboring. First, cases of the disease have now been reported from all continents and a steadily increasing number of countries. By the first designated World AIDS Day, 1 December 1988, the World Health Organization (WHO) indicated that 124,114 cases had been notified from 142 countries, that somewhere between 5 and 10 million people had already been infected by HIV, and that roughly 1 million new AIDS cases could be expected by 1992. Second, AIDS is a global issue insofar as the ordinary indifference of viruses to national frontiers is aggravated by the long latency period of HIV and its unwitting dissemination in the wake of international mobility for business, educational, and recreational purposes. Similarly, although increasingly less significantly for participants from the developed world, the international trade in blood and blood products that may carry the virus establishes a channel of reciprocal national concern. Third, the management of the disease requires, now and for the foreseeable future, the distribution around the world-system of many different kinds of resources, most of them exceedingly costly by the primary recipients' standards: the technical apparatus of research, diagnosis, treatment, and prevention (cell-lines, test kits, condoms, drugs), specialized health advisers and personnel, funds for local prevention programs, and the publications and conferences disseminating knowledge about the disease itself. Finally, AIDS is an international issue insofar as it has rapidly become a focus of intervention by international agencies, both global (WHO) and regional (Council of Europe).

Emphasis has lain on the interdependence of nations in managing a common health emergency, oriented by a standardized set of guidelines for response procedures and united in the effort to eliminate a disease traceable to a (controversially located) single point of origin.[2] Underlining the shared features of the epidemic, however, risks obscuring the extent to which, viewed comparatively, "the AIDS problem" is also a heterogeneous collection of national problems manufactured from the very different understandings, epidemiological profiles, management strategies, and economic consequences of a (broadly similar) viral pathology. This book is an attempt to capture those differences by describing the responses to AIDS in nine countries over its first eight years of incidence. Comparative analysis of health issues is not common in the social sciences and has been almost entirely absent in discussion of AIDS.[3] Our ambition is not to add to the programmatic calls for what might or could or should be done. Rather, by examining what *has* been done, we aim to contribute to the understanding of why, in different kinds of political systems, confronted by different epidemiological profiles of AIDS and displaying contrasting mixes of state, market, and community responsibilities in managing public issues, deliberate choices to act, or to refuse to act, were made. In the rest of this chapter we identify some of the common constraints shaping the responses of the principal actors (governments and local authorities, medical professionals, people with AIDS, voluntary organizations). The body of the book is taken up with the single-country chapters, which examine national sequences of actions and controversies up until late 1988. In the "Conclusion" we compare the most salient features of those responses and offer some suggestions as to how they might best be explained.

RESPONDING TO WHAT?

It can hardly be stressed too strongly that most policies on AIDS throughout the period this book covers have had to be designed and executed in conditions characterized at best by extreme uncertainty and at worst by plain ignorance. Clearly that dimension has not always been—and, in circumstances when rapid action is desired, cannot always be—acknowledged in the public domain. The absence or limitation of knowledge has permitted convictions and nostrums as strident in their claims to truth as they are poorly founded in fact. More subtly, the extent of ignorance has been disguised by recourse to richly metaphorical, and varyingly inappropriate, descriptors from previous epidemics—a creative technique that has been imaginatively, if not in all details convincingly, explored by Susan Sontag.[4] But previous epidemics, of which those metaphors were once literal descriptions, do not provide a simple history lesson for direct application to management of HIV infection, as historians have pointed out.[5] The pathology and transmission routes of HIV are very different from those of cholera, plague, and smallpox; contemporary political and scientific institutions are immeasurably more powerful than their pre-twentieth-century predecessors; and the contemporary understandings of privacy, freedom from discrimination, and civil liberty have drastically transformed the constraints on responses, even by comparison with the thinkable options for confronting the cholera epidemics of the nineteenth century. The past is indeed another country for AIDS; and knowledge of its terrain offers very limited guidance for us now.

Mutability and uncertainty characterize all aspects of the AIDS problem, from the level of the pathogen itself, to its clinical description, to its distribution over time in human populations. Investigations of HIV suggest that its strains are highly variable and its structure highly mutable, even within the body of an individual patient. Indeed, the medical prehistorians of AIDS are currently divided on the length of time that HIV has inhabited human beings: Has it been present for no more than a century in small groups in Africa, whose social isolation in remote areas limited the scope of infection, or benignly occupying the human body for centuries and turned lethal only by the pathogenic side effects of changes in sexual mores, in both more and less developed worlds after 1945, and the formation of a critical mass of promiscuous carriers to ensure its widespread dissemination?[6] The evasiveness and complexity of HIV have damaging implications for the tasks of devising effective drug therapies and vaccines and thus emphasize the urgency of the need to restrict and police known transmission routes through individual behavioral change and effective public response. So, beyond the current scientific uncertainties about the nature of HIV pathology, it is worth emphasizing the twin features of instability and diversity in the public identification of the phenomenon to which response is made: the changing definitions provided by the most influential source of definitions, the Centers for Disease Control (CDC), and the shifting contrasts in patterns of transmission routes in different countries.

The definition of AIDS and the procedures for its identification have been progressively expanded since the name AIDS was first established in late 1982. The acronym freed the disease from association with the social category indicated explicitly by its immediate predecessor, the Gay Related Immune Disease (GRID), and euphemistically by its synonyms, ACIDS (Acquired Community Immune Deficiency Syndrome) and CAIDS (Community Acquired Immune Deficiency Syndrome).[7] The initial definition of AIDS by the Centers for Disease Control was restrictive, marking the disease simply by the presence of Kaposi's sarcoma and a few opportunistic diseases, notably *pneumocystis carinii pneumonia* (PCP). The scientific consensus on a single viral cause for the syndrome, eventually unifying the (French) LAV and (American) HTLV-3 designations as HIV, led the CDC in 1985 to refine its definition for national reporting, essentially by extending the range of opportunistic diseases regarded as indicative of AIDS for patients who had tested seropositive. In 1987 the CDC revised its definition once more to take account of new knowledge about the course and consequences of HIV infection: the list of diseases indicative of AIDS was further increased, and presumptive, rather than laboratory, diagnoses for those indicator diseases were accepted.

Despite the claim that the revisions would have little effect on retrospective figures and prospective reporting, the findings from local studies that have compared the use of the definitions suggest otherwise. Cases deriving from all types of transmission routes show substantially increased numbers. In San Francisco, primarily among the gay community, the revised definition increased the number of reported AIDS cases by 19 percent; a multicenter reexamination of hemophiliac records across the United States produced a 22 percent increase; among ivdu (intravenous drug-using) cases in Spain an increase of 16.7 percent was recorded, and nearly half (43.6 percent) of the 10,747 ivdu-associated AIDS cases reported to the CDC in 1988 would not have met the pre-1987 case definition for the disease.[8] Apart from marking the uncertain scope of the syndrome, shifts in the definition of AIDS have direct practical implications for forecasting and response—implications that are likely to be rendered more uncertain by the yet-to-be-traced pathogenicity of a related HIV virus, named HIV-2, discovered in West Africa in 1985.

Directly related to the synchronic difficulties of identifying the syndrome is the task of diachronic identification of the stages marking the progress of HIV infection and the rates of progress of infected patients through them. In 1986 the CDC reaggregated the previous penumbra of diseases (AIDS, AIDS Related Complex, lymphadenopathy syndrome) into a linear classification marked by four major stages into which patients could fall according to the clinical expression of disease. In the following year a specific scheme to apply to children of up to 13 years, who had not been easily incorporated into the classes designed for adult patients, was established. Although competing classifications—notably the Walter Reed staging classification—had already been developed, the WHO and most of its membership adopted the CDC proposal. While it is accepted that to reach a particular stage is an irreversible passage, the inevitability and pace of progression have not yet been clearly established. The initial optimistic assessments that progression from infection to death was the fate of only a small minority of patients have been supplanted by much more sombre estimates, suggesting that since roughly three in every four seropositives will develop AIDS or an AIDS-related condition within six years of infection, "we should regard progression to clinical AIDS after infection with HIV as the norm rather than the exception."[9] The extent to which the chances of progression between successive stages can be deliberately modified by changes in sexual behavior, drug therapies, and self-care is too early to assess. For most countries, therefore, responses have had to be framed without the guidance of clear estimates of the likely course of the disease in individuals and without the possibility of calculating at all accurately the human and financial demands on the medical professions, health systems, and national budgets.

The second set of differences in the publicly identified "AIDS problem" concerns its forms in the developed and less developed worlds. Two dimensions need emphasis. First, the definitions of the disease itself, and the procedures for its recognition, are distinct. The early experience of using the CDC definition in African countries where sophisticated laboratory tests were not possible stimulated the WHO in 1985 to devise a case definition for developing countries based on clinical evidence and maternal history only. Direct comparison between the CDC and WHO definitions, however, has suggested that considerable discrepancies between the cases classifiable as AIDS could develop. In one study 42 percent of the sample of African children who counted as AIDS cases by the CDC definition fell outside the WHO definition.[10] Not only have the difficulties in health services and testing facilities weakened African countries' capacities to assess the actual scale of HIV infection, but the restricted scope of the definition in practical use, compounded by the differences in the set of opportunistic diseases characterizing infection in Africa and the West, has reduced still further the publicly identified dimensions of the epidemic. The implications for the

Table 1.1
Global Distribution of AIDS 1986–1989

Continent	1986*		1989†	
	Cases	Countries reporting	Cases	Countries reporting
Africa	1,069	10	21,322	46
Americas	29,273	33	99,752	42
Asia	68	9	338	23
Europe	3,694	23	19,196	28
Oceania	344	2	1,286	6
TOTAL	34,448	77	141,894	145

Notes: *latest figures reported to WHO at 14 November; †latest figures reported to WHO at 29 February.

Sources: WHO, Weekly Epidemiological Record 61, no. 47 (21 November 1986): 362; WHO, Weekly Epidemiological Record 64, no. 9 (3 March 1989): 61-62.

reliability of estimates, forecasts, and scale of responses—as well as the problems of making effective international comparisons between the rates of incidence of AIDS in countries using different definitions—are clear.

Second, the contrasts in the nature of the AIDS problem are emphasized by a further difference: the significance of particular transmission routes and the social profile of AIDS cases that they generate. From the beginning, of course, uncertainties over the possible paths for HIV transmission, and the relative riskiness of particular routes, have accompanied the development of the epidemic. Not surprisingly, the progressive revelation of categories of infected people, and of the different paths by which the virus had reached them (semen, blood and blood products, infected mothers, bone transplantation), allowed plenty of public speculation about other, about to be definitely confirmed routes. Leaving aside the claims that lacked any shred of evidence, many questions on transmissibility had not been satisfactorily resolved during the 1980s. Could infection be transmitted through saliva in contact with abraded skin? Could women and men transmit the virus to each other with equal ease? What degree of safety was achieved by a substantial reduction in, rather than elimination of, numbers of sexual partners? How risky, relatively, were different sexual practices?

What became clear, as the epidemiological evidence accumulated, were the marked differences between the dominant patterns of transmission in single societies. The numbers of cases reported from all continents between 1986 and 1989 are set out in Table 1.1, which shows both the rapid geographical spread of AIDS (the number of countries reporting cases to the

Table 1.2
Countries Reporting Largest Numbers of AIDS Cases 1986–1989

Continent	1986*		1989†	
	Countries	Cases	Countries	Cases
Africa	Tanzania	462	Uganda	5,508
	Zambia	217	Tanzania	3,055
	Central African Rep	202	Kenya	2,732
	Kenya	101	Malawi	2586
	Uganda	29	Burundi	1,408
Americas	USA	26,566	USA	99,752
	Canada	755	Brazil	4,709
	Brazil	754	Canada	2,196
	Haiti	501	Haiti	1,661
	Mexico	161	Mexico	1,64
Asia	Japan	21	Japan	97
	Israel	6	Israel	76
	Thailand	3	Quatar	21
	Hong Kong	2	Philippines	20
	Turkey	2	Turkey	17
Europe	France	997	France	5,655
	West Germany	715	Italy	3,008
	United Kingdom	510	West Germany	2,885
	Italy	367	Spain	2,165
	Spain	201	United Kingdom	2,049
Oceania	Australia	322	Australia	1,168
	New Zealand	22	New Zealand	104
	-		Papua New Guinea	8
	-		Fr. Polynesia	3
	-		New Caledonia	2

Notes: *latest figures reported to WHO at 14 November; †latest figures reported to WHO
at 29 February.

Sources: WHO, Weekly Epidemiological Record 61, no. 47 (21 November 1986): 362; WHO,
Weekly Epidemiological Record 64, no. 9 (3 March 1989): 61–62.

WHO doubling in little more than two years) and the high rate of increase
in reported cases (a fourfold increase in twenty-seven months).

The rapid increase in diagnoses has been accompanied by changes in the
list of countries reporting the largest absolute numbers of cases. Table 1.2
sets out the five most affected countries for each continent over the same
period, indicating that, with the exception of Oceania, there have been at
least revisions, and sometimes significant replacements, in the hierarchy of
national incidences of the disease.

Three macro-patterns, characterized by their dominant transmission
routes, have been identified by the WHO to simplify the global incidence
of AIDS.[11] Pattern 1 is distinguished by transmission primarily through gay

and intravenous drug-using (ivdu) groups and characterizes the industrial-ized nations: the Americas (North and South), Western Europe, and Aus-tralia. Pattern 2 is marked by heterosexual transmission, shows roughly equal incidence among men and women, and is principally to be found in sub-Saharan Africa and the Caribbean. Pattern 3 is a residual category, indicating countries into which infection has primarily been introduced from outside through sexual contact or blood products and which have only a small, but perhaps growing, behavioral base for local reproduction: Eastern Europe, North Africa, the Middle East, Asia, and the Pacific area outside Australia and New Zealand.

Two features of that tripartite classification need to be brought out before it can serve as an accurate guide to the specific versions of the AIDS problem to which the nations in the respective categories had to respond. First, it conceals very different epidemiological profiles of AIDS within single pat-terns. Among Pattern 1 countries, for example, Australia and Italy in mid-1988 show contrasting extremes of dominance by, respectively, gays (87 percent of all cases) and ivdus (64 percent of cases). The locally most salient transmission route is thus quite distinct, although it is not yet explained; and it offers not only different prognostic uncertainties but also partly discrete bundles of problems for micro-management. Moreover, the causes and patterns of infection even within those two categories are far from clear, leaving uncertain the importance of the virus' transmission by both sexes among promiscuous ivdus (relative to shared contaminated equipment) and between predominantly homosexual and heterosexual communities through full bisexuals.

Second, the changing international and domestic location of infection must be emphasized in order to capture the significant contours of AIDS. As Table 1.1 shows, while the United States continues to contribute the largest single number of national cases, the rate of increase among the African countries of Pattern 2 is much the most rapid. In the continent as a whole a twentyfold increase in cases was recorded for the years 1986–1988 alone, and the representation of African countries in the ten most affected nations doubled from two (Tanzania, Zambia) to four (Uganda, Tanzania, Kenya, Malawi). No doubt the exceptional increase in cases is to be attributed to better detection and reporting as well as to the progression to full AIDS by patients who had been silently infected earlier than in the West. Nevertheless, it remains likely that HIV infection is in fact more extensive and progressing more rapidly in Pattern 2 than in Pattern 1 coun-tries, not least because of the dominance of the transmission route between heterosexuals.

The shift in the international location of infection toward the less devel-oped world appears to be accompanied by a parallel shift toward the poorer and more socially disadvantaged groups in the developed world. In the United States, for example, blacks and Hispanics, especially in poor urban areas, contribute disproportionately to the profile of AIDS cases:[12] similar increases in the concentration of AIDS in relatively more deprived social groups and regions are reported or anticipated for several countries covered in this book. It seems likely that the progressive drift downwards in the social order is associated both with the growing significance of the ivdu transmission route in the developed world and with the greater difficulties of reducing the risks of infection among its participants by comparison with the gay community. Expansion of that path will steadily expose to infection hitherto relatively less affected social categories, notably women, and will therefore lead to a further recharacterization of the problem and the appropriate responses.[13] AIDS may have been first recognized in its guise as the scourge of an affluent, choice-exercising, rapidly mobilizable social group in some of the richest communities in the world; it may yet finish as one more lethal determinant of restricted life-chances among the relatively and absolutely unfree.

In sum, the context for policy formation on AIDS was marked by scientific uncertainties and controversies, continuing redefinition of the scope of the syndrome, and epidemiological evidence pointing to changes in the centers and dominant transmission routes of HIV. The controversies have of course been continuously refuelled by the flood of information. The years 1982–1988 have been marked by a probably unprecedented concentration of effort to reduce the lack of knowledge and to disseminate internationally the results of research. Four international conferences on AIDS were held between 1985 and 1988, the last drawing several thousand presentations; 1,414 references to the acquired immune deficiency syndrome had been registered on Medline between 1983 and 1986; and no fewer than twelve current international journals, newsletters, and bibliographic updates are devoted exclusively to AIDS.[14] Those advances in the scientific knowledge of AIDS pathology have, however, simultaneously revealed our effective ignorance about the social aspects of risk-increasing behaviors and the consequences of the postwar lack of concern to fund investigations into behavioral research on sexually transmitted diseases.[15] In all societies the dimensions, forms, and social distribution of sexual preference and activity remain almost entirely uncharted, as do the patterns of involvement in intravenous drug use. The difficulties of acquiring that sort of information, and the extent of micro-surveillance required to ensure its reliability, increase still further the uncertainties in selecting appropriate responses to AIDS. They also indicate clearly one set of reasons for the inevitability of ethical and legal controversy over positive proposals for intervention.

DILEMMAS OF RESPONSE

Given that the single continuing certainty about HIV infection has been the lack of any cure, responses in different nations can be placed according to the ways in which they have chosen to deal with the only partly known. Perhaps the fundamental dilemma pits the achievement of sufficiently speedy interventions against the engendering of fear and mistrust by too hasty and dramatic a response. Ideally, appreciation of the need for rapid action is matched by consensus from all sections of the population on specific measures. Realistically, the nature, urgency, and resolution of the problem look different to different groups, no matter how apparently monolithic civil society and how authoritarian the political regime. The array of measures actually debated, adopted, or rejected reflects a fragile, continually renegotiated compromise between, on one hand, taking, and encouraging others to take, actions demanded by the current knowledge on HIV transmissibility to manage present cases of infection and to prevent future ones and, on the other, avoiding responses that are ineffective now and that encourage the infected to distrust all health care and information-gathering institutions. The particular issues that enable us to compare national responses can be grouped under three broad headings: the policing of national boundaries; the policing of internal transmission routes; and the education of specific and general populations. We will deal with each in turn.

The first dilemma of response concerns the policing of the traffic of human beings and vehicles of infection (notably blood and blood products) across national frontiers. In the knowledge that not all HIV carriers can be picked up through testing (since antibodies may appear some months after infection) and that infection cannot be established by even a close lay inspection, governments can theoretically consider all options between banning entry to all foreigners, nationals living abroad, and contaminable products and maintaining whatever open-door policy is currently in place. In practice, among the countries that have introduced new regulations, the nature of boundary reinforcement has varied quite widely. Perhaps the most drastic forms have surfaced in South Africa and India. In South Africa migrant workers from the frontline states who are infected with HIV are being deported after the introduction of compulsory screening for black immigrant workers.[16] In India, in addition to the refusal of enrollment to foreign students without an HIV clearance certificate and the mandatory testing of all visitors who intend to stay for more than three months, the Indian Council of Medical Research has proposed that sexual relations with any foreigner be made a criminal offense carrying a fine and prison sentence.[17] Other countries have also marked out foreign contacts for special surveillance but in less extreme ways. Many North African and Middle East societies (Algeria, Iraq, Morocco, Syria) have made compulsory the testing of all returning nationals; the Soviet Union tests foreign students and selected other citizens; China has banned the import of blood products and limited the occasions on which its citizens can meet foreigners; and many countries, including the United States, insist on all immigrants being tested for HIV, thus adding one further test to the routine medical check commonly demanded of all long-term visitors.[18]

Whatever general pressures there may be to externalize the primary source of pollution, no general trend toward autarchy has occurred beyond the precautions of requiring evidence of an HIV-negative test. The temptation to use clearly punitive measures against foreigners to convince domestic populations that their health is the primary governmental concern has been generally resisted, perhaps not least because of the obvious costs. Good relations with the countries affected by any ban may be put at risk; tourist income (amounting in Tanzania, for example, to the second largest source of foreign revenue) and an essential supply of migrant labor may be forfeited; and academic and professional staff may decide not to go abroad for essential training or may not return. In the case of blood products, since Western countries can hardly afford to do without the nonnational supply, the development of an accurate test by 1985 has provided a convenient local method to eliminate whatever contaminated quantities had not been picked up by testing at the point of donation. To ensure that the blood supply is indeed entirely safe has been one of the principal objectives of the WHO Global Program.

More significant in controlling the spread of disease, and certainly more controversial, is the gamut of measures to track and eliminate HIV infection within national borders. The issues that they raise include some of the enduring problems in the control of public health, which have been given renewed life by the distinctive pathology of AIDS and—in most of the countries described in this book—by contemporary legal and moral aspects of privacy and social diversity. In most countries, too, the combination of democratic politics and saturation by the mass media has ensured wide publicity for the range of opinions on the issues and their resolution. The familiar principal dilemma concerns the balance of obligations toward the infected and toward the community at large. As Walters puts it: "How can we control the epidemic and the harm that it causes without unjustly discriminating against particular social groups and without unnecessarily infringing on the freedom of individuals?"[19] The question poses itself at every point in the sequence from tracking the infection to dealing with the particular cases detected to deciding on the methods to secure desired consequences.

Since HIV infection is publicly invisible yet privately transmissible in its early—perhaps prolonged—stages in individuals, the identification of the virus in carriers can only be to some degree invasive. Merely registering diagnosed AIDS cases entails the certainty of permitting exactly the kind of silent spread of HIV that occurred in the late 1970s; no country where an AIDS case has been recorded has failed at least to discuss doing something more. Since the procedure for the detection of HIV antibodies became commercially available in 1985, the obvious technique has been to test individuals and to screen entire groups. The choices present themselves in sequence. Should the test be administered to individuals, specific groups, or entire populations? Should it be administered (1) only with explicit consent, (2) as an unspecified component of a set of tests to which an individual gives overall, but unspecific, consent, (3) as a condition for admission of an individual to some further benefit, or (4) without consent? Should the testing be anonymous or confidential? Should it be administered once, twice (after the necessary interval to allow for cases of very recent infection without antibodies at the first test), or regularly?

The public health objectives that inform choices at each of those points are essentially two: the gathering of reliable and full data to inform research, predictions, and policy, and the detection of infection to inform carriers and allow an active response for their own benefit and for the protection of others. Achievement of both objectives is of course limited, and may be undermined by the practical possibilities of carrying out tests, by the legal status of behavior likely to encourage infection, and by the beliefs among target groups who recognize themselves as such that participation will bring benefits but no harm to themselves or valued others. Not surprisingly, therefore, as the chapters below show, decisions on the use of the test and the particular circumstances for its use display a wide range of variation. The effects on participation probably vary equally, as no doubt does the relative efficacy of adopting one set of procedures rather than another for its administration.[20] None of our cases shows a refusal to make use of the test at all. But none has gone as far as Cuba, which, having decided to test the entire national population as well as foreigners staying for more than three months, had tested 3.23 million Cubans (31 percent of the entire population) by December 1988, identified 264 seropositives, and confined them all to a special sanatorium for life.[21] The specific decisions over subjects to be tested (everyone requesting it, drug addicts receiving public treatment, pregnant women, applicants for marriage licenses, patients in hospitals, members of the armed forces, prison inmates, and so on) vary considerably: in some cases early decisions to enforce the test on particular groups, for example mandatory premarital testing in Louisiana, have already been found to be costly and probably counterproductive and have therefore been reversed.[22] Moreover, the demands of medical and paramedical organizations to permit verification of the degree of risk their members must run in operations and hospital care have added increasingly vocal and powerful support for the routine testing of everyone crossing hospital thresholds.

Once seropositive individuals have been identified, a further set of choices presents itself, concerning not only the individuals themselves but also their known sexual or needle-sharing partners. Should the cases of seropositivity be made notifiable, as AIDS cases are in many—but not all—countries? Should notifiability include the patient's name and address or be anonymous? Should the infected themselves be isolated and compelled to submit to compulsory treatment of some kind—perhaps in trials for experimental drugs? Should their partners be notified, either by the infected case ("patient referral") or by health officials ("provider referral")?[23] If HIV carriers are unwilling to inform their partners themselves, should they be held legally liable for failure, or should the task of informing those at immediate risk pass obligatorily to doctors and health administrators? Should partners be compelled to undergo an HIV test or be quarantined for a specific period to permit confirmation or exclusion of their infection? What conditions should govern the future interaction of infected people with their partners— explicit admission of HIV status to partners, prohibition on (sc. eventual legal accountability for) sexual practices of a risky kind, a ban on all further sexual activity? In different countries those issues for decision are raised or remain dormant, arouse passionate controversy or wide consensus, pass swiftly into law or return ceaselessly to haunt the debating fora of politicians, medical professionals and people at particular risk. In each case the practical responses to those questions, necessarily entailing a ranking of the perceived interests of infected, likely to become infected, and potentially infectable individuals, will influence the course of the epidemic itself. According to the decisions taken, trust between the differently positioned categories will be maintained or destroyed, the traces of infection rendered as visible as possible or driven underground, and knowledge at individual or epidemiological levels increase or diminish in life-saving or lethal ways.

Finally, decisions on the methods to be used in securing the desired outcomes of the above options need to be confronted. Essentially the choice has lain between persuasion through education and obligation through law. Positive use may be made of the law in several directions. First, AIDS may simply be declared to fall under existing disease legislation and its panoply of rights and obligations. Sweden, for example, declared AIDS a sexually transmitted disease in November 1985, placing an obligation on people who believe they may be infected to consult a doctor, who must examine them and report positive results to the health authorities. One consequence of AIDS has indeed been to reveal that in many countries extensive legal powers to deal with health emergencies lay largely forgotten on the statute books and could simply be applied without modification.[24] Second, the behavior of people diagnosed as HIV-positive or suffering from AIDS may be brought specifically under legal sanction, so that deviation may result in house arrest or compulsory detention in (special sections of) prisons or camps. In Cuba and Korea, for example, the prevention strategy has determined that all seropositives be isolated; in West Australia, HIV carriers believed to be spreading AIDS may be placed under house arrest or imprisoned. Third, existing legislation may be extended explicitly to cover AIDS, notably by inclusion in the lists of occupational diseases and of the conditions to which antidiscrimination provisions apply. Thus, France and Norway have incorporated AIDS into the schedule of diseases which can be acquired at the workplace and for which compensation is provided. In Australia, the state of Victoria made discrimination on the grounds of HIV status illegal in 1988, and recommendations have been made that the federal government create a legislative model for adoption by all states.[25]

Equally important, laws that inhibit the efficacy of prevention or that have the (unintended) effect of discouraging contact between the probably infected and the health services may be repealed. On the first count, the relevant prohibitions concern the content of educational and advertising programs and the legality of the sale of condoms. On the second count, the principal candidates are laws prohibiting homosexual acts, drug use, and prostitution, which in many countries deter participants from approaching any authority able to facilitate prosecution for the manner in which they are likely to have become infected. To our knowledge no country has in fact decriminalized such activities in response to the spread of AIDS. Considerable debate on the desirability of decriminalizing at least some aspects has occurred in many places: New York City, for example, has long considered revising the illegality of possession of syringes; the three Australian states (Queensland, Western Australia, and Tasmania) where anal intercourse is an offense carrying a penalty of up to twenty-one years' imprisonment have been urged to repeal their laws; and, in the case of prostitution, it is not generally illegal in those places, notably the cities of central Africa, where it is most significant in spreading infection. Of course in many societies an informal strategy of nonapplication of such laws may be followed, so that their impact may be weakened without alarming the segments of the population who believe that such laws are necessary for reasons that quite override their eventual consequences for AIDS prevention. But in most cases the simple existence of formal legal sanctions is a significant obstacle to the development of minimal trust.[26]

The degree to which in any particular society the legal system is used to formalize the relations between all parties in the transmission and management of HIV infection depends on two factors: the prior role of the law in medical matters, and the extent of trust between the organized representatives of those parties. Recourse to law as a means of establishing powers and redressing harms is much commoner in some societies than others. In the United States, where the courts have played a significantly greater role in all aspects of medical practice than elsewhere, AIDS has already prompted considerable litigation on issues of discrimination in the workplace and restrictions on access to housing, life insurance, and schooling. In January 1988 the first successful claim for negligence was brought against a doctor who had failed to diagnose AIDS in a female patient.[27] More such cases will certainly follow and will lead to more extensive formalization of the obligations and rights of medical staff and patients in respect of AIDS management. But the extent to which, in any particular society, the interests of differently situated parties are defined, elaborated, and seen to be in conflict with others' interests, depends principally on the degree of organization of such parties and the relationships between their representatives.

Given the absence of a cure for AIDS, the primary response in all countries has necessarily been educational, directed at the achievement of "safe sex," elimination of needle-sharing, and inculcation of a sense of individual responsibility. Education may be provided individually, as in the case of the counseling to precede and follow testing, or collectively, as in the extensive media campaigns directed toward target groups or the general public. A comparison of the educational activities undertaken in different countries should therefore identify the audiences specifically addressed and the contents of the messages directed to them. The extent to which publicly owned media might be used to address particular groups such as gays and ivdus has been a continuing matter for controversy among the organized groups claiming to speak for entire communities; and—determined in part by the outcome of such controversies—the amounts of resources and efforts devoted to more narrowly focused local campaigns through institutions in contact with groups at especial risk have shown great variation within and between single societies.

The nature of the information and exhortation presented in educational programs is similarly shaped by the balance of power between competing groups of disease-definers, usually limited by legal restrictions on the naming of parts and practices. The first AIDS advertising aimed directly at gay men in Britain, for example, was reported as unlikely to use the national press for fear that the detailed advice on safe sex would infringe the Obscene Publications Act.[28] Within such limits public messages may be presented in deliberately dramatic or gently informative ways, reinforcing or weakening in more or less subtle fashion the boundaries between social categories, and legitimating or undermining existing patterns of prejudice. Grim Reapers, beautiful ballerinas, and close-to-copulating couples represent some of the choices among visual and symbolic vehicles believed effective in transmitting messages about safer sex. Great, even extravagant, hopes have been placed on education, although in itself, without substantial accompanying changes in the material availability of resources such as condoms and clean needles, it is no more the panacea for AIDS than it was for other sexually transmitted diseases earlier this century.[29] Countries differ considerably in the extent to which they put such hopes to the test by evaluating the actual reception and effects of information campaigns with a view to future improvements.[30]

WHO RESPONDS?

Schematically, the agents of response are both international and national. The most important international organization is of course the WHO, although some regional bodies have also begun to formulate advice and provide assistance for their constituent members. In 1986, for example, the European Parliament called on the Commission of the European Communities to increase support for AIDS research, establish an international data base, and initiate a Europe-wide educational campaign on AIDS.[31] The response by WHO began with an informal meeting on the characteristics of AIDS in November 1983, followed by the organization of surveillance of AIDS cases. The first collaborative center on AIDS was established in Paris in April 1984 to solicit and collate information from national bodies; by December 1987 a further twenty-nine centers had been added to cover each region of the globe. Information on AIDS was produced in many publications and disseminated through international conferences. A Global AIDS Program (GPA) was launched in 1986 to provide bilateral assistance and enable member states to draw on resources provided by international organizations such as the European Economic Community and by national development agencies in the First World. The funding available to the program has grown very rapidly from U.S. $500,000 and 2 people in 1986 to U.S. $50 million and a staff of some 230 by 1988.[32] In February 1987 a Special Program on AIDS was established with an initial budget of $29 million to be spent on initiatives to prevent new infections, provide care to the already infected, and link national and international campaigns against the disease. By mid-1988 the first WHO-sponsored meeting of health ministers to discuss AIDS prevention strategies had taken place, a World AIDS Day (December 1) had been designated, and 151 of WHO's 166 member states had applied for technical and financial support from the organization.[33] The importance of the unprecedentedly rapid and extended international response by the WHO is of course attributable to the difficulties encountered by national authorities in responding adequately or in ensuring that the most effective prevention strategies are actually adopted.

Actors in the national arena of response come from the four distinctive bases for social order: the state, market, association, and community.[34] The government and its legal powers and administrative organizations; the private actors in the pharmaceutical, blood, sperm and human milk bank, and insurance businesses; the formal representatives of medical professions, groups designated at high risk, and scientific expertise; and the spontaneous demonstrators for action and exclusion—all may contend to influence responses. Their interests in obtaining and using knowledge about infection in general and about individual HIV carriers are distinct and may be diametrically opposed. Societies can be distinguished not only by their quite different mixes of the four principles of order but also by the degree of formal organization and coordination within and between them. Those distinctions run not just between West, East, and less developed worlds but deeply within them.

Governments have of course had the central role in responding to AIDS—a role that has become more significant as the need for continuing national education has become more evident, the array of services proposed for the more varied and increasingly dependent set of AIDS sufferers (children, ivdus) more extensive, and the demand for legal formalization of sociomedical obligations more common. Nonetheless, governments have had to work under powerful constraints, not the least of which is the difficulty of devising and debating policies that may give implicit recognition to, perhaps endorsement of, activities outside the units (heterosexual families) on which positive state intervention in the area of sexuality has traditionally (and bureaucratically) been grounded. The most direct ways of publicly demonstrating the emergency status of AIDS are to establish new institutions with specified exceptional powers, to revise laws that render contact with high-risk groups difficult, and to provide substantial funding for education and research. AIDS can thus be extracted in the most visible way possible from the everyday foliage of misfortune and ill health with its accompanying routine institutional processes. On all three counts, however, the 1980s have proved an unfavorable context for that kind of task.

In the West, expansion in the responsibilities of the state has everywhere been at least questioned and in most countries not merely halted but reversed. Proposals to relax the legal sanctions against homosexuality, drug use, or prostitution have to struggle against a return to private life and "family values" after the political effervescence of the 1970s. Special funding programs must make their way in a climate of reduced spending on public health care and an emphasis on the need for research to attract financial support from private sources. Such financial constraints can lead to the paradoxical transfer of funds from sexually transmitted disease (STD) programs to AIDS programs at a time when the risk of HIV infection among heterosexuals has been definitively and strongly correlated with the presence of other STDs.[35] In Eastern Europe the further decline in the legitimacy of the communist regimes, prompted by a combination of economic woes, ethnic mobilization, and domestic dissent (most notably, Solidarity in Poland), has reduced the possibility of trust-inspiring central initiatives. In the less developed world political elites must commonly struggle not only with parallel problems of legitimacy marked by clear ethnic or territorial limits but also with the hard decisions on the allocation of chronically insufficient resources among a wide range of preventable, but currently lethal, diseases. In the face of dire prophecies for the future effects of AIDS, it is easy to forget that here and now tetanus, measles, whooping cough, and diphtheria together kill 352,000 children annually in Nigeria, 85,000 in Zaire, and 61,000 in Kenya; that leprosy numbers some 10 million victims worldwide, primarily concentrated outside the West; and that an estimated 5 million children of preschool age die each year in Africa from the direct and indirect effects of malnutrition.[36]

Difficulties for governments in initiating responses may be accompanied by serious problems of coordination among the levels of political authority and the jurisdictions of relevant state agencies. Statutory responsibilities for health education and disease prevention may be split up among an array of federal, regional, and city authorities, with no agreed or effective point for the collection of data, issuing of commands, or standardizing of responses.[37] Where federal structures coincide with ethnic or linguistic divisions, delays and inconsistencies in responses are especially likely. Indeed, the extent of direction needed may itself be a matter of dispute, with arguments insisting on the need to maintain local flexibility masking the simple determination not to confront publicly divisive issues or to shoulder increased financial burdens. Since, in Western societies at least, AIDS cases are mostly concentrated in a few large centers, the impact of the health costs associated with the disease will fall very unequally on city budgets. In the case of the United States, it has therefore been argued that while the overall economic impact of AIDS will be no greater than that of any other serious disease and will not constitute a crippling national burden, its consequences for the municipal health budgets of San Francisco and New York will be much more serious.[38] Furthermore, since ivdu AIDS patients generally require more hospital care than other categories, the overall costs will also reflect the relative importance of that transmission route in any particular national profile. In all societies, of course, the health-cost burden on the public purse will be determined by the ratio of financial responsibility for health care between governments and private insurance.

Involvement of the private sector in AIDS issues primarily concerns research and production of drugs and testing kits, the collection and sale of blood and blood products, and the provision of financial resources (life insurance, mortgages, superannuation) to HIV carriers. As the dispute between Gallo and Montagnier shows, the economic dimensions of research competition are very great.[39] Shilts' account of the delays in response by private American blood banks to the emerging evidence on AIDS transmission through blood is well known; but similar cases have been reported elsewhere. In Japan, for example, approval for clinical trials and marketing of heat-treated blood coagulants was deliberately delayed—and is alleged to have resulted in the infection of many of the country's hemophiliacs with HIV—so that a Japanese manufacturer could catch up with foreign competition.[40] Although routine testing for HIV antibodies has succeeded in eliminating blood as a vehicle for infection in the West, it is not easy to prevent contamination at the point of collection in societies where selling blood is a strategy for economic survival, as the case of Brazil shows. Private suppliers of goods and services to the health industry are subject to extensive government regulation; but the desirability of taking decisions in areas such as the refusal of life insurance to gays or to HIV carriers out of private hands by legal prohibitions remains at present a matter of debate. Likewise, in the United States, the benefit of waiving the ordinary rules governing the clinical tests of experimental drugs in order to accelerate discovery of a cure for AIDS is a controversial issue of negotiation among health departments, drug manufacturers, and people with AIDS—just as the ordinary procedures of peer review in assessing scientific articles for publication were temporarily set aside to ensure more rapid circulation of early information about AIDS.[41]

Responses to AIDS among associations display the consequences of the significantly different relations of single associations with governments and with one another. It is likely that medical professionals (surgeons and doctors) still constitute the most organized and powerful groups, despite the increasing erosion of medical autonomy by health administrators, by the professionalization of paramedical occupations, and by the recognition of self-help organizations among patients. In the case of AIDS the power of the medical profession to set the agenda for disease management in narrowly medical terms and to monopolize advice to governments is increased by the continuing uncertainties of HIV pathology but constrained by the capacity of the designated risk groups to mobilize publicly around competing definitions of priorities in rights and responses. That capacity varies by risk group, by country, and by issue.

In Western societies ivdus are the least easily mobilizable category, although the example of Amsterdam demonstrates that grass-roots organizations to involve drug users in education programs and needle-exchange schemes can be created with official support.[42] Nonetheless, even where organization among ivdus and (often unofficial) collaboration with health personnel is possible at the municipal level, the illegality of injecting drugs makes it impossible for its (ex-)practitioners to achieve the status of official contributors to national policy. Similarly, because most HIV-infected women belong to the ivdu category in the West, a major barrier exists to the mobilization of already organized feminist groups in defense of the specific interest of women with AIDS. In the less developed countries, the low level of feminist organization and the solid concentration of HIV infection among prostitutes ensure similar consequences in reducing the likelihood of forceful representation on behalf of women as a specific risk group. Moreover, where prostitution is a substantial accompaniment to the economically essential tourist industry—as it is in Asian countries such as Thailand and the Philippines—strong pressures exist to prevent publicity-generating debates on the extent and risk of infection among the women who participate.[43]

Gay groups in affluent Western cities have shown by far the most successful self-organization in responses to AIDS. Not only have substantial changes in sexual behavior been achieved, but influence on government policy, collaboration with epidemiologists for research purposes, willingness to serve as guinea pigs for experimental drugs, and establishment of support structures for infected patients have marked the community's response.[44] On occasion the influence on official policy making by gay groups has appeared to be so significant as to lead to charges that the government has culpably ignored the health interests of the community at large in favor of the civil rights of the major risk category.[45] It seems clear that the power of gays to influence the substantive content of national and local responses to AIDS depends on the extent of pre-AIDS community organization, the legal status of homosexual activities, and the socioeconomic composition of the category's members.

One set of arenas where the cooperation and conflict between public authorities and representatives of specific interest groups can be tracked is in the array of new institutions that governments create to advise on and manage aspects of HIV infection. The creation of such bodies is itself a signal of the importance given to the epidemic, and their membership and activities constitute a condensed symbol of the perceived urgency of coordinating all participants. By mid-1988 WHO reported that more than 150 countries had established national AIDS committees;[46] and many more specific coordinating bodies have been created in developed and less developed worlds. However, countries show considerable variation in their urgency to establish new institutions, the powers accorded to them, the relations with existing health structures, and the extent to which different groups are represented in their membership. Not only is the perception of the scale of the emergency indicated by the need to circumvent existing institutions and routines; but the degree of participation encouraged from medical, scientific, journalistic, legal, and high-risk categories in determining the shape of the response is publicly displayed.

THIS BOOK

The following chapters indicate how the spread of HIV infection has been followed, represented, and managed in nine countries between 1982 and 1988. The sample includes countries from all three macro-patterns of transmission routes but focuses in particular on Western countries grouped together as Pattern 1. This selectivity has been determined in good part by the dominant position of those countries in generating knowledge about AIDS and providing the most substantial epidemiological research on their own populations. The particular salience given to Europe will, we hope, redress the bias, common in the North Atlantic Anglophone academy, toward identification of the West with the United States and the UK in the analysis of AIDS, but also show how widely the understanding and management of an infectious disease can vary in societies too frequently considered as a homogeneous cultural and institutional bloc.

The single chapters do not seek to cover all aspects of responses to AIDS nor to include detailed examination of all groups whose activities would need to be included in a full comparative account. Responses and demands by medical and paramedical organizations occupy a smaller place than they probably deserve; and the space given to particular cultural, political, and economic features varies not only with the profile of infection in each society but with the disciplinary background of each contributor. The very juxtaposition of different national sequences of reactions and responses should raise further questions about the range of options in principle open to the major social and political actors and about the reasons for the adoption or rejection of the measures considered. In the "Conclusion" we shall compare the patterns of responses in more detail and suggest some of the directions in which their explanations might be sought.

NOTES

1. The fall of the Duvalier regime in Haiti in 1986 is the case cited; R. J. Evans, "Epidemics and Revolutions: Cholera in Nineteenth-Century Europe," *Past and Present* 120 (August 1988): 123.

2. The early political controversy over the origin of HIV in Africa has now subsided somewhat, although the scientific debate continues. For a recent survey of transmission among Africans and from Europeans in Africa to Africans, see A. Ona Pela and Jerome J. Platt, "AIDS in Africa: Emerging Trends," *Social Science and Medicine* 28, no. 1 (1989): 1–8.

3. Tony Coxon, "Review Essay: Social Science and AIDS," *Sociology of Health and Illness* 10, no. 4 (December 1988): 613.

4. Susan Sontag, *AIDS and Its Metaphors* (New York: Farrar, Straus and Giroux, 1989).

5. See, *inter alia*, the essays in *Social Research* 55, no. 3 (1988), "In Time of Plague: The History and Consequences of Lethal Epidemic Disease."

6. Disputants on the two sides include, respectively, R. Gallo and L. Montagnier, "AIDS in 1988," *Scientific American* 259, no. 4 (October 1988): 25–32; and M. Grmek, *Histoire du SIDA* (Payot: Paris, 1989).

7. R. Shilts, *And the Band Played On* (Harmondsworth: Penguin, 1988), p. 138.

8. For the impact of the 1987 revision, see G. W. Rutherford et al., "Impact of the Revised AIDS Case Definition on AIDS Reporting in San Francisco," *Journal of the American Medical Association* 259, no. 15 (15 April 1988): 2235; Jeanette K. Stehr-Green et al., "Potential Effect of Revising the CDC Surveillance Case Definition for AIDS," *The Lancet* (5 March 1988): 520–521; J. M. Gatell et al., "Tuberculosis and the New CDC Definition for AIDS," *The Lancet* (9 April 1988): 832; MMWR Weekly Report, "Acquired Immunodeficiency Syndrome Associated with Intravenous-Drug Use," *Journal of the American Medical Association* 261, no. 16 (28 April 1989): 2314.

9. A. R. Moss et al., "Seropositivity of HIV and the Development of AIDS or AIDS-Related Condition: Three Year Follow Up of the San Francisco General Hospital Cohort," *British Medical Journal* 296 (12 March 1988): 745–750.

10. T. Jonckheer et al., "AIDS Case Definitions for African Children," *The Lancet* (17 September 1988): 690.

11. See J. M. Mann et al., "The International Epidemiology of AIDS," *Scientific American* 259, no. 4 (October 1988): 60–69.

12. Samuel R. Friedman et al., "The AIDS Epidemic among Blacks and His-

panics," *Milbank Quarterly* 65, Supplement 2 (1987): 455–499. See also Chapter 2 below.

13. For an overview and forecast of the impact of AIDS on women, see Beth Schneider, "Women and AIDS: An International Perspective," *Futures* 21, no. 1 (February 1989): 72–90.

14. For the growth in publications concerned with AIDS up to 1987, see Sarat Roberts, Louise Shepherd, and Jenny Wade, "The Scientific and Clinical Literature of AIDS: Development, Bibliographic Control and Retrieval," *Health Libraries Review* 4 (1987): 197–218.

15. William W. Darrow, "Behavioural Research and AIDS Prevention," *Science* (25 March 1988): 1477. Ignorance of sexual practices makes the task of modeling the spread of AIDS and its demographic impact very difficult and prevents the development of any single agreed approach.

16. *Nature* 332 (31 March 1988): 386. White immigrant workers are not tested.

17. *Nature* 333 (23 June 1988): 697.

18. For some details on the measures introduced by different countries, see *WorldAIDS*, no. 1 (1989): 11–12.

19. LeRoy Walters, "Ethical Issues in the Prevention and Treatment of HIV Infection and AIDS," *Science* 239 (5 February 1988): 597.

20. Little appears to be known about the degrees of trust encouraged by particular decisions on the procedures for conducting tests. In one enquiry, in Oregon (United States), the availability of anonymous, rather than confidential, testing increased the demand for testing by 125 percent among gay men but only by 17 percent among ivdus; Laura J. Fehrs et al., "Trial of Anonymous Versus Confidential Human Immunodeficiency Virus Testing," *The Lancet* (13 August 1988): 379–381. The authors do not say whether homosexual acts are illegal in Oregon, so that it is impossible to assess the extent to which the change reflects a reduced sense of risk of violations of confidentiality and eventual prosecution.

21. *New Scientist* (18 February 1989): 65.

22. *The AIDS Letter*, no. 12 (April-May 1989): 6. Illinois was then reported as being about to repeal a similar requirement, which had only been introduced in January 1988.

23. WHO, "AIDS: Consensus Statement from Consultation on Partner Notification for Preventing HIV Transmission," *Weekly Epidemiological Record* 64, no. 11 (17 March 1989): 77–82. The CDC has recommended contact tracing since 1985, as has the U.S. Surgeon-General.

24. See, for the United States, Nancy Ford and Michael Quam, "AIDS Quarantine: The Legal and Practical Implications," *Journal of Legal Medicine* 8, no. 3 (1987): 353–396.

25. Department of Community Services and Health, *Report of the Working Panel on Discrimination and Other Legal Issues—HIV/AIDS*, Consultation Paper No. 2 (Canberra: Commonwealth of Australia, 1989), p. 5.

26. Sanctions may also directly inhibit AIDS management in many ways. Health workers may be incriminated for aiding and abetting prostitution in educating about AIDS; pharmacists may face criminal charges for selling syringes for nonmedical purposes; condom distribution in jails where more than three people occupy single cells may be considered to amount to encouraging obscene acts in public.

27. *The Lancet* (2 April 1988): 779. For a successful action brought by a nurse

against medical staff for negligence in Italy, see below p. 157.

28. *The AIDS Letter,* no. 12 (April-May 1988): 8, quoting the senior program officer of the Health Education Authority.

29. Allan M. Brandt, *No Magic Bullet: A Social History of Venereal Disease in the United States since 1880,* 2nd ed. (New York: Oxford University Press, 1987), p. 369.

30. It is often hard to distinguish the effects of mass educational campaigns about AIDS from the heightening of awareness gained through general media publicity. Evaluations of programs targeted on particular groups are commoner than assessments of national impacts; where governments do more than ask for an opinion from the advertising agencies funded to carry out the campaign, the results are not always encouraging. See, for example, S. Mills et al., "Public Knowledge of AIDS and the DHSS Advertisement Campaign," *British Medical Journal* 293 (1986): 1089–1090.

31. *Official Journal of the European Communities,* no. C 88 (14 April 1986): 83–84.

32. Most of that allocation comes from voluntary contributions earmarked for AIDS rather than from the regular operating budget of the WHO. In 1989 the GPA expects to receive only U.S. $800,000 (0.25 percent) from the regular budget but— thanks to the volume of specific voluntary contributions (c. U.S. $90 million)—will account for 16.6 percent of the total funds made available to the WHO; S. Kingman, "AIDS Brings Health into Focus," *New Scientist,* no. 1665 (20 May 1989): 19–24. The suggestion that AIDS is *directly* drawing WHO funds and personnel away from other urgent health issues is therefore inaccurate.

33. Mann et al., "International Epidemiology of AIDS," p. 69. Visits had been made to 137 countries to provide technical evaluation and had led to the creation of short-term national plans in 106.

34. For discussion of their properties, see Wolfgang Streeck and Philippe C. Schmitter, "Community, Market, State—and Associations? The Prospective Contribution of Interest Governance to Social Order," *European Sociological Review* 1, no. 2 (1985): 119–138.

35. "The two things not to do are to take the resources for AIDS prevention away from the general budget to control sexually transmitted diseases and to isolate the programmes to prevent AIDS from those to control sexually transmitted diseases." P. Piot and M. Laga, "Genital Ulcers, Other Sexually Transmitted Diseases, and the Sexual Transmission of HIV," *British Medical Journal* 298 (11 March 1989): 624.

36. *New Internationalist* 169 (March 1987): 4.

37. For a description of the U.S. response in this vein, see Sandra Panem, *The AIDS Bureaucracy* (Cambridge, Mass.: Harvard University Press, 1988).

38. David E. Bloom and Geoffrey Carliner, "The Economic Impact of AIDS in the United States," *Science* 239 (5 February 1988): 604–609. Given the uncertainties about the actual scale of HIV infection and progression from infection to AIDS, costings of most dimensions of the disease must remain highly speculative; Bloom and Carliner themselves cite seven studies in which the estimates for the cumulative total costs of personal medical care to December 1991 ranged from $6.3 billion to $45.4 billion (Table 1, p. 605).

39. For an examination of the U.S.-French dispute, resolved—despite continuing controversy—by the agreement at the presidential level in 1986, see S. Connor and S. Kingman, *In Search of the Virus* (Harmondsworth: Penguin, 1988).

40. *Nature* 331 (18 February 1988): 552. The Japanese government has subsequently agreed to provide compensation to hemophiliacs who develop AIDS in the form of a monthly allowance of U.S. $1,440; an annual allowance of U.S. $640 will be paid to HIV-infected hemophiliacs who do not develop AIDS.

41. Panem, *AIDS Bureaucracy,* p. 111.

42. See H. Moerkerk, "AIDS Prevention in the Netherlands: Intravenous Drug Users as a Target Group," in WHO, ed., *AIDS Prevention and Control. Papers from the World Summit of Ministers of Health on Programmes for AIDS Prevention, London, 26–28 January 1988* (Oxford: Pergamon Press 1988), pp. 62–65. Elsewhere self-organization has proved much more difficult; S. Friedman et al., "AIDS and Self-Organization among Intravenous Drug Users," *International Journal of the Addictions* 22, no. 3 (1987): 201–219.

43. For details of infection and (lack of) organization among prostitutes in Africa and Asia, see Schneider, "Women and AIDS," passim.

44. For a summary of gay behavior changes and their consequence for rates of infection, see Anne M. Johnson, "Social and Behavioural Aspects of the HIV Epidemic—A Review," *Journal of the Royal Statistical Society* A 151, Part 1 (1988): 99–114.

45. See the Australian case in Chapter 9 below.

46. Mann et al., "International Epidemiology of AIDS," p. 69.

AIDS Policies and Practices in the United States

THE EPIDEMIC IN THE UNITED STATES

Since AIDS was first recognized and named in 1981, the Centers for Disease Control have recorded more than 82,000 reported cases of diagnosed disease.[1] But because only cases of full-blown AIDS are reported to the CDC, the great burden of disease in its asymptomatic and early symptomatic stages goes largely unrecorded. Mortality rates are extremely high—approximately 90 percent for those diagnosed in 1983 or earlier. "AIDS is now the leading cause of death in New York City among men aged 25 to 44 and women aged 25 to 34. In 1986, mortality from AIDS was the eighth leading cause of years of potential life lost before the age of 65 in the United States."[2] Experts have predicted approximately 365,000 cases and 263,000 deaths by 1992.[3] These projections and the public fear of contagion have propelled AIDS to the top of the biomedical and public health agenda.

Of the 82,000 cases recorded by the end of 1988, 32,000 were reported in 1988 alone.[4] Males outnumber females nine to one, and the great majority of the cases have occurred in the age groups from 20 to 50. Perhaps the most striking feature of the demographic profile is the disproportionately high rates among blacks and Hispanics. In both of these populations, their percentage of the AIDS caseload—27 percent for blacks and 15 percent for Hispanics—is approximately twice as large as their percentage of the U.S. population. Among women and children the figures are even more alarming: 51 percent of women with AIDS are black and 20 percent are Hispanic,[5] while 53 percent of children with AIDS are black and 23 percent are Hispanic.[6] Also alarming is the number of infected infants and the impact of the disease on major epicenters like New York and San Francisco. "Recent data from New York City indicate that 1 of every 66 infants born between November 1987 and February 1988 tested positive for HIV antibodies, reflecting the prevalence of HIV infection in women of childbearing age in that city."[7] New York City and San Francisco account for about 30 percent of the reported cases since 1981, but other cities are reporting increasing numbers, for example, Los Angeles 6,010, Houston 2,578, Newark 2,460, Washington 2,382, Miami 2,161, and Chicago 2,128,[8] and small cities and rural areas are beginning to report cases.

Gay and bisexual men continue to bear the major brunt of this epidemic. ["In San Francisco, approximately 50 percent of the male homosexual population is infected with the virus, suggesting the possible future devastation of a large component of the city's population."[9] In 1988 gay men constituted 56.7 percent of the caseload, but this figure is significantly lower than their 64.5 percent share in 1987.[10] An important fact is the apparent decline in new infections. "Evidence from epidemiologic studies in San Francisco suggests that by 1988 less than 2 percent of seronegative homosexual men were being infected annually."[11] In countless interviews and anecdotes gay men themselves testify to remarkable changes in sexual behavior, for example, higher rates of abstinence or sexual exclusivity, avoidance of anal intercourse, and much more frequent use of condoms.[12] Their words are given credence by the indirect evidence of drastically reduced rates for sexually transmitted diseases among gay men.[13] In smaller cities and towns outside the major urban epicenters of HIV disease, changes in sexual behavior may be slower to occur. In these communities gay men are often quite "closeted," denying to the outer world their true sexual identity and to themselves their true risk of AIDS. Where such deception is enforced by social intolerance and discrimination, establishing and maintaining a long-term mutually monogamous homosexual relationship is extremely difficult, and many gay and bisexual men resort to anonymous and high-risk sexual encounters.

[Intravenous drug users, the second largest proportion of the AIDS caseload, constitute the population currently of greatest concern to public health officials. In 1988 they were 30.2 percent of the cases reported, up from 24.6 percent in 1987.[14] "The prevalence of HIV infection among IV drug users varies by geographic area; rates range from 50 to 60 percent in the New York City area to below 5 percent in most areas of the country other than the East Coast."[15] Among the more than 1 million IV drug users in the United States over three-fourths are male, and most of them have their primary sexual relationship with a woman who is not an IV user. This bridge of viral transmission to the heterosexual population has already begun to be evident in the increasing number of cases among women and their infants. Of course, the risk of transmission within IV drug use comes from the sharing of needles contaminated with infected blood, but the risk of sexual transmission is increased by the practice of women exchanging sex for drugs and by the orgiastic sex that sometimes occurs in places where drug users are injecting cocaine or smoking "crack" (a cheap, potent, and highly addictive form of cocaine).

Sharing needles is both a necessity and a ritual among many IV drug users. Ethnographers have reported that the bonding of needle-sharing begins very early in an IV user's career and carries heavy symbolic and even erotic overtones.[16] Furthermore, in many jurisdictions possession of a hypodermic needle without a doctor's prescription is a felony offense. Rather than carry such paraphernalia on their person IV drug users will make use of drug houses or "shooting galleries" where they can rent or share a needle.

IV drug users are often called "junkies," and in the popular image they are hopeless addicts who have no will or desire to exercise self-control. But some researchers and drug treatment outreach workers have found that many IV users are aware of the threat of AIDS and have made efforts to reduce their risk. A lively black market exists for "clean" needles (although their sterility cannot be guaranteed), some users claim they have stopped sharing needles or at least have greatly reduced that practice, and a few are beginning to use condoms. Public health authorities and local community drug treatment organizations have in some localities begun to distribute small bottles of bleach for cleaning needles and have tried to educate users to the necessity of thoroughly sterilizing their paraphernalia. New York City, after years of acrimonious debate, has begun a pilot program to distribute sterile needles,[17] and the small city of Tacoma, Washington, has adopted a program of needle distribution.[18] The compulsive behavior inherent in heroin and cocaine addiction continues, however, to be a thorny problem for disease control.

In the earliest years of the epidemic in the United States, the overwhelming predominance of homosexual transmission created a false image of AIDS as a gay disease, one from which heterosexuals were in effect immune. This stereotype still has some power today, although most people are now aware that the virus does not discriminate. The prevalence of HIV infection within the heterosexual majority is unknown. For partial data we must turn to various population segments that have been tested for other reasons, for example, military recruits, blood donors, some persons admitted to hospitals, and some clients at STD clinics, prenatal clinics, and drug treatment centers. When we combine all of these data, each set of which is biased in its own peculiar way, the overall prevalence is considerably less than 1 percent.[19] Looking at reported cases of AIDS, we see that the proportion attributable to heterosexual transmission in 1988 was 4.8 percent, an increase of 14 percent over the 1987 proportion of 4.2 percent.[20] Much of this increase is probably occurring among women, especially those who are partners of infected male IV drug users.[21]

Because of their multiple sexual contacts female prostitutes are also believed to be at heightened risk of infection and transmission. Strangely enough, however, the data so far do not bear out this hypothesis. Instead, studies show that HIV infection among prostitutes is clearly correlated with IV drug use and not with sexual transmission.[22] Many prostitutes report the frequent use of condoms with their customers, but many also say that they do not use condoms with their steady sexual partner even if the person is HIV-infected.[23]

The mistaken notion that AIDS strikes only gay men is based on a further denial that specific high-risk behaviors identified with gay men do not also occur among heterosexuals. But the most risky sexual act, anal intercourse, is not uncommon among heterosexual couples;[24] and having multiple heterosexual partners has been shown in one study to result in HIV infection.[25] Actually, "there are very poor data available on the sexual behavior of the American populace."[26] The notorious Kinsey reports are forty years old and methodologically flawed. A new national survey of 20,000 respondents is scheduled for completion in mid-1989, but until then one must rely on impressionistic information. With a high divorce rate and easy access to birth control, the American way of sex and courtship has become more liberal. Many people begin having intercourse during their adolescent years and usually with more than one partner. This pattern continues into early adulthood, and because many people find themselves divorced and single in their middle years, sexual adventures are renewed. Even in the era of AIDS these patterns persist because the social and cultural motivators are still very powerful.

The brightest spot in an otherwise gloomy picture concerns the risks associated with transfusions and blood products. The combination of the enzyme-linked immunoassay (ELISA) and Western blot tests for blood screening and the sterilization of blood products through heat treatment has effectively eliminated this source of HIV risk. Because no screening system can be 100 percent foolproof, it is estimated that annually out of 10 million units of transfused blood 100 will be HIV-infected. But since "approximately half of transfusion recipients die of other causes relatively soon after receiving blood, the number of infections directly resulting from transfusion would be even smaller."[27]

FUNDING FOR RESEARCH, EDUCATION, AND SERVICES

Through the early years of the epidemic politicians, public health officials, leaders of the blood-banking industry, and even leaders of the newly emergent gay communities were extremely reluctant to face the prospect of a devastating infectious disease that is blood-borne and sexually transmitted.[28] Part of that reluctance was no doubt based in the evident fact that the group at highest risk in these early years was a population of homosexual males who had multiple sexual partners. The dominant view of the heterosexual establishment was that persons with AIDS were suffering the consequences of their deviate lifestyle. The AIDS issue was avoided from the White House on down to the local level. Leaders of the blood-banking institutions were fearful that AIDS hysteria would undermine public confidence in the safety of the nation's blood supply, and thus they continued to deny the possibility of blood-borne transmission even after the first several transfusion-based cases appeared. Within gay community organizations and the gay media a battle raged over whether to recognize the killer in their midst and openly confront the issues of sexual behavior and disease or aggressively to deny the stigma and sexual repression that AIDS added to their already difficult lives.

Additional problems of organizational structure and inadequate funding created blockages in action:

It is hard to imagine that any one time is convenient for a health emergency to occur, but the early 1980's were clearly ill suited for it. Faced with inflation and unemployment, a conservative administration began to cut domestic spending. The swing to fiscal conservatism was accompanied by a move to transfer the authority and the revenue base for many programs from the federal government to the states. The new management at [the Office of Management and Budget within the White House] mandated overall government retrenchment, with the result that [the Centers for Disease Control] and [the Food and Drug Administration] lost 25 to 30 percent in operational costs, capital expenditures and personnel. In [fiscal year 1982] CDC alone reduced its personnel approximately 30 percent.[29]

Reductions in funding intensified the competition between health agencies, and the in-fighting was further accentuated by internal reallocations to fund AIDS programs. The federal health establishment is a many-headed bureaucratic system with no one in effective control. In American politics this kind of pluralism is tolerated, sometimes celebrated, and even potentially advantageous in the normal give-and-take of competing interests. But when an emergency appears, the lack of coordination and authority can stymie even the well-intentioned. Who determines the overall strategy, sets the priorities, and ensures that always limited resources are allocated appropriately and expended effectively? In the emergency of AIDS, from the beginning and to date, the answer has been no one.

Until very recently federal funding for AIDS activities was a constant struggle.[30] The Reagan administration's budget allocations for AIDS were always much lower than the requests by health agencies or the demands of nongovernmental groups and organizations. Congress was more responsive to the messages of alarm coming from the health establishment, the AIDS constituency, and the public at large. Each year congressional leaders were able to increase the AIDS budget and in the process chastise the White House for its negligence in the face of a public health emergency.[31] Then, in late 1986, the influential Institute of Medicine published a thorough report entitled *Confronting AIDS: Directions for Public Health, Health Care and*

Research, which recommended that the federal government do the following:

1. Undertake a massive media, educational, and public health campaign to curb the spread of HIV infection.
2. Begin substantial long-term and comprehensive programs of research in the biomedical and social sciences intended to prevent HIV infection and to treat the diseases caused by it.

Within a few years these two major areas of action should each be supported with expenditures of $1 billion a year in newly available funds not taken from other health or research budgets. The federal government should bear the responsibility for the $1 billion in research funding and is also the only possible majority funding source for expenditures of the magnitude seen necessary for education and public health.[32]

Armed with this authoritative assessment, liberal Democrats, particularly those from constituencies with relatively high AIDS prevalence, were able to get very substantial increases in budgets for AIDS activities. In the fall of 1988, the first comprehensive AIDS funding legislation passed Congress.[33] The law called for $1 billion to be committed to speeding up biomedical research on cures and vaccines, developing care and treatment networks, and expanding risk reduction programs. With this appropriation more than 700 new federal employees will be hired to expedite the review and approval process for new drugs and to carry out educational programs. Because some AIDS funding was approved under other legislation, the total for the fiscal year beginning 1 October 1988 was $1.5 billion. In the budget proposals for fiscal year 1990 the outgoing Reagan administration has projected a 13 percent increase in AIDS funding, but at the expense of cutting support for government-funded health care programs.[34] At this time it is unclear whether the new administration under President Bush will substantially alter the Reagan proposals, but the pressures for lowering the federal budget deficit are intense, and budget-cutting has become politically popular in Washington, D.C.

Many states have developed some funding for AIDS activities, but the sums are, in most cases, small by comparison with the federal budgets. Most cities and counties are too strapped for funds generally to make major commitments to a specific health problem. Instead, they rely on state and federal funds for any unusual projects.

Charitable trusts and foundations are the repositories of vast amounts of wealth, but only very recently have these organizations begun to support AIDS programs. The exception has been the Robert Wood Johnson Foundation, which has funded a multimillion-dollar program to provide community-based services to persons with AIDS in some of the highest prevalence urban areas. In December 1988, "the fund announced that it

was giving $16.6 million to 54 community, health, and chur
tions, including four universities, for AIDS projects. Four out ⟨
selected for awards were outside the three epicenters of HIV infecᴛᴜᴄ.
York, San Francisco and Los Angeles."[35] Some new foundations have beeɴ
formed specifically to fund AIDS work. Examples are the American Foundation for AIDS Research, the San Francisco AIDS Foundation, and the
Chicago AIDS Foundation. These organizations have been greatly assisted
in their fund-raising by the support of celebrities from the entertainment
industry, but many thousands of small donations have come from local
communities and individuals.

PUBLIC HEALTH LAW AND POLICY

In the United States, protection of the public health is primarily a state
and local concern. The legal authority for public health laws is derived from
a state's inherent and constitutionally reserved powers to govern, or its
"police powers," as they are called. These confer upon a state the ability
to promulgate "reasonable laws necessary to preserve the public order,
health, safety, welfare, and morals" of its citizenry.[36] State authority is
limited only to the extent that the federal government chooses to legislate
in the area or "preempt" state efforts and the extent to which state action
interferes with constitutionally protected substantive and procedural individual rights.

The federal government has chosen to regulate the public health only in
regard to the entry of diseased persons into the United States from a foreign
country, the movement of infected persons from one state to another, and
the protection of military personnel.[37] The AIDS regulatory programs implemented by the federal government thus far have been of this nature. In
1985 the Defense Department began testing all new recruits for HIV antibodies; persons testing positive are not inducted. It subsequently began
screening all active-duty personnel, but without an absolute requirement of
discharge from the armed forces.[38] The Bureau of Immigration and Natu-
ralization Services administers HIV antibody tests to all immigrants, refugees, and illegal aliens applying for legal status.[39] Screening of employees
is also done by the Peace Corps, Job Corps, and Department of State.[40]

Historically the principal public health response of the states to infectious
or contagious disease has been first to identify those individuals who are
infectious through voluntary or compulsory testing, screening, and reporting, and then to control the spread of the virus by restricting the contact
between infectious and noninfectious individuals through isolation and
quarantine. Statutes on the books as many as 150 to 200 years prior to the
first diagnosed cases of AIDS gave state and local health officials broad
authority to take whatever measures are necessary within a state to prevent
the spread of disease. For example, a Massachusetts statute passed in 1797

gave local public health authorities power to "take care and make effectual provision in the best way they can, for the preservation of the inhabitants, by removing such sick or infected person or persons, and placing him or them in a separate house or houses, and by providing nurses, attendance, and other assistance and necessaries for them."[41] More recent versions, such as the one in force in Illinois from 1877 to the present, direct the state department of health to investigate the causes of dangerously contagious or infectious diseases, especially when in epidemic form; declare, enforce, and modify quarantine; adopt, repeal, and amend rules and regulations, including regulations to identify which diseases would be considered communicable; and make sanitary inspections for the preservation and improvement of the public health.[42] Other state public health statutes are specific to individual diseases such as venereal disease and tuberculosis.[43]

For the majority of states with broad public health laws, no additional statutory authority has been needed to protect the public against the spread of AIDS. These public health agencies have the authority, if not the resources, to institute programs of AIDS education, counseling, testing, treatment, and personal control. Other states, without preexisting authority, have, through the passage of legislation, expanded the scope of their coverage to include AIDS and, in some instances, ARC (AIDS-related conditions) and HIV infection. The typical progression has been for a state to create a task force or study commission to examine various aspects of AIDS. After a period of review states have, to the extent needed, sought various types of enabling legislation. Educating and counseling the public on how to prevent transmission of the virus has often been the first priority, followed by the appropriation of special funding and the creation of pilot projects to provide for patients' medical, mental health, and social service needs. Voluntary testing programs have been established. As a last step regulatory measures have been added or strengthened,[44] often with public health authorities and legislative bodies at odds with one another over the kinds of measures that are most appropriate for the control of the spread of the disease and the extent to which the interests of infected and high-risk persons should be protected.

New regulatory measures have mandated the reporting of AIDS, ARC, and HIV infection and the control of infectious persons.[45] Although AIDS, as defined by the CDC, is a reportable condition throughout the country, ARC and HIV infection are not. Several states, including Arizona, Colorado, Florida, Idaho, Illinois, Minnesota, Montana, South Carolina, and Wisconsin, passed laws either specifically requiring the reporting of ARC and of positive HIV antibody tests or requiring the reporting of any case related to a variety of diseases, including AIDS.[46] Colorado, Idaho, and Kentucky enacted statutes that extend state isolation and quarantine authority expressly to persons with AIDS or the HIV virus. Alabama, Connecticut, Indiana, Minnesota, and North Carolina laws give health officers the authority to restrict or confine persons with communicable diseases who are endangering the public health. Florida, Illinois, and Rhode Island adopted sexually transmissible disease (STD) control acts that allow public health authorities to first designate AIDS, ARC, and HIV infection as an STD, and then under certain circumstances quarantine persons to prevent the spread of the disease.[47]

The Florida statute is illustrative of the typical disease control process that must be followed. Physicians are required to report all diagnosed cases of AIDS and ARC or be subject to a fine of $500 per offense. Diagnosis of the disease must be based upon diagnostic criteria of the Centers for Disease Control. The Florida Department of Health and Rehabilitative Services (HRS) is authorized to interview persons who are infected or suspected of being infected. The act allows for the compulsory apprehension, examination, and treatment of persons suspected of being infected with or exposed to a sexually transmitted disease following a court hearing and issuance of a warrant.[48]

Provision is also made for the quarantine of persons or places as a result of the "probable spread" of a sexually transmitted disease. Before quarantine can be imposed, an order from a judge must be obtained following a hearing on the matter. At the hearing, HRS must prove by clear and convincing evidence that the public's health is significantly endangered by the person with the STD or by the place where significant sexual activity likely to spread the disease is undertaken; that all other reasonable means of correcting the problem have been exhausted; and that no less restrictive alternative exists. Information disclosed during the hearing is strictly confidential and must be sealed by the court from disclosure.[49]

In addition to the general disease control statutes, other specialized public health laws and policies have been adopted. Of these, statutes and policies requiring mass HIV screening and the testing of various populations have been common. The screening of blood and blood products for the HIV virus to ensure their safety is now a universal standard of practice in the United States. By November 1982 it was known that the AIDS virus could be passed through blood transfusions. By March 1983 the Public Health Service had recommended that persons in high risk groups not give blood. Routine screening of blood and blood products began in January 1985 when the ELISA test became available commercially. Shortly thereafter the Food and Drug Administration (FDA) amended blood donor regulations to require that each unit of blood and blood products be tested and records of test results maintained. State legislatures, with the support of public health officials and most interest groups, also acted quickly in passing laws to require testing of blood and donated materials, including organs and semen, and to make it a criminal offense to donate blood or blood products while knowingly infected with the virus.[50] The Defense Department's screening of recruits and military personnel, although controversial at first, has become accepted practice. Further, as shown by the blood and military screening programs, the accuracy of currently marketed HIV antibody tests compares favorably with other medical diagnostic tests, quieting the fears of many about false positive and false negative test results.[51]

But attempts to require mass HIV screening and testing of other populations have not been as successful, and the proper role for HIV testing continues to be one of the most controversial public policy issues. The general sentiment among public health professionals has been that the screening of populations not engaged in high-risk sex or IV drug use is unlikely to produce a public health benefit. At a conference convened by the Association of State and Territorial Health Officers, public health officials issued a consensus recommendation that "HTLV-III antibody tests should not be used for involuntary screening of any individual or group. Use of serologic testing is not appropriate, for example, as a precondition for employment, evidence of insurability, admission to hospitals, or admission to schools."[52]

On the other side, state legislators responding to the fears of their constituents have shown strong interest in instituting HIV screening of marriage license applicants, sex offenders, and those in a hospital setting, as well as a lesser interest in screening diverse populations such as food handlers and school children. Two states, Louisiana and Illinois, actually established premarital AIDS screening requirements. The Louisiana testing requirement was repealed a year later,[53] and there is strong support within the state for repeal of the Illinois provisions as well.[54] Utah went a step further and banned marriages altogether of persons with AIDS.[55] A small number of states now require individuals convicted of sex crimes and drug offenses to be tested.[56] Most common are statutes, like the ones passed in Nevada, Illinois, and Florida, that mandate that prostitutes submit to HIV antibody testing.[57] Currently three jurisdictions conduct mass screening of all new prison inmates. A number of others test selected prison populations.[58] Proposals to test food handlers, health care workers, and school children have often been debated, but have not passed.

The principle of confidentiality is well recognized in public health law and has broad-based support. But even though virtually all states have provisions in their general public health statutes to safeguard the confidentiality of information reported to their public health departments, there has been considerable disagreement over whether confidentiality protection should be expanded to include confidentiality of HIV test results and the diagnosis of AIDS or ARC.[59] A number of states have protected the privacy rights of persons with AIDS and added AIDS-specific confidentiality provisions to existing laws or passed new laws on the subject.[60]

Whether or not informed consent should be obtained in advance of HIV testing has also been widely debated. It is common practice for physicians to order batteries of laboratory tests for their patients without detailed explanations of each test or specific consent other than that inferred from the patient's general consent to treatment. Physicians' organizations and lobbying groups have generally opposed informed consent requirements that would impinge upon their ability to direct their patients' diagnosis and treatment. But because there have been numerous accounts of patients being tested without their knowledge or consent and then being subjected to loss of insurance benefits or other forms of discrimination, there has also been strong support for requiring informed consent in advance of HIV testing.[61] A few states have supported the right of persons with AIDS to direct their own medical care and mandated that informed consent be obtained before HIV testing can occur.[62]

Most public health laws passed in response to the AIDS epidemic are constitutional and enforceable over the civil liberties interests of the individuals regulated by them. Courts, called upon to review the application of public health laws, have established a tradition of deferring to the judgment of state lawmakers and local health agencies, provided the laws serve a legitimate state purpose and reasonably achieve that purpose. Critical questions are whether there is a medical or disease control justification for the measure being taken and whether adequate procedural protections are provided. State legislative bodies and public health officials cannot legally bow to the unsubstantiated fears, biases, negative attitudes, or intolerance of the public or others. And when public health authorities act to restrict the rights of an individual, they must follow the kinds of procedures incorporated in the Florida STD statute discussed previously.[63]

Persons with HIV infection have been vulnerable to discrimination. They have lost their jobs, homes, insurance, and health care without good medical or social reason. Their primary protection against discrimination has been statutorily based. Section 504 of the federal Rehabilitation Act of 1973 bans discrimination against the handicapped by entities receiving federal funds. As interpreted by the U.S. Supreme Court in *School Board of Nassau County v. Arlines*,[64] a case involving the dismissal of a school teacher with infectious tuberculosis, policies excluding children with AIDS from school or of dismissing or refusing to hire employees with AIDS are violative of the act.[65] Most states have similar statutes prohibiting discrimination against the handicapped, and several state courts have already found that they apply to AIDS and, in some instances, HIV infection. Many apply to the private sector as well as the public sector and are broad enough in scope to cover discrimination in employment, housing, and access to health care. A few cities have enacted statutes or ordinances explicitly banning discrimination against persons with HIV infection. Several jurisdictions have gone so far as to ban the use of HIV tests for insurance purposes.[66]

The use of antidiscrimination laws in the AIDS context is new. Few court cases define the limits of their application. A great deal of confusion exists at both the federal and state level over whether specific laws apply to AIDS,

ARC, and also HIV infected individuals who are symptom-free. There is also a lack of uniformity among the states, with some states outlawing discrimination in multiple settings and others in none. A climate of fear has developed as AIDS discrimination has been documented throughout the country. Discrimination is so extensive that many people will not voluntarily submit to an HIV test. Fear has been a major constraint to wide acceptance of many potentially effective public health measures.[67] Because a successful health policy depends upon the cooperation of potentially infected persons, numerous groups, including the President's Commission on the HIV Epidemic, have called for the enactment of a federal statute specifically designed to prevent discrimination on the basis of HIV infection or AIDS. According to prominent American Bar Association leaders testifying before the Presidential Commission on the HIV Epidemic, "AIDS presents a national emergency which must be dealt with through national policy. This is not a case where each state can be left to deal with the issue as best it can."[68]

STRENGTHS AND WEAKNESSES OF THE HEALTH SYSTEM

Looming on the horizon of the epidemic is the prospect of financial bankruptcy for many health care institutions with increasing numbers of indigent AIDS patients. Huge shortfalls in payment for patient care are anticipated. This problem is created by the grossly inadequate patchwork of health insurance coverage in America. The principal government program to fund health care for the indigent, Medicaid, is already badly underfunded and fails to cover the actual cost of care. Although federal funding for AIDS has been greatly increased, only 5 percent is committed to patient care.[69] Privately purchased health insurance is not a solution for AIDS costs, because the insurance companies are determined to keep AIDS patients off their rolls.[70] They are demanding that new applicants for insurance be tested for HIV infection, and if found positive, rejected for coverage.[71] In many cases insured persons with AIDS who make insurance claims are denied benefits on the grounds that their HIV infection occurred prior to their becoming a policy holder. Some companies are denying insurance to anyone who fits a certain demographic profile or lives in a neighborhood with a significant percentage of gay residents.[72]

The cost of care is inflated because of a lack of housing or home care for ambulatory AIDS patients and a lack of long-term care/nursing home beds for bedridden patients.[73] Patients who have nowhere else to go simply stay in the hospital, being forced to choose the most expensive alternative. This problem has become especially acute among infants with AIDS whose parents are unable to care for them because of their own illness. New York City may be a harbinger for the rest of the nation. "On any given day,... 5 to 6 percent of the 35,000 hospital beds are filled by patients who are medically cleared for discharge but cannot find a nursing home bed or a home attendant."[74] The San Francisco approach of providing volunteer home help to persons with AIDS has kept health care costs much lower, but this alternative is already reaching its limits.[75] As the epidemic grows and the pool of volunteers is exhausted, the demand for care outside the hospital must be met by paid health care professionals and institutions. The federal Department of Health and Human Services recently provided $2.8 million to twelve organizations to develop care and service programs for children with HIV disease. Another nineteen facilities have received a total of nearly $7 million to construct nonacute care intermediate and long-term care facilities.[76]

These newest efforts do not meet the growing need for such facilities. The increasing number of AIDS patients who are drug users and/or poor is creating a patient population with more medical complications and less ability to pay.[77] New medications and treatment modalities are more medically effective but also more expensive. For example, the antiviral AZT can cost $8,000 to $10,000 per patient per year. As our ability to treat AIDS improves and patients' life spans are lengthened, the lifetime cost of care per patient also increases.

In several important dimensions, the health care professions are not adequately meeting the challenge of this epidemic: "The acuity of disease of persons with HIV infection, the complexity of their physical and psychosocial needs, the high fatality rate, and the fear of exposure to HIV, along with low salaries and understaffing in many facilities, create a potential for considerable stress, burn-out turnover, and dramatic projected shortages for the delivery of HIV patient care in the near future."[78] At a time when the complex and intensive needs of AIDS patients are creating a heightened demand for skilled nursing care, the nation is facing a shortage of nurses. "In the hospital setting alone, the vacancy rates for registered nurses exceed 13 percent."[79] Enrollments in nursing schools are down and the projected needs for the next decade far exceed the projected supply. Because of low salaries and little opportunity for career advancement, many nurses are leaving the profession. Added to these structural disincentives is the fear of HIV infection.

Physicians also are concerned about the personal and professional risks that AIDS poses. Some physicians are quick to refer elsewhere any patient that they suspect is HIV-infected. A survey of 258 doctors in New York City found that 25 percent believed it would be ethical to refuse to treat an AIDS patient.[80] Surgeons are demanding that their patients be tested for HIV infection prior to surgery and if infected be given alternative nonsurgical treatment.[81] In 1987 the American Medical Association adopted a policy statement opposing on ethical grounds the refusal to treat HIV-infected patients, but the debate continues within the medical profession. Physicians often complain that they are not technically qualified to treat AIDS patients, and indeed very few medical education programs are providing adequate training regarding the multifaceted problems presented by AIDS:

Several training efforts are currently under way.... Health Resources and Services Administration has provided approximately 10 grants to develop AIDS regional education and training centers... to prepare community primary care providers to diagnose, counsel and care for Persons with AIDS and other HIV-related conditions. ... In addition, the National Institute of Mental Health has awarded contracts to 21 institutions (universities, professional associations, and volunteer organizations) to provide comprehensive training for health care providers and trainees (medical students and residents) in the medical and psychiatric complications of AIDS, as well as in the ethical, psychological, and prevention-related behavioral aspects of the disease.[82]

While these programs are laudable, they will not adequately meet the longer-term needs for thousands of professional medical providers who are able, and, more important, willing to care for HIV-diseased patients.

Prevention of HIV transmission among IV drug users cannot be adequately accomplished without large-scale programs of drug treatment.[83] At the current time drug treatment programs are underfunded and understaffed, so much so, in fact, that drug users who want to enter treatment must wait up to six months for an opening. Approximately 10 percent of the nation's IV users are in drug treatment at any one time. Neighborhood groups often oppose the establishment of treatment centers in their communities. Drug treatment counselors need additional training and support to provide AIDS risk reduction education to their clients and to handle the tough issues of disease and death that some of their clients are facing. All of these problems could be substantially solved with increased funding, but some basic treatment barriers remain. No single treatment modality has been remarkably successful, and rates of recidivism are high. For heroin users the substitution of methadone is touted by many as the best approach, but for users who inject cocaine no such substitute exists.[84] Furthermore, the criminalization of drug use makes drug users outlaws, leery of dealing with any governmental authorities, even those in public health roles.

EDUCATIONAL PROGRAMS

It is commonplace now to hear health officials refer to AIDS education as "our only vaccine." In June 1988, the Office of Technology Assessment, an agency of the U.S. Congress, released a report entitled *How Effective Is AIDS Education?* It outlines the types of educational efforts already undertaken and then evaluates their effectiveness. The federal government has conducted two national public information campaigns itself. October 1987 was declared AIDS Awareness Month, and the many activities and media messages were the springboard for an ongoing campaign called "America Responds to AIDS." Under this rubric the Public Health Service has sponsored conferences, produced educational materials, and placed AIDS prevention messages on radio and television. More recently, in May 1988, the Surgeon General, as the nation's chief health spokesperson, mailed to all U.S. households a special report on AIDS, describing in clear terms the nature of the disease and recommending specific prevention measures for individuals.

Federal dollars are also combined with state and local government funding for similar programs at local levels. The production and distribution of brochures, posters, and other media messages has become a regular practice. These materials are supplemented by more creative efforts directed at specific high-risk populations. In Ohio, for example, AIDS educators put safer sex messages on cocktail napkins in gay bars and trained the bartenders in these establishments to give out knowledgeable risk reduction advice to their customers. To avoid the right-wing political pressure that comes with the use of governmental funds, many of these more innovative projects have been backed by private fund-raising. But another major institution, the Roman Catholic Church, has in many of its dioceses opposed any educational campaign that promotes the use of condoms. This opposition in major urban areas with high AIDS prevalence, such as New York City, Philadelphia, and Los Angeles, forces AIDS prevention programs into distracting political struggles. Nevertheless, in cities and towns across the nation public health officials and citizen volunteers continue to promote AIDS prevention through speeches to local groups, workshops for high-risk individuals, and a myriad of aural and visual messages.

How effective is all this educational activity? Nobody knows, at least from a formal evaluation point of view. In fact, methodologically rigorous evaluation of AIDS education programs is very rarely done, perhaps because in many cases it is impossible to control some of the most significant variables. Changes in knowledge are demonstrable, as are changes in attitude. Indeed, many studies have shown that AIDS education is effective in these psychological dimensions. An encouraging finding is that more accurate knowledge is positively correlated with more tolerant attitudes toward those who are infected. But what evidence we have indicates that changes in knowledge and attitudes often do not substantially affect behavior, especially in the use of condoms.

AIDS education too frequently relies on fear-generating techniques in the hope of convincing people to make behavioral changes. But a great deal of research indicates that generating fear is not an effective educational strategy unless it is combined with information on what the individual can do to reduce the fear engendered and with the means (devices, services, personal skills) to do what is recommended.[85] These two necessary components, especially the latter, are often neglected or missing in AIDS education. For example, promotion of condoms must be accompanied by availability and information on how to use them. Persons who are convinced and ready to adopt safer sex practices often have great difficulty convincing their sexual partners to make the necessary changes. Heterosexual women who must rely on their partner to wear a condom are often fearful of emotional or even physical fights if they insist on this practice.

Racial and ethnic minorities present cultural and language barriers to effective educational programming. Establishment educators need to work through local minority leaders and organizations, but these people often shy away from involvement with AIDS issues. Even though blacks and Hispanics have exceptionally high AIDS prevalence rates, denial is also prevalent in these communities. Given their historical experience of prejudice and discrimination, it is easy to understand why they resist identification with yet another stigmatizing trait. Hostility to homosexuality is sharply evident in these groups, and drug use is an embarrassing reality, the effects of which are well known and roundly condemned. The prominence of religious institutions generates heavy-handed moralizing about AIDS without providing any clear and constructive discussion about risk reduction.

Despite these difficulties some educational approaches have been effective. One-on-one counseling, with intensive follow-up, has helped individuals and couples to adopt safer practices. Even more effective are community-based efforts to change the social norms and mores of sexual behavior. As safer sex becomes the socially valued norm, individuals change to be in conformity. This process has been observed in some of the larger urban gay communities and probably accounts for the drastically decreased incidence rates of HIV infection among gay men. But large numbers of people engaging in risky behavior are not members of an AIDS-conscious cohesive community, so from a society-wide perspective AIDS-related behavior change is a longer, slower, more massive project.

Although no one can say from scientifically conducted evaluations that public information campaigns and other educational techniques are effective, it is known that they were a significant part of the long-term change in the American norms and mores regarding smoking. And since education is "our only vaccine," these efforts must be pursued. One hundred and thirty-seven educational programs have already been funded by the federal government alone. Hundreds of local efforts backed by other resources are also under way. Over the last several years, AIDS has been by far the biggest health news story in the popular media, and much of the coverage has been basically sound on the biomedical and epidemiological facts. The most mundane truth about education is that we learn through repetition and redundancy, by receiving the same message through many different channels. AIDS education must be introduced into every setting possible, especially those where people are dealing with issues potentially related to AIDS, for example, family planning, reproductive health, substance abuse, fitness and wellness, maternal and child health, and sex education. AIDS education must be made a part of a broader community health effort, embedded in the information and means to a healthier life in general. This comprehensive approach is more realistic in its recognition of the social context of multiple risks, especially among poor people where many serious, even life-threatening, community health problems need to be confronted.

PREDOMINANCE OF GAY ORGANIZATIONS

When the definitive history of the AIDS epidemic in America can finally be written, it will document the tremendous efforts made by gay men individually and in organizations to confront, struggle courageously against, and at last conquer this disease. Certainly no other segment of American society has made comparable contributions and sacrifices. Despite an early period of denial, gay men can now be found centrally involved in every aspect of AIDS work.

To be gay in America is to be socially illegitimate. Anti-sodomy statutes exist in twenty-six of the fifty states, and although they are very rarely enforced, their constitutionality was recently upheld by the U.S. Supreme Court. In some more local jurisdictions statutes exist forbidding discrimination on the basis of sexual preference, but whenever such measures come up for debate, anti-gay sentiment is voiced in the strongest and most righteous terms. Social psychological research indicates that many heterosexuals fear homosexuals, considering them dangerous. In such a cultural climate it is not surprising to find discrimination against gays in employment, housing, social services, education, and law enforcement. The reactions from gay men have ranged from complete concealment and elaborate deception to complete disclosure and an open expression of their basic identity. This latter choice has been facilitated by the development of gay communities in many of the larger cities, where social life is organized around bars, social clubs, religious organizations, and community cultural activities. Gays have also begun to exert their power through political organizing at the national and local levels and through gay-oriented legal defense organizations.

In the contemporary context of AIDS, the heterosexual majority has reacted with ambivalence to the gay community. Never before have heterosexuals learned so much about the very existence and the experience of gay life. In many AIDS activities heterosexuals have been forced to work closely with gay men, and prejudice and stereotypes often crumble in the face of cooperation and friendship. But AIDS has also added a weapon to the arsenal of bigotry. Many heterosexuals say that they are protecting themselves against AIDS by avoiding any social contact with gays. Heightened fear gives rise to more acts of discrimination, and gay organizations report alarming increases in anti-gay violence.

Particularly at the local level, many of the most active AIDS organizations are also gay organizations. In New York City, for example, the Gay Men's Health Crisis was formed by a few gay activists in the living room of a gay writer.[86] At first committed to fund-raising, it rapidly developed into a multifaceted service organization.[87] Other gay communities soon followed suit: in Los Angeles with the L.A. AIDS Project, in Atlanta with AID Atlanta, and in St. Louis with Effort for AIDS, to name but three. In San Francisco, many already existing gay organizations turned their attention to the threat of AIDS.

Voluntary organizations are a prominent feature of American society and culture. Most of these voluntary organizations are quite weak, with no structure of real authority to take action and very little money in their treasuries. Nevertheless, Americans know how to form these organizations and how to create an administrative shell for the group; they have lived in and formed such groups from the time they were children.

So when AIDS appeared, AIDS organizations sprang up spontaneously and quickly, then struggled to be effective. Frequently these groups have very few paid staff (and those are paid poorly), relying on volunteers to carry out the mission of the group. Their continuing dependence on volunteers is both a strength and a weakness. By using volunteers one can stretch the dollars to provide more services, and the central presence of many volunteers assures that the organization will not lose touch with the community it wants to serve. But volunteers, whose lives are filled with other demanding activities, are often hard to mobilize effectively when they do not have the necessary skills to deliver the services, some of which may be psychologically or technically complex. Resources must be expended to train volunteers, yet turnover among them is often quite high, especially in AIDS work, where fear, grief, and a sense of personal vulnerability can be very burdensome.

What have these organizations actually done? One is tempted to answer, everything. They have been the principal and in many locales the only purveyors of clear, explicit, and culturally appropriate education for risk reduction, especially among the gay population. Through the use of telephone hotlines, articles in the media, posters, pamphlets, and innumerable discussions they have advocated the adoption of safer sex techniques, especially promoting the use of condoms.

In many practical ways, these organizations have directly assisted those who are ill or who are otherwise distressed by HIV disease. Finding or providing housing, financial aid, legal assistance, and counseling and support are major services. Many persons with AIDS are able to live at home if they can get some help with daily tasks and some companionship and social support. Home help is provided by thousands of volunteers in hundreds of cities and towns. These efforts are usually led by and largely staffed by gay men. As AIDS takes its terrible toll, gay men are also volunteering for support services in hospices.

Political pressures are brought to bear on national and local service providers and policy makers through gay establishment organizations like the National Gay and Lesbian Task Force, which also has chapters in many of the states, and anti-establishment activists like ACT UP (AIDS Coalition to Unleash Power), a New York group that engages in confrontational politics. Begun by gay men, ACT UP has gained power and influence as it has opened its membership to women, blacks, and Hispanics.[88] In fact, throughout the many grassroots AIDS organizations, women, both lesbian and heterosexual, have provided countless volunteer hours of service. And many AIDS organizations, although basically gay identified, provide all of their services to any person in need regardless of their sexual orientation.

As these organizations have grown and matured, the established institutions have looked to them as vehicles to carry out programs of education and service provision. In AIDS funding, local, state, and federal dollars have been targeted to "high-risk groups" and mandated to go to local organizations. This practice is due in part to the American belief in the efficacy of the nongovernmental sector. Public health educators within the funding bureaucracies also believe that they must work through community organizations to be credible and culturally acceptable. Funding local organizations has also been convenient for government agencies that do not have the will or the capability to conduct AIDS programs themselves. For the organizations these dollars have become their lifeline, but the funds often come with strings attached. Repeatedly, local organizations have gotten into trouble or had to compromise the content of their educational messages in order not to offend the sensibilities of some legislator or bureaucrat. The most egregious example of this political pressure is the Helms amendment, a measure forced through Congress by Senator Jesse Helms which forbids federal funding for any AIDS educational materials or programs that implicitly condone or promote homosexuality. Thus efforts to teach people how to lead a healthy gay sex life cannot be supported by federal funds.

OTHER VOLUNTARY ORGANIZATIONS

Some work is beginning among IV drug users. In New York City, local nongovernmental drug control organizations have been the impetus for the city government's recently initiated pilot program to distribute sterile needles. These groups simply announced that in order to save lives they were going to defy the law and hand out free sterile needles to IV users along with AIDS risk reduction education. Outreach workers on the street, many of them former drug users, are going into drug houses to talk to people about the risk of needle-sharing, hand out bleach sterilization kits, and warn against sexual transmission of HIV.

In hundreds of communities across the nation local AIDS task forces or coalitions have formed, bringing together representatives from public health, medicine, education, religion, and social services. Sometimes such a group may have an official status, but more often the membership is voluntary. In places where the gay community has not been able to assume the major burden for AIDS activities, these organizations have often taken on these tasks or seen to it that some agency in the community does so. Their principal contribution now and in the future will be in mobilizing established community institutions to recognize and deal with the burgeoning problems of the epidemic. Many existing civic and religious organizations are beginning to develop an AIDS activities component. These groups are especially important in minority communities where the credibility of governmental authorities is often suspect.

Business corporations are owners of great wealth and wield enormous influence politically and in the lives of their employees. They also tend not to see themselves as social entities, preferring to shift social responsibilities to governmental and nonprofit organizations. The AIDS epidemic is, however, beginning to intrude on the economic singlemindedness of American businesses. Most Americans get their life and health insurance coverage through their employers, and AIDS is inflating the premium payments, thus creating higher costs for business. The turmoil created in the workplace by irrational fears of casual contact transmission generates tension and lowers productivity. With rare exceptions, most businesses are just beginning to develop policies, especially in the personnel area, regarding AIDS and to provide AIDS education to their employees.[89]

CONCLUSION

As we near the end of the first decade of the AIDS epidemic, the United States still does not have a national AIDS policy or a coordinated strategy for combatting this public health threat. Under heavy political pressure the Reagan administration appointed a Presidential Commission with many of its members representing right-wing views to investigate the epidemic and recommend policies and practices. To the surprise of many, the commission's final report laid out a blueprint for action that was scientifically sound, politically sensitive, and far-reaching in its critique of current efforts and its call for major reforms. But nearly all its recommendations require greatly increased spending on research, education, drug treatment, and training of health care providers in addition to financial support for the care of AIDS patients.[90] President Reagan was distinctly cool in his response to the commission's findings. President Bush, on the other hand, has been rhetorically much more receptive, even to the point of endorsing the commission's call for federal legislation outlawing discrimination against persons who are HIV-infected. He has not made any commitments, however, to the increases in funding necessary to implement the commission's strategy.[91]

Meanwhile the harsh realities of the epidemic are forcing people to rethink some basic practices, institutional arrangements, and values. For example, the life-threatening circumstances of AIDS patients have created a demand for major revisions in the protocols and acceleration in the processes for approving new experimental medical treatments.[92] Health care providers are confronting major ethical dilemmas in their desire to avoid treating HIV-infected persons. AIDS has exposed the gross inequities and gaping inadequacies of the American way of financing health care, especially for indigent patients.[93] AIDS has made clear the long-standing need for positive, plain-spoken, comprehensive sex education for adolescents and for many adults, including health care professionals. Finally, the disease of AIDS will not be conquered until a majority of Americans change their discriminatory behavior toward sexual, racial, and ethnic minorities. As more gay men fall ill from HIV infection, perhaps acquired years ago, and as the epidemic of viral transmission expands among blacks and Hispanics, the white heterosexual majority must abandon its historical pattern of hostility and neglect toward those who are "different," and instead conquer fear with compassion.

NOTES

1. United States AIDS Program, Center for Infectious Diseases, "AIDS Weekly Surveillance Report," (Atlanta: Centers for Disease Control, 26 December 1988).

2. Institute of Medicine, National Academy of Sciences, *Confronting AIDS: Update 1988* (Washington, D.C.: National Academy Press, 1988), p. 52.

3. AIDS Program, Centers for Disease Control, "Quarterly Report to the Domestic Policy Council on the Prevalence and Rate of Spread of HIV and AIDS— United States," *Morbidity and Mortality Weekly Report* 37 (16 September 1988):552.

4. "AIDS Weekly Surveillance Report," 26 December 1988.

5. *Report of the Presidential Commission on the Human Immunodeficiency Virus Epidemic* (Washington, D.C.: National Academy Press, 1988), p. 52.

6. Institute of Medicine, *Confronting AIDS: Update 1988,* p. 52.

7. Ibid.

8. "AIDS Weekly Surveillance Report," 26 December 1988.

9. Institute of Medicine, *Confronting AIDS: Update 1988,* p. 52.

10. "AIDS Weekly Surveillance Report," 26 December 1988.

11. Office of Technology Assessment, Congress of the United States, *How Effective Is AIDS Education?* (Washington, D.C.: U.S. Government Printing Office, June 1988), p. 11.

12. W. Winkelstein, Jr., M. Samuel, N. S. Padian, J. A. Wiley, W. Lang, R. E. Anderson, and J. A. Long, "The San Francisco Men's Study. III. Reduction in Human

Immunodeficiency Virus Transmission among Homosexual/Bisexual Men, 1982–6," *American Journal of Public Health* 76 (1987):685–689.

13. Centers for Disease Control, "Continuing Increase in Infectious Syphilis—United States," *Morbidity and Mortality Weekly Report* 37 (29 January 1988):35–38.

14. "AIDS Weekly Surveillance Report," 26 December 1988.

15. Office of Technology Assessment, *How Effective Is AIDS Education?*, p. 18.

16. Don C. Des Jarlais, Samuel R. Friedman, and David Strug, "AIDS and Needle Sharing Within the IV-Drug Use Subculture," in Douglas A. Feldman and Thomas M. Johnson, eds., *The Social Dimensions of AIDS: Method and Theory* (New York: Praeger, 1986), pp. 111–125.

17. Bruce Lambert, "New York to Begin Giving Free Needles to Narcotic Addicts," *New York Times*, 12 August 1988.

18. Jane Gross, "Needle Exchange for Addicts Wins Foothold Against AIDS in Tacoma," *New York Times*, 23 January 1989, p. Y8.

19. Institute of Medicine, *Confronting AIDS: Update 1988*, pp. 47–49.

20. "AIDS Weekly Surveillance Report," 26 December 1988.

21. Office of Technology Assessment, *How Effective is AIDS Education?*, p. 30.

22. Centers for Disease Control, "Antibody to Human Immunodeficiency Virus in Female Prostitutes," *Morbidity and Mortality Weekly Report* 36 (27 March 1987):157–161.

23. Office of Technology Assessment, *How Effective Is AIDS Education?*, p. 30.

24. William H. Masters, Virginia E. Johnson, and Robert C. Kolodny, *Human Sexuality* (Boston: Little, Brown, 1982), pp. 52–53, 289, 302–303.

25. Centers for Disease Control, "Positive HTLV-III/LAV Antibody Results for Sexually Active Female Members of Social/Sexual Clubs...Minnesota, "*Morbidity and Mortality Weekly Report* 35 (14 November 1986):697–699.

26. Office of Technology Assessment, *How Effective Is AIDS Education?*, p. 25.

27. Institute of Medicine, National Academy of Sciences, *Confronting AIDS: Directions for Public Health, Health Care and Research* (Washington, D.C.: National Academy Press, 1986), p. 54.

28. Randy Shilts, *And the Band Played On: Politics, People, and the AIDS Epidemic* (New York: St. Martin's Press, 1987).

29. Sandra Panem, *The AIDS Bureaucracy* (Cambridge, Mass.: Harvard University Press, 1988), p. 87.

30. Peter S. Arno and Karyn Feiden, "Ignoring the Epidemic: How the Reagan Administration Failed on AIDS," *Health/PAC Bulletin* (December 1986):7–11.

31. Shilts, *And the Band Played On*; Panem, *AIDS Bureaucracy*; Office of Technology Assessment, *Review of the Public Health Service's Response to AIDS* (Washington, D.C.: U.S. Government Printing Office, February 1985).

32. Institute of Medicine, *Confronting AIDS*, pp. 33–34.

33. Irvin Molotsky, "Congress Passes Compromise AIDS Bill," *New York Times*, 14 October 1988, p. A12.

34. Associated Press, "Reagan's Last Budget: $1.5 Trillion," *State Journal-Register* (Springfield, Ill.), 10 January 1989, p. 1.

35. Liz McMillen, "Robert Wood Johnson Foundation Pursues New Plan to Be More Responsive to Nation's Health Problems," *Chronicle of Higher Education*, 4 January 1989, pp. A30–A32.

36. Kenneth Wing, *The Law and the Public Health* (Ann Arbor: Health Administration Press, 1985), p. 19.

37. See Nancy Ford and Michael Quam, "AIDS Quarantine: The Legal and Practical Implications," *Journal of Legal Medicine* 8 (September 1987): 365–367.

38. M. R. Herbold, "AIDS Policy Development Within the Department of Defense," *Military Medicine* 151 (1986): 623–627.

39. Larry Gostin and Andrew Ziegler, "A Review of AIDS-Related Legislation and Regulating Policy in the United States," *Law, Medicine and Health Care* 15 (Summer 1987): 9; "HIV Tests for Immigrants, Illegal Aliens to Begin," *AIDS Policy and Law* 2 (September 1987): 2.

40. Gostin and Ziegler, "Review of AIDS-Related Legislation," p. 9; "Job Corps Planning to Screen Its Trainers for AIDS Virus," *New York Times*, 17 December 1986.

41. Act of June 22, 1797, ch. 16, GEN. LAWS OF MASS. (1822). The current version can be found at MASS. GEN. LAWS ANN ch. 111, sec. 95 (West 1983).

42. ILL. REV. STAT. ch. 111 1/2, par. 22 (1987).

43. CAL. HEALTH AND SAFETY CODE sec. 3180 et seq. (Deering 1982).

44. Gostin and Ziegler, "Review of AIDS-Related Legislation," pp. 6–8.

45. An indirect vehicle for disease control has been the criminal prosecution and conviction of HIV-infected individuals who knowingly put others at risk for transmission of the virus. Criminal cases have been brought all over the country against HIV carriers for transmitting or attempting to transmit the virus. Three different means are being used. First, traditional criminal charges such as attempted murder, manslaughter, assault, aggravated assault, nacrotics use, possession of drug paraphernalia, sodomy, and prostitution have been brought to punish or deter the AIDS offender. Second, a large number of states have relied upon already existing public health laws that make it a crime for a person willfully to expose another to a contagious disease. And third, a few states have recently enacted AIDS-specific offenses; some are tied to prostitution and others pertain to high-risk behavior in general. Several additional models for AIDS offenses have been proposed. There are, however, a number of evidentiary and practical problems connected with each of these approaches that make reliance on these means ineffective. Nancy Ford and Michael Quam, "AIDS and Criminal Liability," paper presented at the annual meeting of the American Public Health Association, Boston, Massachusetts, November 1988. See also Thomas Fitting, "Criminal Liability for Transmission of AIDS: Some Evidentiary Problems," *Criminal Justice Journal* 10 (Fall 1987): 69–97.

46. Gostin and Ziegler, "A Review of AIDS-Related Legislation," p. 10.

47. Kathleen Sullivan and Martha Field, "AIDS and the Coercive Power of the State," *Harvard Civil Rights-Civil Liberties Law Review* 23 (1988): 144–145, note 18. Contact notification is a common feature of public health venereal and sexually transmitted disease laws. Statutes give public health officials the power to inquire about the previous and current sexual partners of the infected person. Relying on the person's cooperation, the laws do not give public health authorities the power to compel disclosure of partners' names. In some states, contact notification provisions now extend to the sexual and needle-sharing partners of HIV-infected individuals. Typically the partners are notified and encouraged to have serologic testing performed. See, e.g., ILL. REV. STAT. 1987, ch. 111–2, par. 7405 (1987).

Physicians also have a professional obligation to warn third parties who have had

intimate contact with HIV-infected persons. In some states the duty to warn endangered third persons is either a statutory or common law obligation. There is a
great deal of debate over whether such warnings should occur when patient confidentiality would be breached as a result. There is general sentiment, however, that
at a minimum health care professionals should encourage seropositive patients voluntarily to notify their partners. Institute of Medicine, *Confronting AIDS: Update
1988*.

48. FLA. STAT. ANN. secs. 384.25–27 (West Supp. 1987). See also Ford and
Quam, "AIDS Quarantine," pp. 378–381.

49. FLA. STAT. ANN. sec. 384.28–29 (West Supp. 1987).

50. Gostin and Ziegler, "Review of AIDS-Related Legislation," p. 8.

51. Eight different tests have been licensed for antibody detection and are commercially available, seven enzyme-linked immunoassay (ELISA) tests and one Western blot test kit. Institute of Medicine, *Confronting AIDS: Update 1988*, p. 71.
Common medical practice is to perform an ELISA test initially. If the results are
positive for the virus a second ELISA test is performed, followed by a Western blot
test should the second ELISA test also be positive.

52. Public Health Foundation, *Guide to Public Health: State Health Agency
Programmatic Response to HTLV-III Infection* (Washington, D.C.: Public Health
Foundation, 1986), p. 18.

53. LA. REV. STAT. ANN. sec. 9:229–9:333 (West 1965 & Supp. 1989), repealed by 1988 La. Acts 345, sec. 2, eff. July 1, 1988, and 1988 La. Acts 808, sec.
82, effective July 18, 1988.

54. ILL. REV. STAT. ch. 40, par. 204(b) (1987). See I. Wilkerson, "Prenuptial
AIDS Screening a Strain in Illinois," *New York Times*, 26 January 1988, p. A1;
Bernard J. Turnock and Chester J. Kelly, "Mandatory Premarital Testing for the
Human Immunodeficiency Virus: The Illinois Experience," *Journal of the American
Medical Association* 261, no. 23 (16 June 1989): 3415–3418.

55. The statute reads, "The following marriages are prohibited and declared void:
(1) with a person afflicted with acquired immune deficiency syndrome, syphilis, or
gonorrhea that is communicable or that may become communicable..." UTAH
CODE ANN. 30–1–2 (1984 & Supp. 1988). The Utah statute, because it bans the
marriage of antibody-positive individuals, cannot survive a constitutional challenge.
Banning a marriage for an indefinite period interferes with a person's fundamental
right to marriage as established by the U.S. Supreme Court in the 1977 case of
Zablocki v. *Redhail*, 434 U.S. 374 (1977).

56. Institute of Medicine, *Confronting AIDS: Update 1988*, p. 77.

57. Ibid, p. 78. See also Gostin and Ziegler, "Review of AIDS-Related Legislation," p. 9.

58. These states are Colorado, Nevada, and South Dakota. Iowa and Missouri
had testing programs that they have discontinued. Most systems test for HIV infection only of high-risk group members, when medically indicated or as a part of
a blind epidemiological study. U.S. Department of Justice, *AIDS in Correctional
Facilities: Issues and Options* (Washington, D.C.: National Institute of Justice,
1987), pp. xx–xxi.

59. Bernard Dickens, "Legal Rights and Duties in the AIDS Epidemic," *Science*
239 (1988): 581. See also Morton Winston, "AIDS Confidentiality and the Right
to Know," *Public Affairs Quarterly* 2 (April 1988): 91–104.

60. Larry Gostin and William Curran, "AIDS Screening, Confidentiality, and the Duty to Warn," *American Journal of Public Health* 77 (March 1987): 364. See also Gostin and Ziegler, "Review of AIDS-Related Legislation," p. 13.

61. Institute of Medicine, *Confronting AIDS: Update 1988*, p. 72.

62. One state, Illinois, enacted an informed consent requirement as a part of a larger AIDS Confidentiality Act in 1987. As a result of the lobbying efforts of the Illinois Medical Society the following year, the informed consent requirements were weakened to the point that they are now meaningless. Informed consent is no longer required when "in the judgement of the physician, such testing is medically indicated to provide appropriate diagnosis and treatment to the subject of the test, provided that the subject of the test has otherwise provided his or her consent to such physician for medical treatment." ILL. REV. STAT. ch. 111 1/2, par. 7308 (1987 & Supp. 1988).

63. See Ford and Quam, "AIDS Quarantine," pp. 367–378.

64. 107 U.S. 1129 (1987).

65. One recent federal appellate court held that Section 504 specifically covers AIDS in finding that a public school teacher with AIDS could not be dismissed because of his illness. *Chalk* v. *U.S. District Court for the Central District of California*, 840 F. 2nd 701 (9th Cir. 1988). Courts have held likewise in a number of cases involving the exclusion of children with AIDS from classroom settings. See *Robertson* v. *Granite City Community Unit School District No. 9*, 684 F. Supp. 1002 (S.D. Ill. 1988).

66. Dickens, "Legal Rights and Duties," pp. 581–582.

67. Institute of Medicine, *Confronting AIDS: Update 1988*, pp. 63–64.

68. "Toward a National AIDS Policy," *American Bar Association Journal* 74 (1 July 1988): 123.

69. William Booth, "No Longer Ignored: AIDS Funds Just Keep Growing," *Science* 242 (1988): 859.

70. D. E. Bloom and G. Carliner, "The Economic Impact of AIDS in the United States," *Science* 239 (1988): 604–610; Office of Technology Assessment, U.S. Congress, *AIDS and Health Insurance* (Washington, D.C.: U.S. Government Printing Office, 1988).

71. E. R. Shipp, "Insurance Concerns Seek AIDS Test," *New York Times*, 1 February 1987, p. Y19.

72. A. Philipson and G. Wood, *AIDS Testing and Privacy: An Analysis of Case Histories* (San Francisco: mimeo, 1987); Bloom and Carliner, "Economic Impact of AIDS."

73. Bruce Lambert, "New York Approves a Ward for AIDS in a Nursing Home," *New York Times*, 12 August 1988, p. Y24; Michel Marriott, "New York City Picks Eight Sites to House Homeless AIDS Patients," *New York Times*, 31 October 1988, p. Y16.

74. Howard W. French, "Poor Overwhelm New York Hospitals," *New York Times*, 4 December 1988, p. Y22.

75. Peter S. Arno, "The Nonprofit Sector's Response to the AIDS Epidemic: Community-Based Services in San Francisco," *American Journal of Public Health* 76 (1986): 1325–1330.

76. "HHS Announces Grants for Services to Children with AIDS," *The Nation's Health*, January 1989, p. 23.

77. Institute of Medicine, *Confronting AIDS: Update 1988*, p. 109.

78. *Report of the Presidential Commission,* p. 23.

79. Ibid.

80. R. N. Link, A. R. Feingold, M. H. Charap, K. Freeman, and S. P. Shelov, "Concerns of Medical and Pediatric House Officers about Acquiring AIDS from Their Patients," *American Journal of Public Health* 78 (1988): 445–459.

81. M. Carol Pogash, "Bad Blood," *Image (San Francisco Examiner),* 15 January 1989, pp. 9–17.

82. Institute of Medicine, *Confronting AIDS: Update 1988,* p. 102.

83. *Report of the Presidential Commission,* pp. 94–102.

84. Stephen C. Joseph, "A Methadone Clone for Cocaine," *New York Times,* 11 January 1989, p. Y25.

85. Shilts, *And the Band Played On.*

86. R. F. Soames Job, "Effective and Ineffective Use of Fear in Health Promotion Campaigns," *American Journal of Public Health* 78 (1988): 163–167.

87. Anne-Christine d'Adesky, "ACT UP's Unruly Democratic Spirit," *In These Times,* 20 July–2 August 1988, p. 18.

88. Richard Dunne, "New York City: Gay Men's Health Crisis," in John Griggs, ed., *AIDS: Public Policy Dimensions* (New York: United Hospital Fund of New York, 1987), pp. 155–169.

89. Marilyn Chase, "Corporations Urge Peers to Adopt Humane Policies for AIDS Victims," *Wall Street Journal,* 20 January 1988; p. 31; Dirk Johnson, "Corporations Seek Policy for AIDS in the Workplace," *New York Times,* 15 October 1987, p. Y13; Nancy L. Merritt, "Bank of America's Blueprint for a Policy on AIDS," *International Business Week,* 13 March 1987, p. 65.

90. *Report of the Presidential Commission.*

91. Julie Johnson, "Bush Is Urged to Be a Leader in the Fight on AIDS," *New York Times,* 2 December 1988, p.Y9; Julie Johnson, "The Bush View on AIDS: Money Will Tell Much," *New York Times,* 29 January 1989, p. E24.

92. Gina Kolata, "Alliance of AIDS Advocates Would Speed New Drugs," *New York Times,* 26 November 1988, p. Y7; Lawrence K. Altman, "Mainstream Medicine Joins Growing Debate about Drug Approval," *New York Times,* 6 December 1988, p.Y23; Mark Gevisser, "AIDS Movement Seizes Control," *The Nation,* 19 December 1988, pp. 677–680.

93. Bruce Lambert, "Flaws in Health Care System Emerge as Epidemic Rages," *New York Times,* 8 February 1989, p.Y1.

Responding to AIDS in Brazil

INTRODUCTION

Since registration of the earliest confirmed cases in 1982 and 1983, the rapid spread of AIDS in Brazil has become the focus of increasing attention both at home and abroad.[1] By 1986 the number of reported cases of AIDS in Brazil had surpassed the numbers reported by both Haiti and France, and since that time, even with increased reporting from the nations of Central Africa, Brazil has consistently ranked among the leaders on the list of nations reporting cases of AIDS to the World Health Organization. By April 1989, with as many as 6,202 cases and 3,119 confirmed deaths, as well as a rate of increase in reported cases running as high as 100 percent per year, the epidemic had spread into virtually every region of the country.[2] Perhaps even more troubling, for any number of reasons, the problem of underreporting has been widespread, and the Ministry of Health in Brasília has itself estimated that the number of unreported cases in the country as a whole probably ranges somewhere between 30 and 100 percent of those officially recorded.[3]

Even in the face of such statistics, the fact remains that in Brazil, as in so many other countries, the spread of AIDS has yet to become a significant focus of official attention. The federal government has largely failed, for a number of different reasons, to allocate sufficient resources or to define a coordinated national program to combat the epidemic. As in other countries, the lack of adequate government action in the face of the epidemic has thus intensified the need for concrete action on the part of the voluntary sectors of Brazilian society. Yet even here, while some important steps have been taken, a complex set of social, cultural, and historical forces has tended, until quite recently, to limit the effect not only of the government response, but of civil society responses as well.[4]

Although the record of relative inaction and neglect that has characterized what we might describe as the social history of AIDS in Brazil clearly shares much in common with the history of AIDS in the United States, the countries of Western Europe, and many of the nations in Central Africa, it has nonetheless been shaped by a specific set of circumstances that emerge as at least somewhat distinct, particularly when compared with the cases of these other nations. Analyzing the forces that have shaped the response to AIDS in Brazil must thus be understood as centrally important not only as the first critical step toward the development of more informed and effective policies in Brazil itself, but also as fundamental to the broader project of developing a comparative analysis of the international AIDS pandemic. Precisely because the struggle against AIDS depends so heavily upon the development of global cooperation, on what has been described as an internationalist approach to disease control, perhaps the greatest contribution that the social sciences can make lies in the heightened understanding that they can potentially offer of the significant differences that have marked both the spread of AIDS itself and the diverse responses of particular societies seeking to confront it.[5]

THE SHAPE OF AIDS IN BRAZIL

Although cases of AIDS had begun to be diagnosed in Brazil as early as 1982, little public attention was given to a disease that was perceived as afflicting only the wealthy homosexual population of the United States.[6] It was not until June 1983, with the death of a leading fashion designer, that AIDS began to draw the attention of the Brazilian media. Even then, however, because the designer, like the other early Brazilian victims of AIDS, was himself a well-known and well-to-do homosexual who spent much of his time in New York, the focus of this increasing attention was directed less at understanding the disease than at classifying and categorizing its victims.[7]

Even before AIDS had become statistically significant in Brazil, then, it had become the subject of media attention and, by extension, a topic of conversation in daily life.[8] Playing on a complex, and sometimes contradictory, set of beliefs related to emotionally charged subjects such as sexuality and death, the discussion of the disease was almost invariably carried out less in terms of objective knowledge of scientific information than in terms of misinformation or partial information.[9] Between 1983 and 1985, an image of AIDS and its victims was gradually constructed in Brazilian popular culture that was only loosely based on available epidemiological information, but that would prove to be perhaps the most powerful force

shaping the Brazilian response to the epidemic for years to come. Throughout this period, the vast majority of AIDS victims were perceived to be well-
to-do individuals who enjoyed the luxury of dividing their time between
Rio de Janeiro or São Paulo and foreign centers such as New York or Paris.
Even more important, they were almost uniformly identified as homosexual
males whose sexual conduct was characterized by its high degree of promiscuity. The extent to which this image of the AIDS victim as a wealthy,
promiscuous, homosexual male in fact represented epidemiological reality
was rarely raised, even by medical experts and public health officials, as the
spread of AIDS in Brazil was perceived through its peculiar lens.[10]

Countering this image with a more empirically grounded understanding
of the epidemiology of AIDS in Brazil would prove to be a particularly
difficult task for a number of different reasons. On the one hand, access to
fully trained medical doctors has traditionally been limited both in rural
areas and among the poorer sectors of more heavily urbanized areas in
Brazil, and even where modern medical facilities are available, the complicated symptomatology of AIDS has made the accurate diagnosis of the
disease notoriously difficult.[11] On the other hand, the weight of prejudice
and discrimination has often caused both patients and doctors to resist
reporting AIDS cases, and even after 1986, when notifying public health
officials of cases of AIDS became compulsory, it is likely that the stigma of
the disease itself has continued to cause a significant degree of underreporting.[12] Even in light of these problems, however, state health organizations in Rio de Janeiro and São Paulo have been registering cases since 1984,
and statistics compiled by the Ministry of Health in Brasília have offered
at least some sense of an epidemiological reality that diverges sharply from
the view of AIDS that has been constructed in the popular imagination (see
Tables 3.1–3.5).

What is perhaps most striking about the epidemiological picture that has
emerged since 1986 is in fact the diversity that it seems to represent in the
face of the relatively uniform vision of the epidemic (and of its victims) built
up in popular culture. As of April 1989, while by far the highest number
of cases could still be found in heavily urbanized areas such as São Paulo
(3,843 cases, or 62 percent of the total number of cases reported in Brazil
as a whole) and Rio de Janeiro (948 cases, or 15.3 percent of the total
number of reported cases), the spread of the epidemic had already reached
virtually every region of the country (see Table 3.5).[13] No less striking, while
the sexual transmission of the AIDS virus has continued to constitute the
single most significant factor in the spread of the disease (accounting for
4,326 cases, or 69.8 percent of the total number of reported cases), only
2,598, or 41.9 percent of the total number of AIDS cases in Brazil, were in
fact listed as homosexual males. Another 1,210 cases, or 19.5 percent of
the national total, were classified as bisexuals, while 518, or 8.4 percent of

Table 3.1
Brazil: AIDS Cases and Deaths 1980–1989*

Year	No. of cases	No. of deaths
1980	1	1
1981	-	-
1982	7	7
1983	25	20
1984	117	93
1985	454	314
1986	901	561
1987	1,890	1,053
1988	2,498	987
1989*	309	83
Total	6,202	3,119

Note: *Preliminary data through 1 April 1989.

Source: Ministério de Saúde, 1989.

the total number of cases, were linked to heterosexual transmission. Finally, 1,237 cases, or 19.9 percent of the national total, were tied to transmission through the use of intravenous drugs and the transfusion of contaminated blood or blood products (see Table 3.2).

The picture that emerges from the statistical data recorded by the federal government, then, is far more varied than the popular image of the epidemic might suggest. While the importance of homosexual practices in the spread of the AIDS epidemic in Brazil can hardly be denied, it is equally impossible to characterize AIDS in Brazil solely along these lines. And while the federal government has failed to compile statistical data on the social background of AIDS patients, at least one study carried out by independent researchers in the state of Rio de Janeiro has analyzed the occupations and residences of AIDS victims, and suggests that, far from being a disease limited to the elite, well-to-do sectors of Brazilian society, the epidemic in fact cuts across class and status boundaries, taking its greatest toll on members of the lower-middle and lower classes.[14] This hardly seems altogether surprising, of course, in a society that has traditionally failed to resolve even the most basic health problems of the poor—and in which the widespread existence of homelessness, children earning their living in the streets, and both female and male prostitution for survival are common facts of daily life. Increas-

Table 3.2
Brazil: AIDS Cases by Category of Transmission and Sex 1980–1989*

Category of transmission	Males Number	%	Females Number	%	Total Number	%
Sexual transmission	**4,175**	**74.0**	**151**	**26.8**	**4326**	**69.8**
Homosexual contact	2,598	46.1	--	--	2,598	41.9
Bisexual contact	1,210	21.5	--	--	1,210	19.5
Heterosexual contact	367	6.5	151	26.8	518	8.4
Blood transmission	**913**	**16.2**	**324**	**57.5**	**1,237**	**19.9**
IV drug use	507	9.0	182	32.3	689	11.1
Transfusion	213	3.8	142	25.2	355	5.7
Hemophilia	193	3.4	--	--	193	3.1
Perinatal transmission	**33**	**0.6**	**51**	**9.1**	**84**	**1.4**
Undefined or other	**518**	**9.2**	**37**	**6.6**	**555**	**8.9**
Total	5,639	90.9**	563	9.1**	6,202	100.0

Notes: *Through 1 April 1989; **Proportional distribution by sex. Male/female ratio 10:1.
Source: Ministério de Saúde, 1989.

ingly, it would appear, regardless of the stereotypes and prejudices ingrained in the popular view of AIDS in Brazil, the reality of the epidemic is in fact the reality of Brazilian society as a whole. The face of AIDS is the face of Brazil.[15]

SOCIAL AND CULTURAL CONTEXTS

If the picture that has gradually begun to emerge of the AIDS epidemic in Brazil differs, in a number of significant ways, from the stereotypes that have marked the popular discussion of the disease, it has offered only limited insight into the social conditions that have actually structured the development of the epidemic. In order to understand more fully not only the spread of the disease, but also the ways in which Brazilian society has

Table 3.3
Brazil: Percentage of AIDS Cases by Category of Transmission and Year 1980–1989

Category of Transmission	1980	1982	1983	1984	1985	1986	1987	1988	1989*
Sexual Transmission	100.00	100.00	91.67	81.03	82.43	79.43	68.78	65.67	71.31
Homosexual Contact	--	71.43	54.17	56.03	51.80	50.51	42.43	37.44	31.97
Bisexual Contact	100.00	28.57	37.50	20.69	26.13	23.66	19.83	16.65	25.41
Heterosexual Contact	--	--	--	4.31	4.50	5.26	6.52	11.59	13.93
Blood Transmission	--	--	4.17	12.07	10.81	13.14	20.94	22.78	19.67
IV drug use	--	--	4.17	0.86	1.13	3.66	10.66	15.65	14.75
Transfusion	--	--	--	--	3.15	5.37	7.62	4.97	1.64
Hemophilia	--	--	--	11.21	6.53	4.11	2.65	2.16	3.28
Perinatal Transmission	--	--	--	--	0.23	0.57	1.27	1.82	.82
Undefined or other	--	--	4.17	6.90	6.53	6.86	9.01	9.73	8.20

Note: *Through February 1989.

Source: Data provided by the Ministry of Health, Division of Sexually Transmitted Diseases and SIDA-AIDS.

Table 3.4
Brazil: AIDS Cases by Age and Sex 1980–1989

Age Group (years)	No.	%	Sex Male No.	%	Female No.	Total %
Less than 1	33	0.6	38	6.7	71	1.1
1 to 4	28	0.5	29	5.2	57	0.9
5 to 9	32	0.6	11	2.0	43	0.7
10 to 14	41	0.7	3	0.5	44	0.7
15 to 19	136	2.4	26	4.6	162	2.6
20 to 24	547	9.7	94	16.7	641	10.3
25 to 29	1,056	18.7	120	21.3	1,176	19.0
30 to 34	1,275	22.6	91	16.2	1,366	22.0
35 to 39	974	17.3	49	8.7	1,023	16.5
40 to 44	654	11.6	42	7.5	696	11.2
45 to 49	384	6.8	19	3.4	403	6.5
50 to 54	171	3.0	13	2.3	184	3.0
55 to 59	117	2.1	11	2.0	128	2.1
60 and older	95	1.7	14	2.5	109	1.8
Unknown	96	1.7	3	0.5	99	1.6
Total	5,639	100.0	563	100.0	6,202	100.0

Note: Through 1 April 1989.

Source: Ministério de Saúde, 1989.

responded to it, we must ultimately turn to a wider social and cultural context—in particular, to the beliefs and practices that structure both sexual interactions or contacts and the exchange of blood and blood products. In Brazil, as in other societies, it is through sexual exchanges, on the one hand, and contact with infected blood, on the other, that transmission of the AIDS virus takes place; yet the ways in which such contacts take place are anything but random, and understanding the specific character and development of AIDS in Brazil depends on some understanding of the ways in which such practices are socially and culturally constituted.[16]

Table 3.5
Brazil: AIDS Cases and Rates per Million Population, by Region and States or
Territories, 1980–1989

REGION States & Territories	Cases No.	%	per million pop.
BRAZIL	6,202	100.0	46.6
NORTH	46	0.7	6.5
Rondônia	6	0.1	8.6
Acre	4	0.1	11.5
Amazonas	7	0.1	4.1
Roraima	1	0.0	10.0
Pará	24	0.4	5.9
Amapá	3	0.0	14.4
Tocantins	1	0.0	1.1
NORTHEAST	470	7.6	12.2
Maranhão	15	0.2	3.3
Piauí	13	0.2	5.4
Ceará	64	1.0	11.1
Rio Grande do Norte	33	0.5	15.8
Paraíba	24	0.4	8.1
Pernambuco	162	2.6	24.3
Alagoas	31	0.5	14.1
Sergipe	18	0.3	13.9
Bahia	110	1.8	10.5
SOUTHEAST	5,077	81.9	87.3
Minas Gerais	238	3.8	16.5
Espírito Santo	48	0.8	21.3
Rio de Janeiro	948	15.3	75.6
São Paulo	3,843	62.0	132.6
SOUTH	420	6.8	20.6
Paraná	96	1.5	12.0
Santa Catarina	47	0.8	11.7
Rio Grande do Sul	277	4.5	33.1
CENTRAL-WEST	189	3.0	21.3
Goiás	55	0.9	12.6
Mato Grosso	34	0.5	23.8
Mato Grosso do Sul	35	0.6	22.3
Distrito Federal	65	1.0	42.7

Note: Through 1 April 1989.

Source: Ministério de Saúde, 1989.

Nowhere is this more evident than in the case of sexuality. While the discussion of AIDS in Brazil has been carried out largely in terms of categories such as "homossexualidade" (homosexuality), "bissexualidade" (bisexuality), and "heterossexualidade" (heterosexuality), these categories are in fact highly problematic within the context of Brazilian sexual culture. While they are clearly the most salient classifications structuring the sexual universe in the United States and much of Western Europe, they are actually quite recent importations in Brazil. They certainly do exist in Brazilian culture, particularly in the discourse of the medical sciences, but they are not, by any means, the categories that most Brazilians use to think about the nature of sexual reality. On the contrary, their impact has generally been limited to a relatively small segment of Brazilian society: an educated elite drawn principally from the middle and upper classes in the most modern urban areas.[17]

Traditionally, categories such as "homossexualidade" and "heterossexualidade" have in fact been far less significant within the ideological structure of Brazilian sexual culture than what we might describe as notions of "atividade" (activity) and "passividade" (passivity). Particularly among males from the popular sectors of Brazilian society, the so-called active partners in same-sex interactions, for example, do not necessarily consider themselves to be either "homossexual" (homosexual) or "bissexual" (bisexual)—designations that are more commonly reserved, if they are used at all, for the perceived "passive" partners in these interactions. While a heavy stigma has always been attached to male passivity, activity in occasional same-sex sexual relations has been relatively unproblematic.[18] Indeed, there would even seem to be a certain possibility for the negotiation of active and passive sexual performances in same-sex interactions, and same-sex sexual relations do not, by any means, preclude sexual interactions with the opposite sex predicated on the assumption of male activity and female passivity. In short, while sexual roles (like partners) may vary, they tend to be far more significant than sexual object choice in the construction of sexual identity.[19]

A product of this particular configuration of the sexual universe, then, has been a certain fluidity in the construction of sexual relationships that is itself certainly reflected in the epidemiology of AIDS in Brazil, with its unusually high (19.5 percent of the total number of cases) level of transmission through bisexual contacts. What we might describe as a sexual subculture focused on same-sex interactions has been a part of Brazilian urban life since at least the early part of the twentieth century, and has become increasingly visible over the course of the past three decades.[20] The boundaries of this subculture have been relatively flexible, however, and it has been organized less around a shared "identidade homossexual" (homosexual identity) than around a set of quite diverse same-sex desires and practices. What might be described (even if with a certain degree of exaggeration) as the relative uniformity of the gay subculture in the United States, for example, is altogether absent in Brazil, where a plurality of classifications and identities come together without ever forming a single, clearly defined social group. "Michês (hustlers), "travestis" (transvestites), effeminate "bichas" (literally, "worms," but perhaps best translated as "queens"), self-consciously masculine "bofes" (studs or trade), "sapatões" (dykes), "sapatilhas" (baby dykes or femme dykes), and any number of other figures all intermingle in the space of this subculture, and the variations on these different genres respond fully to the striking class and regional differences that so profoundly mark the nature of social life in Brazil. To a far greater extent than in the gay communities of the United States or Western Europe, however, participants in the complicated world of this subculture (known collectively, and principally among themselves, as "entendidos"—literally, "those who know or understand" the particular workings of the subculture) have tended to both enter and exit with relative ease, often living the vast majority of their lives outside of its boundaries. And their relationships with members of the opposite sex, within the socially sanctioned norms of sexual life in Brazilian society, are often even more significant to their conceptions of self than are their occasional excursions into this alternative sexual territory.[21]

Gradually, over the course of the past decade, this relatively diverse, alternative subculture has clearly felt the influence of the gay liberation movement in countries such as the United States and France (the two societies that have perhaps had the greatest impact on Brazilian cultural life). Particularly among members of the middle class in Brazil, the notion of an "identidade gay" (gay identity) has exerted a certain attraction (indeed, the middle-class gay has been added to the profusion of sexual classifications), and the possibility of a "movimento homossexual" (gay liberation movement) has been explored as a distinct political option. But the model offered up by the experience of the gay communities in Europe and the United States has failed to affect significantly the lives of the vast majority of even those individuals who are involved in same-sex interactions. And while numerous gay organizations have formed in cities throughout the country, their membership has almost always been limited and their existence tenuous at best. Relatively little has been built up in the way of a clearly defined "comunidade gay" (gay community) with its own institutions, publications, and the like.[22]

This configuration has been particularly important in Brazil, of course, with the emergence of the AIDS epidemic. The existence of this distinct sexual subculture has provided a space for the spread of the epidemic, while at the same time giving it its own unique character and directionality: its early emergence among males involved in same-sex relations along with its rapid development among males involved in relations with both the same and the opposite sexes. Among certain segments of this subculture, such as the travestis, for instance, who almost uniformly have little choice but to earn their living through prostitution, and whose clients are frequently otherwise involved in sexual relations with women, limited studies indicate a rate of HIV-1 infection as high as 38 percent.[23]

At the same time that the particular form of this subculture has partially defined the spread of the epidemic, however, it has also influenced the ways in which Brazilian society has responded to it. Indeed, the general lack of a clearly defined community with its own institutional structure and self-identified constituency has severely limited the ability of the population that has experienced the greatest risk of HIV-1 infection both to act on its own behalf and to exert political pressure for action on the part of the state. The kinds of education and information campaigns mounted by gay groups in the United States or the countries of Western Europe, along with the important activities of voluntary organizations committed to the care and treatment of AIDS patients, have been almost unknown in Brazil, and the pressure politics necessary to counteract government inactivity in these other countries have been largely impossible in a setting where gay political groups are both very limited and factionalized. While some groups (such as Atobá in Rio and the Grupo Gay de Bahia in Salvador) have become involved in AIDS education and have focused on AIDS as a significant issue, others have not, and there has emerged little in the way of a broader coalition of organizations or cooperation between different groups.[24]

Just as the social construction of the sexual universe has left its own distinct mark on the development of AIDS in Brazil, the specific practices that have determined the flow of blood have also shaped the development of the epidemic and the ways in which Brazilian society has been able to respond to it.[25] The lack of effective regulation and control over the supply of blood is a long-standing problem in Brazil. In part, of course, this lack of an effective regulatory system is the result of certain fairly easily understandable limitations in the more general public health system—limitations that are themselves linked to the complicated problems of economic development. At the same time, however, the problem can also be tied to a culturally constituted ideological system in which blood donation is valued not as a humanitarian act but as a source of income. As much as 70 percent of the blood that is collected and processed in the state of Rio de Janeiro, for example, is in the hands of private commercial organizations using paid blood donors.[26] Blood donation has thus traditionally been the province of the poorest sectors of Brazilian society (the same sectors, of course, that have the least access to adequate medical care), and an entire class of "professional blood donors" who sell their blood in order to meet the most minimal conditions of material existence has become an integral part of the Brazilian blood market.[27]

The extensive commercialization of the blood supply, together with a lack of rigor in government regulation of the blood industry in Brazil, has traditionally led to high incidence of transfusion-associated infectious diseases such as syphilis, hepatitis, and Chagas disease. It is estimated, for example, that as many as 20,000 new cases of Chagas disease are caused each year in Brazil by transfusions of infected blood.[28] And the already significant problems associated with the blood supply have only been accentuated, of course, by the emergence of AIDS. In Rio de Janeiro, for example, one recent study of 100 beggars found that 70 percent were professional blood donors—and that 7 percent were HIV positive.[29] One out of every five cases of AIDS reported in Rio is due to contaminated blood; and while blood transmission accounts for 19.9 percent of the cases of AIDS in the country as a whole, only 11.1 percent of the total number of cases are linked to the use of intravenous drugs: hemophiliacs and other recipients of contaminated blood and blood products account for 8.8 percent of the total number of cases that have been reported thus far.[30]

Although the gravity of this situation has led to government decrees aimed at ensuring that blood banks test for HIV-1, such testing is relatively costly, and government regulations have been widely ignored. In contrast to the United States and the countries of Europe, the government seems to have been relatively powerless to enforce its own decrees and prevent their cir-cumvention; and precisely where the enforcement of regulations related to blood screening has been the most rigorous, as in states such as Rio de Janeiro and São Paulo, it seems to have simultaneously given rise to an entire network of clandestine blood banks run for profit by racketeers who fiercely resist government regulation. In Rio de Janeiro alone, while nearly a dozen clandestine blood banks have been shut down over the course of the past year, the director of the state health inspection unit has estimated that more than thirty others have thus far escaped detection.[31] And as in the case of the population involved in same-sex sexual practices, there exists little in the way of organized political pressure groups capable of pushing for more effective control of the blood supply. Associations representing hemophiliacs have been active, and there seems to be far greater public sympathy for the plight of AIDS patients infected through blood transfusions (who are frequently portrayed as "innocent victims" in contrast to individ-uals infected through their own willful sexual behaviors), but their ability to really influence the political process in any significant way has been limited at best, and their impact has probably been no greater than that of the few gay liberation organizations that have focused on AIDS as a social and political issue.[32]

Brazil, of course, is an immensely diverse country, and the shape of the AIDS epidemic varies to some degree in different areas—just as AIDS in San Francisco differs in important ways from AIDS in New York, and AIDS in Kinshasa differs from AIDS in rural parts of Zaire. While HIV-1 trans-mission through intravenous drug use remains limited (11.1 percent of the total number of cases) in Brazil as a whole, for example, in areas of the city and state of São Paulo where drug use has been particularly significant, the proportion of cases linked to this mode of transmission has been much higher, ranging between 15 and 23 percent of the cases reported.[33] Still, the general pattern of the epidemic throughout the country has tended to reflect both the relatively fluid and open-ended nature of sexual contacts, particularly among males, and the blatant commercialization of blood and blood products. And the same social and cultural context that has so significantly structured the epidemiology of AIDS in Brazil has simultaneously shaped (and, to a great degree, limited) the ways in which the society as a whole has begun to confront the continued spread of the disease. This general social and cultural context has, in turn, been complicated still further, however, by yet another set of circumstances: by a specific historical moment, and, in particular, a complicated set of social and political transformations that have profoundly influenced the ways in which Brazilian society has responded to the AIDS epidemic. Perhaps even more than the factors that we have examined thus far—or, at the very least, interacting with them— it is this historical context that has shaped what we might describe as the politics of AIDS in Brazil.

THE POLITICS OF AIDS

The emergence of the AIDS epidemic in Brazil between 1982 and 1984 coincided with the development of a social, political, and economic crisis that has been accurately described as probably the worst in Brazilian history. The first cases of the disease were reported in 1982 and 1983, during the last of five military governments that had ruled the country since the coup of 1964, and the continued spread of the epidemic has been played out against the backdrop of the country's tentative, and at times tenuous, return to civilian rule. At the same time, the economic crisis, linked to Brazil's immense foreign debt and the politics of both international lending and economic dependency, has generally accentuated already existing problems in the structure of the country's public health system while simultaneously limiting the government's ability to respond to the problems posed by a new epidemic disease. For better or for worse, the politics of AIDS in Brazil has been played out in relation to this wider historical context.[34]

Perhaps the most significant consequence of this historical context has been a widely felt sense, on the part of the Brazilian people, that neither individual citizens nor nongovernment organizations are truly capable of significantly influencing the political process. This sense of a certain political impotence is itself the product of twenty years of authoritarian rule, in which civil liberties and the rights of citizens were widely disregarded, followed by what might be described as a kind of collapse of hope in relation to the return to civilian government. The late 1970s and the early 1980s— a period described by the military rulers themselves as one of "abertura" or "opening" in preparation for a return to civilian rule—were characterized by extensive social and political action. Feminism, the ecology movement, and the black movement all flourished in Brazil during this period of gradual liberalization, as did a number of groups in the movimento homossexual, and there was considerable optimism concerning the political future of the country. Much of this political energy focused, in 1983 and 1984, on the campaign for Diretas Já: the campaign for direct election, by popular vote, of Brazil's first civilian president in more than two decades. While it brought large segments of the population into the streets for demonstrations across the country, however, this campaign for direct elections was ultimately a failure, as the last military government refused to give up its plan for a more gradual return of power to civilian society.

It is difficult to describe, particularly for readers unfamiliar with the psychological effects of life under authoritarian rule, the impact that the failure of the campaign for direct elections in fact had on Brazilian political life. So much energy had been focused on this question that its negative resolution created a kind of void or vacuum in public life, and large segments of the population watched the activities of the new republican government with a high degree of skepticism. A sense of optimism began to surface once again in 1986, when the new administration launched the Plano Cruzado—an economic plan aimed at ending Brazil's spiraling inflation and predicated on the active involvement of the civilian population as watchdogs charged with regulating merchants to ensure compliance with price controls. Once again, however, the ultimate failure of the initiative, the declaration of a moratorium on foreign debt payments, and the return to an inflationary economy transformed the optimism of 1986 into an increasingly bleak pessimism in 1987 and 1988, as members of the politically influential middle class began to give up hope and a widespread exodus to live and work abroad became part of modern Brazilian life.

While these developments seem far removed from the development of the AIDS epidemic, they are in fact intimately tied up with it, as they have profoundly influenced the political climate that has in turn determined AIDS policy. On the one hand, the tensions between holdovers of authoritarianism and hopes for democracy seem to have reproduced themselves in AIDS-related policies, while the economic crisis has further complicated the problem of AIDS funding by severely limiting the available resources for all public health initiatives, thus making the competition for health-related spending all the more extreme. The general sense of despair in civil society concerning the impact that both individuals and groups can have in influencing the political process has, in turn, accentuated the already acute absence of voluntary groups with clearly identified constituencies at risk for the transmission of AIDS, and has limited the level of participation in organizations aimed at influencing AIDS-related public policy. While the role of the state has thus emerged as fundamental to meeting the problems associated with AIDS in Brazil, a whole range of forces seems to have combined to limit the influence that civil society has been able to exert in shaping the policies and activities of the state.

The result of these various circumstances has been an at times frightening climate of prejudice and discrimination on the one hand, linked to delays in government action and the sometimes directionless development of public policy on the other hand. Lack of information and, perhaps even worse, misinformation, have resulted in a whole catalogue of individual cruelties, as persons assumed (correctly or incorrectly) to carry the AIDS virus have quite literally been run out of town or suffered threats of physical violence.[35] Perhaps even more alarming, precisely those individuals and institutions that might be expected to be leaders in AIDS awareness have often been anything but, as individual doctors as well as leading hospitals have often refused to treat AIDS patients, while other medical experts have disseminated inflamatory, alarmist, and sometimes blatantly untrue information that has done little more than incite prejudices against the victims of the epidemic.[36] And the vestiges of an institutionalized authoritarianism have at times been frighteningly evident in the persecution of perceived risk groups such as homosexuals, prostitutes, and transvestites, who have frequently been the victims of police violence legitimized and justified as AIDS prevention activities.[37]

This general climate must be linked, of course, to a series of delays in the development of a national AIDS policy. As in so many other nations, even after the epidemic had clearly become statistically significant, the Brazilian government was slow to take action. Inactivity was justified, at first, by the immensity of Brazil's other unresolved public health problems—a few hundred cases of AIDS seemed relatively inconsequential in comparison to thousands of cases of Chagas disease, malaria, tuberculosis, meningitis, and the like. In addition, the severe financial strains of the current economic crisis have consistently been cited as unavoidable pressures limiting the availability of funding for basic research, educational programs, and the care and treatment of AIDS patients.[38]

As the numbers began to mount, the potential impact of the epidemic became more evident, and international attention began to focus on government inactivity in Brazil. However, the Ministry of Health finally began to take some action. Perhaps most significantly, in May 1985, a government Portaria or Executive Order called for the establishment of a Programa Nacional da AIDS (National AIDS Program) to be elaborated by a new Divisão Nacional de Controle de Doenças Sexualmente Transmissíveis e SIDA-AIDS (National Division for the Control of Sexually Transmitted Diseases and SIDA-AIDS) within the Ministry of Health, and this newly formed unit began work on elaborating an extensive five-year plan aimed at directing Brazil's response to the epidemic between 1988 and 1992.[39]

Even following the formation of a new institutional structure aimed at responding to the epidemic, however, it was only at the end of 1986 that

Table 3.6
Brazil: Stages of State Response

1982 First reported cases of AIDS.

1985 Executive Order establishes the Programa Nacional de AIDS and the Divisão de Doenças
Sexualmente Transmissíveis e SIDA-AIDS of the Ministry of Health.

1986 Executive Order adds AIDS to the list of diseases requiring mandatory notification.

1987 Executive Order requires that all blood donations in the country be screened for HIV.
Executive Order establishes the Comissão Nacional de Controle de AIDS to advise the
Ministry of Health in formulating a national AIDS policy.

1988 Law passed by Congress and signed by President José Sarney requires registration of
blood donors and testing of all blood donations for HIV.

Law passed by Congress and signed by President José Sarney guarantees social benefits
for AIDS victims forced to retire or take a leave of absence from their employment for
reasons of health.

The new Brazilian Constitution prohibits the commercialization of blood and blood
products.

the Minister of Health signed a further order mandating compulsory notification of AIDS cases and making it possible to begin to track the epidemic
nationally (see Table 3.6). However, despite the order, it has been largely
impossible to ensure full compliance on the part of doctors, who often
follow their patients' wishes in failing to record the AIDS diagnosis.[40] In
May 1987, in turn, the Ministry of Health ordered the screening of blood
donations, but the lack of both legal sanctions and an official regulatory
apparatus has made it impossible to enforce effective screening procedures.[41]
Finally, while education and information have been seen as the key to
reducing the spread of the epidemic, it has only been in 1987 and 1988
that a large-scale educational program has begun to be implemented and
that the mass media have been effectively explored as an integral part of
the educational process.[42] And even here, the explicit nature of the information presented has drawn the criticism of conservative forces such as the
Roman Catholic Church, and it has been necessary to revise the educational
campaign, not to increase its effectiveness, but in order to avoid offending
moral sensibilities.[43]

Even up to the present, the lack of comprehensive and efficient policy
initiatives has gone hand in hand with a continued lack of adequate funding
for even the most basic programs. Virtually all major AIDS-related research
in Brazil has had to rely on funding and expertise from external sources

such as the Pan American Health Organization, the Centers for Disease Control, and the National Institutes of Health in the United States—and, as a result, has also had to respond to a research agenda determined in the vastly different social setting of North America.[44] In September 1988, as the spread of the epidemic continued to increase by 100 percent per year, the federal government announced a reduction of 30 percent in AIDS funding for the coming year, leaving the Ministry of Health's National AIDS Program without sufficient funds for basic medicines and blood-testing supplies. While help from private foundations and the international health community has increasingly been made available (and clearly will need to be expanded in the future), a basic commitment to combatting the epidemic has yet to emerge from the government in Brasília, and the Ministry of Health's own AIDS team has been left alarmingly understaffed and underfunded.[45]

At the same time that the history of AIDS has been marked by discrimination, neglect, and official inactivity, however, in Brazil, as in so many other countries, a critical response to this record has gradually begun to emerge, and is itself perhaps the other side of the increasingly widespread lack of confidence in the established institutions of Brazilian society. Indeed, to a large extent this response seems to have depended on a certain kind of disgust in the face of institutional inactivity, and a sense that nothing will be done if individual citizens fail to take matters into their own hands. In a number of fairly limited instances, it has emerged from already existing organizations in the gay liberation movement, such as the Grupo Gay de Bahia or Atobá, which have become increasingly active in distributing educational and informational materials (interestingly, the groups with the greatest sense of the diversity of Brazilian sexual and homosexual culture seem to have been the most active, while those more fully committed to Western European and North American models have generally been less likely to focus on AIDS education). Perhaps even more commonly, however, the rise of AIDS activism has taken shape not within already existing organizations originally founded in relation to other issues, but through the formation of new organizations specifically in response to the many complicated problems raised by the epidemic.

Since late in 1985, when a diverse group of people came together in São Paulo to form GAPA, the Grupo de Apoio à Prevenção à AIDS (Group for Helping the Prevention of AIDS), the first major organization of AIDS activists in Brazil, these new AIDS organizations have increasingly constituted not only the most important critics of government policy, but often, as well, the leaders in AIDS education, in the defense of civil liberties for AIDS victims, and even in the provision of basic care and treatment services for AIDS patients. The formation, membership, and intent of these organizations have all varied, ranging from largely distinct chapters of GAPA, formed in more than half a dozen different cities by diverse groups of individuals whose backgrounds may include gay activism, social work, or health care for AIDS patients, to ABIA, the Associação Interdisciplinar de AIDS (the Brazilian Interdisciplinary AIDS Association), formed by influential intellectuals and researchers, to ARA, the Apoio Religioso Contra AIDS (the Religious Support Group Against AIDS), an ecumenical group formed by liberal religious leaders, to the Movimento Antônio Peixoto (the Antônio Peixoto Movement), formed by people with AIDS along with their friends and loved ones.[46] Perhaps because of such significant differences in their background and composition (along with the kind of factionalism that has traditionally characterized Brazilian politics), there has thus far emerged relatively little in the way of collaboration and cooperation among these diverse groups.[47] Yet taken as a whole, working in their different ways in different areas and in different regions of the country, such groups of AIDS activists have nonetheless emerged over the course of the past two to three years as perhaps the greatest hope for the future.

Already, there is at least some reason for a certain degree of optimism. The pressure applied by such organizations has increasingly brought a more reasoned and reasonable consideration of AIDS into the media, and has gradually begun to shake the largely erroneous popular stereotype of the disease and its victims. In addition, the efforts of AIDS activists seem to have pushed the medical/scientific establishment and the Ministry of Health in the direction of a greater sensitivity in relation to both the nuances of Brazilian sexual culture and the need for an understanding of social diversity in relation to AIDS. Leading representatives of groups such as GAPA, ABIA, and the Grupo Gay de Bahia have been included, for example, along with medical doctors, scientists, and public health officials, in the formation of the Ministry of Health's Comissão Nacional de Controle de AIDS (National Commission for the Control of AIDS). Whatever the limitations of the government's educational and informational programs, they have been planned (if not always effectively carried out) with relatively little of the "moral panic" that has sometimes characterized AIDS education in other countries, and they have largely avoided stigmatizing the members of so-called high-risk groups while at the same time placing central emphasis on reducing discrimination aimed at AIDS victims. While there is obviously much to be done in a situation that is becoming more and more critical with each passing day, the gradual emergence of a critical dialogue between the state and voluntary sectors of Brazilian society offers the possibility, perhaps for the first time, of forging policy initiatives that will truly respond to the reality of the AIDS epidemic in Brazil.

CONCLUSION

Precisely because AIDS is a disease that is spread through socially determined practices, the shape that it takes in any given setting is as much a product of social and cultural structures as it is the result of biological factors. By extension, just as a specific set of social and cultural circumstances shapes the spread of AIDS, it also conditions the ways in which particular societies respond to it—the ways in which they define or interpret the disease, the reactions they have in relation to its victims, the steps they take in order to prevent it, and so on. While the specific case of AIDS in Brazil has drawn somewhat less attention than a number of other cases, it is nonetheless instructive. Precisely because it presents a number of significant differences when compared with other, better-known patterns, it perhaps offers the chance to at least partially rethink, within a comparative framework, our understanding not only of the disease itself, but of its profound social consequences throughout the world.

International epidemiologists have tended to focus on two major patterns of HIV-1 transmission. The first of these patterns places central emphasis on transmission principally through homosexual relations and intravenous drug use, and has been identified in the countries of Western Europe, Australia, New Zealand, and most of North and South America. The second places emphasis on transmission principally through heterosexual relations and transfusions with contaminated blood, and has been identified in the countries of Africa as well as in a number of the nations of the Caribbean.[48] Although Brazil has typically been included as another example of the first of these patterns, a closer inspection of the details of the Brazilian case suggests a number of important differences when compared with both of these patterns or models of HIV-1 transmission.

On the one hand, while a high percentage of the AIDS cases thus far reported in Brazil have been linked to homosexual contacts, intravenous drug use has thus far been somewhat less important than in countries such as the United States or many of the nations of Western Europe. On the other hand, as in the developing countries of Africa and the Caribbean, AIDS cases linked to transfusion with contaminated blood have been common, while heterosexual transmission, though increasing gradually with time, has remained far less significant. In contrast to both of these better-known patterns, AIDS cases in patients classified as bisexuals have been unusually frequent, leaving open the question of just what direction the epidemic will be likely to take in the future. Understanding these differences, in turn, requires some understanding of the specific details of Brazilian life, in particular, its relatively open-ended configuration of the sexual universe, combined with the uncontrolled commercialization of the exchange of blood and blood products. Taken together, these social and cultural factors simultaneously distinguish the Brazilian case from better-known examples in North America or Africa, while at the same time perhaps linking it to any number of other Latin American countries, where similar patterns both in the social construction of sexual life and in the socially determined flow of blood within a capitalist market open up the possibility of what might ultimately emerge as a distinct Latin American pattern or profile of the epidemic.[49]

The specificity of such differences is just as important in turning from the spread and development of the epidemic itself to the ways in which society has responded to it. The same kinds of social factors that condition the transmission of the AIDS virus also influence the ways in which different societies seek to confront it, and, again, the case of Brazil, and perhaps of other Latin American nations as well,[50] is in a number of ways significantly different than those of the major Anglo-American or Western European nations, on the one hand, and the countries of Central Africa and the Caribbean, on the other hand. While homosexual and bisexual sexual contacts have accounted for a particularly high percentage of the reported cases of AIDS in Brazil, the lack of a gay community organized along the lines of such communities in the countries of the fully developed and industrialized West has clearly had a significant impact on the initial response of Brazilian society in the face of the epidemic, and continues to be a significant factor in the particular way in which the politics of AIDS has developed in contemporary Brazilian life. And while the contamination of blood and blood products has been especially significant in Brazil, unlike many of the other countries in the developing world, this has been less the result of economic underdevelopment itself—that is, an absolute lack of necessary resources—than the result of a particular set of social and political forces that have simultaneously transformed blood into a market commodity while undercutting efforts that might regulate or inhibit the highest available profit margin.

These various factors, in turn, must be linked to the particular historical moment—to Brazil's tentative transition from an authoritarian military government to a civilian democracy facing a set of profoundly difficult social and economic problems (again, a transition with parallels in a number of other Latin American nations). While this transition has taken place with what might be described as relative stability when compared with some of the countries (for example, Uganda or Haiti) where the spread of AIDS has been particularly severe, it might simultaneously appear to be disjointed and uneasy at best when compared with the representative democracies of any number of other nations (Australia, France, the United States) faced with the problems raised by the epidemic. As in so many other Latin American nations, the transition from authoritarian dictatorship to tentative democracy has been played out, as well, in the midst of an economic crisis created by the politics of dependency. While the resources available for the fight against AIDS have in no way been as limited as those available in most African or Caribbean nations, their scarcity has nonetheless created a distinct set of pressures that is qualitatively different from that found in the wealthier nations of the fully industrialized West—a set of pressures that has unavoidably shaped the response to the epidemic in a number of highly specific ways. Along with the wider social and cultural context, this historical situation has played a fundamental role in determining both the form of the AIDS epidemic in Brazil and the ways in which Brazilian society has responded to it.

Ultimately, then, the record of relative inactivity in the face of the potentially critical spread of AIDS in Brazil, as well as the hope for a more effective response in the future, must be read against the background of a complex set of social, cultural, political, and economic circumstances. If the face of AIDS is the face of Brazilian society, then the social history of the epidemic is also the history of Brazil itself. As any number of the groups that have begun to organize around AIDS in Brazil have themselves demonstrated, critically analyzing this history, and the specific circumstances that have produced it, is perhaps the first step toward inventing a more effective response in the future. This is no less true as we turn from a single case to the wider context of the international pandemic: understanding the specific forces that have shaped the history of AIDS in different societies, and situating these societies in a comparative framework, is necessarily the first step in seeking to build a more effective global response to the epidemic in the future. It is among the most significant contributions (and, by extension, should be seen as among the most pressing projects) that social researchers can make in responding to what can quite accurately be described as among the most serious problems currently facing the international community.

NOTES

Research on AIDS in Brazil has been supported by a grant from the Wenner-Gren Foundation for Anthropological Research, Inc. Previous field research in Brazil was made possible through grants from the Tinker Foundation, the Center for Latin American Studies, the Department of Anthropology, and the Graduate Division, all at the University of California, Berkeley; the Brazilian Fulbright Commission; and the Wenner-Gren Foundation for Anthropological Research, Inc. For all manner of help and assistance, I would particularly like to thank Professor Gilberto Velho and the faculty and staff of the Departamento de Antropologia of Museu Nacional and the Universidade Federal do Rio de Janeiro, along with Peter Fry, Joan Dassin, and Michael Adams, of the Ford Foundation in Rio, and Lair Guerra de Macedo Rodrigues and Pedro José de Novais Chequer of the Ministério de Saúde in Brasília. Special thanks to Carmen Dora Guimarães, Herbert Daniel, Ranulfo Cardoso Jr., Sílvia Ramos, and Walter Almeida of the Associação Brasiliera Interdisciplinar de AIDS, to Benilton Bezerra Jr., Claudio J. Struchiner, Joel Birman, Jurandir Freire Costa, Maria Andrea Loyola, and Sérgio Carrara of the Instituto de Medicina Social at the Universidade do Estado do Rio de Janeiro, and to Edward MacRae, Luiz Mott, Nancy Scheper-Hughes, Rosemary G. Messick and Vagner João Benício de Almeida. While responsibility for the views developed here is entirely my own, the research would have been impossible without the help and support of many friends and colleagues.

1. See "OMS aletra para risco de epidemia de AIDS no Brasil," *Folha de São Paulo*, 6 December 1986; L. G. Rodrigues and Pedro Chequer, "AIDS no Brasil, 1982–1987," *AIDS: Boletim Epidemiológico* (Ministério de Saúde) 1, no. 9, (Semana Epidemiológica 48–52/1987); Panos Dossier No. 1; *AIDS and the Third World* (London: Panos Institute, 1987).

2. *AIDS: Boletim Epidemiológico* 11, no. 9 (Semana Epidemiológica 9 a 13/ 1987).

3. "AIDS/Um Flagelo Brasileiro," *Manchete*, 37, no. 1895 (13 August 1988): 26–32.

4. For this assessment see Richard Parker, "Acquired Immunodeficiency Syndrome in Urban Brazil," *Medical Anthropology Quarterly* 1, no. 2 (1987): 155–175; ABIA, "The Face of AIDS in Brazil," paper presented at the Fourth International Conference on AIDS, Stockholm, Sweden, June 1988. See also "Programa da AIDS perde Cz$ 900 milhões," *Jornal do Brasil*, 9 September 1988; "Brasil carece de política anti-AIDS," *O Globo*, 21 June 1988.

5. Parker, "Acquired Immunodeficiency Syndrome"; L. C. Chen, "The AIDS Pandemic: An Internationalist Approach to Disease Control," *Daedalus*, 116, no. 2 (1987): 181–195.

6. Parker, "Acquired Immunodeficiency Syndrome," p. 156: Joao Silvério Trevisan, Devassos no Paraíso; *A Homossexualidade no Brasil, Da Colônia à Atualidade* (São Paulo: Editora Max Limonad Ltda, 1986), pp. 248–249.

7. Parker, "Acquired Immunodeficiency Syndrome"; Nestor Perlongher, *O Que É AIDS* (São Paulo: Editora Brasiliense, 1987).

8. ABIA, "Face of AIDS"; Claudia Morães and Sérgio Carrara, "Um Mal de Folhetim," *Comunicações do ISER* 4, no. 17 (1985): 20–27.

9. ABIA, "AIDS no Brasil: Incidência e Evidência," *Comunicações do ISER* 7, no. 31 (1988): 4–8.

10. Even the Ministry of Health has had a role to play in constructing this image. As late as July 1988, the Minister of Health characterized AIDS as a "doença de elite" (disease of the elite), apparently justifying the withholding of resources for diagnosis, treatment, and prevention on the grounds that the middle and upper classes can afford the expense of such services; see "Ministro diz que AIDS ataca a elite," *Folha de São Paulo*, 17 July 1988. More generally see Herbert Daniel, "A Síndrome do Preconceito," *Comunicações do ISER* 4, no. 17 (1985): 48–56; and Jane Galvão, "AIDS: A 'Doença' e os 'Doentes,' " *Comunicações do ISER* 4, no. 17 (1985): 42–47.

11. Parker, "Acquired Immunodeficiency Syndrome," p. 157.

12. A point insisted on by ABIA in its reports cited in notes 4 and 9 above.

13. A description of the spread of AIDS into rural Brazil is provided in Nancy Flowers, "AIDS in Rural Brazil," in Ruth Kulstad, ed., *AIDS 1988: AAAS Symposia Papers* (Washington, D.C.: American Association for the Advancement of Science, 1988), pp. 159–168.

14. Carmen Dora Guimarães et al., "A Questão dos Preconceitos," *ABIA: Boletim 3*, July 1988, pp. 2–3.

15. ABIA, "Face of AIDS." Given the general lack of data on the social back-

ground or class standing of AIDS victims in Brazil, it is difficult to develop an empirically based picture of the epidemic in the country as a whole. Interviews with AIDS researchers and primary care providers throughout the country confirm the results of limited studies (for example, Guimarães et al.) in pointing to the current cross-class dimensions of the epidemic. Since many of the very earliest cases of AIDS in Brazil were in fact recorded in relatively well-to-do individuals who frequently spent extensive time traveling or living abroad, however, it seems clear (even if in only impressionistic terms) that the AIDS epidemic in Brazil, as in nations such as the United States and France, has been a drift socially downwards. This impression is confirmed, as well, by the recent increase in cases of AIDS among IV drug users, who tend to be members of the poorer sectors of Brazilian society.

16. See ABIA, "Face of AIDS"; Parker, "Acquired Immunodeficiency Syndrome"; Parker, "Sexual Culture and AIDS Education in Urban Brazil," in Kulstad, *AIDS 1988*, pp. 169–173.

17. Peter Fry, *Para Inglês Ver: Identidade e Política na Cultura Brasileira* (Rio de Janeiro: Zahar Editores, 1982); Peter Fry and Edward MacRae, *O Que É Homossexualidade* (São Paulo: Editora Brasiliense, 1983). See also Richard G. Parker, "Masculinity, Femininity, and Homosexuality: On the Anthropological Interpretation of Sexual Meanings in Brazil," *Journal of Homosexuality* 11, no. 3–4 (1985): 155–163; Richard G. Parker, "Youth, Identity, and Homosexuality: The Changing Shape of Sexual Life in Brazil," *Journal of Homosexuality* 17, no. 3–4 (1989): 269–289; and the papers cited in the preceding note.

18. Michel Misse, *O Estigma do Passivo Sexual* (Rio de Janeiro: Edições Achiamé Ltda, 1981). It is worth noting that in Brazil, as in many Catholic countries, homosexuality is not a legal offense. Police oppression or harassment of perceived homosexuals sometimes occurs, but is generally predicated not on legitimate legal constraints but on popular prejudices—in particular, on stigmas related to male effeminacy or passivity.

19. For descriptions of Brazilian sexual culture, see the accounts by Fry, Fry and MacRae, Parker, and Perlongher cited above.

20. This is stressed by Nestor Perlongher, *O Negócio do Michê: A Prostituiçao Viril* (São Paulo: Editora Brasiliense, 1987), and by Trevisan, *Devassos no Paraíso*.

21. Perlongher, *O Negócio do Miché*. I illustrate this point in greater depth elsewhere (see the references in notes 4 and 16).

22. For relevant discussions, see Herbert Daniel and Leila Miccòlis, *Jacarés e Lobisomens* (Rio de Janeiro: Edições Achiamé, 1983); Trevisan, *Devassos no Paraíso*; and Perlongher, *O Negócio do Miché*.

23. Rodrigues and Chequer, "AIDS no Brasil."

24. Both in relation to the few gay organizations that do exist as well as in relation to the victims of AIDS themselves, class is very probably an important element here. Gay organizations with a predominantly middle- or upper-middle-class membership have tended to serve more for recreational than political purposes, and the upper-middle-class affiliations of many early AIDS victims may well have limited a collective political response to the epidemic. The more recent spread of the epidemic among the poorer sectors of Brazilian society reinforces the same problem from a different direction, as members of lower classes are less likely to

identify themselves as homosexuals or gays, and, in turn, are less likely to be involved in, or even aware of, the activities of the middle-class organizations.

25. ABIA, "Face of AIDS"; ABIA, "AIDS no Brasil"; See also Sílvia Ramos, "A Metamorfose do Sangue na Hora da AIDS," *Tema Radis* 6, no. 10 (June 1988): 20–21.

26. A. Padilha, "Vigilância Sanitária," *Tema Radis* 6, no. 10 (June 1988: 5.

27. For the economic dimensions see ABIA, "Face of AIDS," 1988, and Bernard Galvão-Castro et al., "Human Immunodeficiency Virus Infection in Brazil," *Journal of the American Medical Association* 257, no. 19 (1987): 2592–2593.

28. ABIA, "Face of AIDS"; Padhila, "Vigilância Sanitária."

29. Maria Inez Carvalho et al., "HIV Antibodies in Beggar Blood Donors in Rio de Janeiro, Brazil," *Memorias do Instituto Oswaldo Cruz* 82, no. 4 (1987): 87–588.

30. *AIDS: Boletim Epidemiológico* 2, no. 3 (Semana Epidemiológica 36 a 39/1988). See also ABIA, "Face of AIDS."

31. See "The AIDS Epidemic in Brazil: Blood Transfusions the Main Concern," *San Francisco Chronicle*, 7 June 1988.

32. Associações dos Hemofílicos (Associations of Hemophiliacs) have existed for some decades, on the national level as well as in each different state. Traditionally, however, they have tended to serve largely as self-help organizations. With the emergence of AIDS, this general orientation has clearly begun to give way to an increasing politicization, and the Associações have been heavily involved in seeking to shape more effective policies for the regulation of the blood supply. Even though a relatively high degree of public sympathy exists for the plight of hemophiliacs in the face of AIDS, however, their relatively limited numbers also limit their potential influence in a political system that rarely responds to the interests of groups that exert no special economic power.

33. See ABIA, "Face of AIDS," and "AIDS/UM Flagelo Brasileiro." It is worth noting, however, that even if the number of cases does not compare to the caseload found in São Paulo, an increase in cases of AIDS among intravenous drug users seems to be occurring throughout Brazil and is clearly one of the significant trends in the current epidemic (see Table 3.3). Virtually no research has been carried out on drug use of any kind in Brazil, and it is thus difficult to evaluate the current situation. While the use of both marijuana and cocaine has become more widespread during recent years in all segments of the Brazilian population, IV drug use seems to be far less frequent and more limited to marginalized sectors of the population such as the urban poor. Intravenous drug use is apparently quite common, however, among at least some groups (such as female and transvestite prostitutes) who are also considered to be at high risk due to sexual practices, and among IV drug users generally needle-sharing is said to be common. It seems likely, therefore, that drug use will continue to become a more important element of the AIDS epidemic in Brazil as time goes on, and that the heterosexual transmission of the AIDS virus will ultimately be linked not only to bisexual practices but to IV drug use as well.

34. ABIA, "Face of AIDS."

35. See the reports in *Veja*, 4 September 1985, pp. 109–110; 9 December 1987, p. 55; and 10 August 1988, pp. 66–76; and *Isto É Senhor*, 14 September 1988, pp. 46–51.

36. In addition to the reports in *Veja*, see Luiz Mott, "Os Médicos e a AIDS no

Brasil," *Ciência e Cultura,* 39, no. 1 (1987): 4–13; "A Multiplicação do Mal: A AIDS se Espalha," *Veja,* 14 August 1985; and Trevisan, *Devassos no Paraíso.* The role of medical professionals in responding to AIDS has of course been diverse, and the irresponsible actions of some individuals should not obscure the active involvement of others who have sought to respond rationally to the epidemic and to influence more effective actions on the part of the government. Until quite recently, however, there has emerged little in the way of collective action aimed at influencing policy, and there seem to be no organizations comparable to the groups of gay physicians found in the United States and France.

37. See Perlongher, *O Que É AIDS*; "Fright Grips Brazil as AIDS Cases Suddenly Rise," *New York Times,* 25 August 1985.

38. On both aspects see Parker, "Acquired Immunodeficiency Syndrome"; Panos, "AIDS and Third World"; and "Verbas para AIDS não acompanham a incidência," *Jornal do Brasil,* 24 July 1986.

39. Ministério de Saúde (Divisão Nacional de Controle de Doenças Sexualmente Transmissíveis), *Estrutura e Proposta de Intervenção,* (Brasília: Ministério de Saúde, 1987); L. G. Rodrigues, "Public Health Organisation in Brazil," in Alan F. Fleming et al. (eds.), *The Global Impact of AIDS* (New York: Alan R. Liss Inc., 1988), pp. 229–232. It remains to be seen, of course, whether or not the detailed plan elaborated by the Divisão Nacional de Controle de Doenças Sexualmente Transmissíveis e SIDA-AIDS will in fact be put into effect, as lack of adequate resources has continued to hinder the implementation of AIDS-related policy ("Programa da AIDS perde Cz\$ 900 milhões"). The country's current economic troubles make it seem unlikely that elaborate initiatives will be possible without extensive international aid.

40. Portaria no. 542, signed on 22 December 1986, added AIDS to the list of diseases requiring mandatory notification in Brazil under an already existing law. Theoretically, at least, failure to comply with this law is thus a legal offense. Enforcing such a law would be practically impossible, however, and the Ministry of Health has therefore sought to encourage voluntary compliance on the part of physicians rather than invoking legal sanctions in cases of noncompliance. As ABIA and the Panos Institute report underline, it is virtually impossible to estimate the number of cases intentionally unreported.

41. Brazil's new Constitution, which went into effect in October 1988, technically outlaws the commercialization of blood and blood products. The Brazilian Congress must now create the necessary legal and regulatory machinery in order to enforce the Constitution, and it therefore remains to be seen whether or not the commercialization of blood can in fact be effectively controlled.

42. The proposed educational program has targeted health professionals, the general public, groups engaging in high-risk behaviors, and adolescents as its key audiences, and has developed a number of highly sophisticated television campaigns; see Lair Guerra di Macedo Rodrigues, "Brazil's Educational Programme on AIDS Prevention," paper presented at the World Summit on AIDS, London, January 1988; "Unico Remédio: Informaçao," *Visão,* 18 February 1987, pp. 36–43. There seems to have been little in the way of research to monitor the effect of the government's campaign, however, and it is therefore difficult to evaluate its success or failure. There is some reason for hope, as at least one limited study conducted by a major newspaper in São Paulo has indicated a significant increase in the use of condoms:

between December 1985 and February 1987, condom use increased from 6 percent to 27 percent among young people between the ages of 15 and 25, and from 17 percent to 49 percent among self-identified homosexual and bisexual adult males. *Folha de São Paulo,* 2 February 1987; Luiz Mott, "A Penetração do Preservativo no Brasil Pós-AIDS," *BEMFAM* (Sociedade Civil Bem-Estar Familiar no Brasil), Publicações Técnicas, 1988, no. 14. Still, it is impossible to know just how widespread these developments really are, or how influential the government's campaign has been in shaping them. A general lack of knowledge concerning the social dimensions of the epidemic makes it difficult effectively to plan educational and informational programs in a society as highly stratified as Brazil, and it seems unlikely that the same basic strategies will be equally effective for the members of different social classes.

43. The response of the Catholic Church, and of religious groups in general, to the problems raised by AIDS in Brazil has generally been highly conservative, and at times even reactionary; see Luiz Mott, "AIDS: Reflexões sobre a Sodomia," *Comunicações do ISER* no. 17 (1985): 20–27. The internal politics of the Church in Brazil are complicated, however, and there is a strong liberal/left faction. These divisions have been reflected in the response of the Church to the AIDS epidemic, and specific policies have varied widely from region to region; Hilary Regan, "Brazilian Bishops Split on Strategies to Control Spreading AIDS Epidemic," *Latinamerica Press* 19, no. 4 (1987): 6. The Ministry of Health has clearly sought to work as closely as possible in collaboration with the Church (Rodrigues, "Brazil's Educational Programme"), sometimes bending to Church pressure and sometimes managing to secure the cooperation of the Church. In early public service announcements on television, for example, the Ministry of Health was forced to drop the use of the term "camisinha"—from "camisinha de Venus" (literally, Venus' little T-shirt), the popular designation for the condom—due to the opposition of religious leaders; the more explicit language has reappeared, however, in recent television announcements, without significant comment on the part of Church officials.

44. The role of economic dependency in AIDS research is complicated enough to warrant a study in its own right. In Brazil, at least, it seems to have raised problems on a number of different levels. The actual focus of research projects sometimes responds to problems that are thus far relatively insignificant in Brazil, while other significant questions (such as the social epidemiology of bisexual transmission of HIV-1) are left altogether unstudied. Collaborative work with foreign institutions also raises its own problems. Some foreign researchers exhibit a rather remarkable degree of misinformation concerning the actual shape of the AIDS epidemic in Brazil, while Brazilian researchers sometimes complain about exploitation in the division of labor established for collaborative projects.

45. For these details see *Jornal do Brasil,* 9 September 1988; *O Globo,* 21 June 1988.

46. The function and organization of these different groups has varied greatly. Some, such as ABIA and some chapters of GAPA, have attained a relatively high degree of sophistication and organization, as well as financial support from international institutions such as the Inter-American Foundation or the Ford Foundation, and have been able to combine the activities of full-time staff members with those of voluntary members. Other organizations, such as the Movimento Antônio Peixoto and, again, some chapters of GAPA, seem to have relied almost solely on the personal

resources of a handful of members and have maintained an almost exclusively voluntary character.

47. This lack of collaboration is perhaps most evident in the complete independence of the different chapters of GAPA. Gradually, however, some degree of cooperation does seem to be emerging between groups such as GAPA and ABIA, as well as between such voluntary groups and state and local health officials in cities such as Rio, São Paulo, and Belo Horizonte.

48. Peter Piot et al., "AIDS: An International Perspective," *Science* 239 (1988): 573–579.

49. See Joseph Carrier, "Sexual Behavior and the Spread of AIDS in Mexico," *Medical Anthropology* 10, no. 213 (1988). Relatively little has been written on the social dimensions of AIDS in Latin America, particularly in comparison to the far more extensive literatures that have emerged on AIDS in the fully industrialized West as well as in the developing countries of Africa. Perhaps not surprisingly, given its incidence and impact, AIDS in Africa has dominated the discussion of AIDS in the Third World. The significant differences both within and between African nations have often been ignored, however, and the fact that AIDS in the Third World has occasionally been treated as nothing more than an equivalent of this very general picture of AIDS in Africa should only highlight the pressing need for comparative research not only in the different African societies, but also in the countries of Asia and, particularly in light of the present discussion, Latin America.

50. Ibid.

AIDS Policy in France: Biomedical Leadership and Preventive Impotence

"New York struggles, Paris continues to dance": thus ran the title of a cover story published on 18 June 1983 by the Parisian left-liberal daily *Le Matin*. With more than 3,500 diagnosed AIDS cases by mid-1988, France had become the third country in the worldwide distribution of known cases only five years after this surprising title. France has played a distinctive role in the social and political history of AIDS for two reasons: French researchers were the first to isolate the virus in 1983, and French hospitals started experimental treatment on a large scale long before pressure from people with AIDS imposed in other countries a shortening of the period that separates experimentation from commercialization of drugs. While there is no doubt that France has played a major role in the biomedical arena, at the same time national preventive strategies on a large scale started late, effectively only in 1987, and in a very timid way. In this chapter I will examine the reasons for this apparently paradoxical situation: biomedical leadership combined with preventive impotence.

EPIDEMIOLOGICAL TRENDS

The first AIDS cases in France were diagnosed in 1981 just after the first description of such cases in the CDC's *Morbidity and Mortality Weekly Report*. In fact, Dr. Willy Rozenbaum arrived at this diagnosis when he encountered a homosexual patient with just the same clinical signs.[1] A few other cases quickly followed, all male homosexuals. With their public health and epidemiological background, Rozenbaum and a few young colleagues expected that the disease would follow a direction similar to the one observed in the United States. At the same time, and according to the dominant

French rationalist and Pasteurian tradition, the "lifestyle hypothesis" never really entered the scientific debate, which was quickly oriented toward the discovery of the agent of transmission.

With almost no support from the political authorities, this small group of researchers and doctors created a small unit of "epidemiological awareness" to collect, exchange, and discuss the international literature and case materials. Along with the few doctors treating the first AIDS patients, the virologist Françoise Brun-Vezinet, the immunologist Jacques Leibowitch, and the psychiatrist Didier Seux joined the group.[2] This first informal AIDS research group rapidly established contacts with the Pasteur Institute. There, the analysis of a lymph node of one of Willy Rozenbaum's patients by Françoise Barré-Sinoussi, who was working in Luc Montagnier's research group, permitted the isolation of the virus then named LAV.

Given the weakness not only of epidemiology as a scientific field, but of the health surveillance administration in France, this informal network of researchers and physicians also became the first national surveillance agency, anticipating the systematic data collection through standardized questionnaire centralized by the Ministry of Health in 1984–1985. Observation soon revealed that the disease was spreading at the same speed as in the United States, with cases doubling every ten to eleven months, and was affecting the same specific groups: male homosexuals and intravenous (IV) drug consumers. A high concentration of cases in the Paris region was also noted.

Since 1984–1985, those epidemiological trends have been confirmed and can be made more specific (see Table 4.1). With 2,758 (57 percent) of all diagnosed AIDS cases, male homosexuals have remained the largest exposed group, although it is notable that their weight in the number of cases diagnosed annually has declined from two-thirds (64.9 percent) in 1985 to just over half (51.9 percent) in 1988.[3] The second largest group comprised the 817 (17 percent) IV drug consumers (including gay ivdus) whose contribution to the annual cases had more than doubled (10.5 percent to 21.5 percent) over the same period. The geographical concentration of AIDS cases was certainly overestimated in the first years of observation. As long as the HIV antibody test was not yet widely available and the medical profession, especially general practitioners, remained poorly informed about this new disease, it was probably underdiagnosed outside the capital. Moreover, well-informed homosexuals living in the provinces and experiencing health problems similar to the ones described in the press as symptoms of AIDS tried to get treatment in Paris in one of the few hospital services with a reputation in the new field. A survey conducted in 1986 in a Paris hospital showed that 16 percent of all treated AIDS patients came from the provinces.[4] Alongside the concentration of AIDS cases in groups similar to the ones most infected in the United States and most other Western European countries, the French epidemiological data show some specific features. First, in the category of male homosexuals, the disease began its spread in the

Table 4.1
France: AIDS Cases by Category of Transmission 1982–1988

Year	Homosexual*	Ivdu†	Haemophiliac	Transfusion	Pediatric	Heterosexual	Unknown	Total
1982	27	-	-	1	-	10	8	46
1983	75	1	-	6	4	31	10	127
1984	202	12	2	16	16	64	20	332
1985	524	64	8	33	39	118	42	828
1986	1162	233	22	108	62	219	93	1899
1987	2169	573	37	249	117	373	222	3740
1988**	2758	817	59	325	128	491	296	4874

Notes: *includes bisexuals; †includes 130 ivdu and homosexual cases; **as at 30
September.

Source: *Bulletin épidémiologique hebdomadaire* 43 (31 October 1988): 170, Table 2.

upper middle classes and then slowly penetrated the lower middle classes. Blue-collar men only entered the statistics in significant numbers in 1986 but have rapidly increased since then. Second, among male homosexuals the disease started its diffusion in Paris, before spreading to very small provincial towns and before attacking larger provincial towns in the same proportions. This advance reflects the logic of the sexual marketplace. Socially isolated homosexuals living in the countryside tend to satisfy their sexual desires in Paris, whereas larger towns represent small self-sufficient marketplaces protected longer from the circulation of the virus.[5] The specific central importance of Paris as a place for sociosexual exchanges accounts for the more even and generalized regional distribution of AIDS in France than in most other large Western European countries, where the disease remains concentrated in specific urban regions. Today Paris and its environs account for only 51.6 percent of all cases.[6]

In the IV drug consumer category, however, AIDS coincides with low social status. This reflects the evolution, observed in the 1970s, of the heroin drug culture from a largely middle-class phenomenon toward an increasing concentration in sectors of the population hit by the long-lasting economic crisis, unemployment, and marginalization. Poorly integrated children of North African immigrant labor form an important segment of this group now facing the risk of AIDS. Also, the sex ratio in this group does not differentiate between men and women. Since drug trafficking and consumption are strictly punished by French law, there are no exact estimates of the French IV drug-consuming population: only those users who seek a cure in one of the existing rehabilitation centers, which can collectively accommodate no more than a few hundred clients, are registered. The most rapid growth rate of infected IV drug consumers is to be found in the Mediterranean Southeast (Marseille and Nice regions), where the epidemic is following the same pattern as in neighboring Italy. Most cases of pediatric HIV infection, amounting to between five and ten cases each week, are linked to the drug consumer group to which one or both of their parents belong.

Finally, the relatively high proportion of AIDS cases from blood transfusion (7 percent) singles out France in comparison to other countries. Since systematic screening was introduced in France at roughly the same time (August 1985) as in other European countries, this phenomenon is hard to explain. From 1983 onwards people belonging to a "risk group" have been asked to abstain from blood donation, and the publicly controlled blood-bank system, with unpaid donors and blood products deriving from French sources, is now considered safe. It can be assumed that the introduction of systematic screening of blood products in mid-1985 stimulated many people at risk to donate blood in order to get a free test for HIV. So the relatively high number of cases due to transfusion might be linked to these contradictory effects of the imposition of blood control and to the traditions of

medical prescription and a more frequent therapeutic use of blood transfusions in France than elsewhere. The proportion of infected hemophiliacs
is estimated at 50–70 percent of a total population of some 5,000 people.

In sum, present trends indicate a displacement from the homosexual to
the IV drug consumer group, a declining concentration of cases in the greater
Paris region, a high incidence in the Mediterranean Southeast, a social
displacement from the higher middle classes to lower social strata, and the
appearance of the first cases with no known risk factor (probably by heterosexual transmission). Given the very early awareness among some health
professionals and researchers of the potential threat represented by AIDS,
how could the situation have deteriorated so rapidly as to give France a
leading position in the disease's incidence worldwide?

HOW TO DEPLOY A "DOUBLE RHETORIC"

From the beginning, efforts at prevention have had the difficult task of
shaping messages according to the specific distribution of infection and the
broader gradient of risk. How can the most exposed groups be rapidly
alerted and persuaded to change their behavior without at the same time
mobilizing medically unjustified repressive reactions among the less exposed
general population? How can messages be clearly formulated to address
marginalized groups without at the same time stigmatizing them? Again
and again debates on specific policy measures have illustrated this dilemma.
For example, in late 1983, when the blood banks asked members of risk
groups to abstain from blood donation, they were accused of discrimination
through their use of this "bad blood rhetoric," even though no legal sanctions were envisaged against members of such groups who continued to
donate their blood. This apparently neutral and technical measure devised
to minimize a health risk lent itself easily to suspicions that it would have
stigmatizing labeling effects.

How difficult it still was in 1984 to develop a targeted information campaign for the gay population can be illustrated by the conflict that developed
between the first French AIDS experts and the Association of Gay Physicians
(AMG). This association was created in 1981 and now has some 240 members. It has close relationships with the gay press and various civil rights
groups. Its main objective is to "sensitize the medical and paramedical
professions concerning specific health problems of homosexuals and to inform the gay community about health issues." The AIDS experts formally
organized themselves in 1983 into the Association for Research on AIDS
(ARSIDA), copying the model of the League Against Cancer. All researchers
from the Pasteur Institute, the National Institute for Health and Medical
Research (INSERM), and hospital doctors working on AIDS joined this
association, which was primarily concerned with prevention and the collection of funds for research. They tried to make formal contact with the

gay physicians and to enroll their gay colleagues in the fight against AIDS, in particular behind their emphasis on the need for prevention. However, in an early document written in 1983, the gay physicians made accusations about the contradictory and exaggerated nature of the information given about AIDS. Such information, their argument ran, could only weaken the gay community. However, only one year later, when more than 150 AIDS cases, almost all of whom were homosexuals, had been registered in France, the AMG's message changed drastically: "Analysis of the data shows that AIDS in France has practically become a gay disease. As far as prevention is concerned, limiting the number of sexual partners, abstaining from blood donation and using condoms seem to be the only reasonable measures."[7]

Long before the public debate became focused on the balance between concern for civil liberties and public protection, the gay community was divided over the issue of how to define AIDS: just another instrument for reversing liberalizing trends and sexual emancipation, or a general health problem that happened to concern gay men more than others? The first of these interpretations prevailed in the gay press before 1984; the second— AIDS as a gay issue—became dominant thereafter. Before 1984 gay activists and media sources accused the general press of homophobic intentions. But once the virus was discovered and its major avenues of transmission identified, gay militancy adapted to this new situation by getting directly involved in campaigning for safer sex.

The gay community in France followed the American model in its evolution in the 1970s, with the emergence of a gay press and a large infrastructure of bars, meeting places, and bathhouses in big cities. At the same time the gay militancy that was generated by May 1968 almost disappeared in the early 1980s along with the general decline of social movements in France. In addition, although homosexuality has been socially repudiated, it has never been a crime in French legislation. In the public discussion over AIDS in France the closing of meeting places such as back rooms or bathhouses never really became an issue. Rather, it was simply assumed that such practices would change under the threat of a deadly disease.

The about-face in the interpretation of AIDS and the consequent redirection of gay activities gave birth to the first voluntary associations specifically concerned with AIDS, Vaincre le SIDA, and AIDES, both created in the spring of 1984. One year later a regional organization was founded in Lyon. Vaincre le SIDA was founded by the gay physician Patrice Meyer, while AIDES was established by Daniel Defert, a friend of the philosopher Michel Foucault, who was a fervent advocate of the gay cause and had died a few months earlier. AIDES was quickly to become the most important voluntary association in the field, recruiting some 200 volunteers each year in the Paris region. In 1988 it was transformed into a national federation with public interest status, an umbrella organization for twenty regional committees, with a particularly important branch in the Marseille area. In the same year Daniel Defert and his association shared with Elizabeth Taylor the Onassis Prize for humanitarian action in the field of AIDS. This public recognition, nationally and internationally, proves how successfully voluntary associations had transformed what had initially been defined as a gay issue into a general issue.

Although often compared to its American counterparts, such as the Shanti project in San Francisco or the Gay Men's Health Crisis in New York, the French voluntary sector has some specific features. Its declared objective is not to become a long-term substitute for the public sector but to put pressure on existing institutions to force them to confront and respond to AIDS. Explicitly, these organizations have no religious leaning. They represent a combination of the different features of a self-help group of the sick, a pressure group in favor of more research funds, and an expert group intervening in public debates. They are at the same time an avant-garde for launching new ideas for the health sector and a public force that the health institutions can use to increase broad support for more resources and reform measures.

The transformation of the AIDS problem from a particular issue into a general cause can be described sociologically as a process of alliance-building between the gay associations and the world of the health professions.[8] For the AIDS experts in search of intermediaries with the groups that were most exposed and most difficult to reach, the voluntary associations with their important gay constituency were ideal partners. At the same time the associations quickly attracted health professionals with reformist ideas dissatisfied with traditional hospital services and doctor-patient relationships. The voluntary associations, particularly AIDES, became the major agencies for promoting day-care services attached to specialized hospital divisions, for organizing psychological and social support, and for encouraging the general medical community to acquire the necessary medical and psychological skills to deal with this expanding disease. In 1986 the first crisis apartments (*appartements de relais thérapeutique*) for AIDS patients were opened in Paris as a result of a joint initiative by a socialist gay group and AIDES. The voluntary associations also became the champions for defending civil liberties and fighting all forms of discrimination and exclusion.

From the alliance between the relatively small group of internationally known AIDS experts and voluntary associations emerged a specific climate that shaped public debates in France between 1984 and 1986, a climate best described by the term "de-dramatization." Its script ran as follows. As a sexually transmitted disease without a cure, AIDS concerns everybody: HIV has no sexual preference. The best instruments to halt the spread of AIDS, which is an "avoidable disease," are self-control and individual responsibility. Safer sex and the use of condoms represent the "only available vaccine." Given that the situations of contagion are well defined, there is no need to exclude HIV-positive people from social life, and no specific regulatory measures are needed. Further research, more and better information, and resistance to all "irrational reactions"—these were the demands formulated by the experts and given impetus by the media. Indeed, France—as the country where the virus had been discovered and which had attracted many American patients in search of experimental cures, among them Rock Hudson—was to show how to cope rationally and scientifically with this disease and how to prevent moralistic overreactions and prejudice. As can be shown from the media treatment of AIDS, this "French" attitude of dedramatization, considered as a rational coping strategy in contrast to the panic created elsewhere, also permitted the expression of feelings of national pride, pride that had been deeply wounded in the controversy resulting from the publication of Robert Gallo and his colleagues of the identification of the HTLV–3 virus long after they had received communication of Luc Montgnier's description of the LAV virus.[9]

On both a general and individual level, scientific optimism and the use of experimental treatments unavailable elsewhere reinforced hope. The scientific solution of the problem, a vaccine and a cure, appeared to be a goal reachable in the near future. This confidence and hope were dramatically damaged in fall 1985 when the Minister of Health, Georgina Dufoix, announced the allegedly promising results of cyclosporine treatment achieved in a Paris hospital. Only a few days later, however, two of the patients under treatment died. That episode highlights a recurrent aspect of the relations between science and politics: in the name of scientific and national prestige, results of a hypothetical nature are announced by political authorities and published in the media rather than in the scientific press, rapidly generating illusions of hope followed by despair.

Despite the consensual climate during the period until 1986, the government was hesitant to take decisive action. No large information campaigns were started, and no great increases were made to research budgets. Only a few administrative measures were taken, notably the compulsory testing of donated blood and blood products in August 1985 and the compulsory—but anonymous—registration of AIDS cases in 1986. On the wider issue of testing, the central "Ethics Committee," a counseling body to the health administration composed of prestigious representatives from medical and biological research and designed to advise the government on such difficult issues as artifical procreation, had published its policy recommendations in 1985. The committee proposed that no testing should be carried out without consent and that test results should be communicated to all seropositives, including blood donors. No specific information campaigns were, however, conceived at that time. Indeed, although rapidly increasing, the numbers of diagnosed cases had not then transformed AIDS into a major public threat. As opinion polls show, few people cared about AIDS before 1986.[10] Only subsequently did AIDS appear among the major identified problems that our society has to face.

The insistence on de-dramatizing and preventing public panic can also be understood from the following alternative perspective. Until 1986 the relative inactivity of the Socialist government in power might well have been a reflection of a doubly motivated desire to keep AIDS out of the political arena and avoid its incorporation in public polemics. First, the government wanted to avoid a legal discussion on an eventual application to AIDS of the existing legislation concerning sexually transmitted diseases. A French law enacted by the Vichy regime in 1942 and copied from the then existing German legislation requires registration and contact tracing. For years, however, this law had remained all but unused even in the case of the most common STD, syphilis. When in 1984 German legislators discussed the application of their own STD legislation to AIDS, French commentators quickly referred to the "Nazi" origin of these measures, thus preventing all debate in France before it could really get started. In consequence, AIDS is not legally classified as a sexually transmitted disease in France.

In the second place, the Socialist government feared the divisive effects of measures such as the liberalizing of the sale of condoms and syringes advocated by the AIDS experts. A Socialist government liberalizing the distribution of condoms and the sale of syringes could be readily suspected of demographic indifference and favoring drug addiction. So, rather than endangering consensus in this very sensitive area, the government preferred inactivity and a wait and see attitude to the certainty of provoking adversarial debates shortly before legislative elections—elections that were regarded, rightly in the event, as likely to be difficult for the Socialist Party.

At a more general level, the two-year phase of de-dramatization recalls the reactions observed by historians in times of large epidemics, when health authorities tended at first to deny the danger in order to prevent collective panic.[11] In the case of AIDS this phenomenon is far from being limited to France. It prevailed in most Western European countries, where government information campaigns started only in 1986 and 1987. All governments, by definition the guardians of the general interest, had a difficult time creating messages and policies adapted to a major public health problem that concerned sexuality rather than working conditions and that affected primarily marginalized and stigmatized social groups.

In such a situation other governments—notably in the Netherlands, Switzerland, and the Federal Republic of Germany—relied very heavily on voluntary organizations with the ability to reach targeted groups for their prevention work. In France the cooperation between government and the voluntary sector was quite limited. Obviously, the representatives of AIDS organizations were accepted as discussion partners and their advice was given a hearing. But the government, traditionally reluctant to delegate power and financial resources to the voluntary sector, followed the same traditional Jacobin pattern in the case of AIDS. An example will illustrate the contrast between France and its European neighbors. In West Germany voluntary associations for AIDS have at their disposal more than five times the financial resources available to AIDES, with its budget of 2 million francs in 1987. In Germany the voluntary sector is subsidized by the government, which supplies almost 90 percent of its resources; in France government subsidies are insignificant, amounting to less than 20 percent. As in other sectors, the French authorities observe the associations' achievements and, in the event that they are judged efficient, integrates them into existing public institutions.

While official collaboration on the policy decision level was limited, it was more easily established in the field of social research projects. In 1985 an annual survey on attitudes and behavior changes in the gay population was begun. Financed by the Ministry of Health and Social Affairs, this project was devised and conducted by a group of sociologists in the National Center of Scientific Research (CNRS) in close cooperation with the widely circulated gay paper, *Gai Pied Hebdo*. The first survey showed that gays were already well informed about AIDS, but that behavior changes remained very limited. For example, only 5 percent of respondents said they used condoms in 1985. It also showed that behavior change depends on self-confidence and that community networks and informal information in the peer group had more influence than the mass media in securing changes in behavior.[12] Obviously adaptation to the risk was still largely inadequate, even in the most exposed groups. It was only to take place after 1986, and the last of these surveys, conducted in the summer of 1988, showed more than 70 percent of gays using condoms. But, somewhat obscured in the overall pattern, social class differences in risky activities remain significant. In 1988 only 2 percent of upper-middle-class gays still have high risk behavior, as against 40 percent of working-class gays.

AIDS AS A NATIONAL CAUSE

Rupture with the de-dramatization phase came after the change of government in early 1986, when a right-center coalition between Gaullists (RPR) and Giscardians (UDR) replaced the Socialists in power. More or less simultaneously, the Second International Conference on AIDS, held in Paris in June 1986, gave wide publicity to AIDS policy issues as well as offering the new Minister of Health, Michèle Barzach, a forum for announcing new measures in a spectacular way: liberalization of the sale of condoms and a widespread information campaign. In the framework of demographic policy measures, the existing legislation prohibited publicity for birth control devices, including condoms, which could be sold only in drugstores. A year later, in the identical context of the International Conference on AIDS in Washington, D.C., in June 1987, the Minister of Health announced an intensive effort to facilitate voluntary testing through the creation of anonymous test sites in all of France's ninety-five administrative areas. In addition, making syringes freely available in mid-1987—they had been obtainable only on medical prescription hitherto—was designed to stop the spread of the virus through needle-sharing among IV drug consumers.

But implementation of these measures took a long time. Several months passed between the Minister of Health's announcement in June 1986 and the final decision to allow publicity for condoms. The first anonymous test site, the establishment of which had been announced in May 1987, did not open its doors until March 1988. Here again the government's actions followed in the footsteps of voluntary associations, which had already created a test site in Paris in mid-1987 and in Lyon a few months later. Even after AIDS had been declared a national cause, it was less the government than the associations who remained the major promoters of social innovations.

No doubt any government aware of and sensitive to potential political disputes would find it hard to devise a policy line both efficient in public health terms and able to prevent polarization. The national information campaign of 1987 provides an example of how the aim of increasing awareness and provoking behavioral change without simultaneously mobilizing fear and irrational reactions was addressed in practice. In trying to manage these conflicting objectives, the French information campaign chose to adopt a low profile and a "minimal message." In the clips shown on public television stations, an ascending red curve was seen while the commentator stated that "AIDS is progressing and progressing." All of a sudden a young person appeared and broke the curve with the words "AIDS won't get me." People were then encouraged to ask for more detailed information brochures concerning the modes of contamination and efficient precautions, in particular condom use. Newspaper advertisements showed the same images and messages. A total of 24 million leaflets were mailed to households, and 13 million brochures were distributed to the general public through the social services, pharmacists, and general practitioners: specific target audiences included the armed forces and the universities.[13] Although no scientific evaluation of this campaign has been made, opinion polls suggest that it had a limited effect on attitudes and even less effect on behavior. In any case, by the time the 1987 campaign was launched, basic information was already well disseminated. The campaign, which lacked an explicit message, did not diminish the exaggerated fears that still existed in France (see "Popular Opinion" section below). By avoiding addressing explicitly the issues of (homo)sexuality, drug consumption, and AIDS-related practices, the campaign no doubt avoided stigmatization, but at best it produced neutral results.

At the same time more targeted efforts took place in high schools and universities. Since sexual education is a very weak subject in France (limited to a few hours in natural history or biology classes), the issue of AIDS entered the school system through conferences by outside speakers, mostly medical doctors, or through videotapes. In Paris an experiment to train pupils themselves as AIDS educators was made on a very limited scale, the hypothesis being that communication about sexual matters in the same age group is more meaningful and effective than "expert advice." This experiment showed encouraging results and was imitated in other regions. However, the national school administration has had a rather reluctant attitude toward AIDS education, as it feared that parents could react negatively to explicit messages about sexuality. Another experiment in youth communication, launched in the rather conservative region of Brittany, tried to use as educational material comics adapted to the 15–18 year age group. But when parents opposed the comics for their explicit sexual scenes and explanations about condom use, the school administration halted the experiment.

As long as the public debate stayed on a relatively general level, consensus was easy to maintain. But once concrete policy measures are taken, they tend to affront moral convictions and polarization becomes likely. In this context the French Catholic Church, which was opposed in principle to condom use, kept a rather low profile. Only in a few places did small groups of fundamentalists, who have since then separated from the Roman Church, campaign hysterically. The circular letter published by the bishops' conference in 1987 was a balanced document reiterating some moral principles but at the same time rejecting all interpretations of AIDS as a punishment from God. It went on to remind all Catholics of their obligation to brotherly love and charity toward the suffering. The text was generally read as a clear position against medically unjustified demands for quarantine.[14]

FROM THE REFUSAL OF COERCION TO POLITICIZATION

Irrespective of its shortcomings, a guiding line giving coherence and continuity to the French AIDS policy of all governments, left or right, can easily be identified: the refusal to employ coercive measures. The few concrete policy measures that have been taken so far (early 1989)—the free sale of condoms and syringes—can rather be labeled "liberal." The only coercive measure that has drawn little criticism is the systematic testing of donated organs, blood, and semen. The debates over testing are the best illustration of this liberal "red line." First formulated in 1985 when systematic testing of donated organs, blood, and semen products was introduced, the official guidelines require informed consent prior to the test and that in all cases the results be communicated to the testee. Consent by donors of blood and semen is taken for granted since they are assumed to know that all blood is tested: HIV-positive donors are therefore systematically informed about the test result, and there should be no exceptions to the rule. It is common knowledge that tests were administered without prior consent in prisons and in the institutions with responsibility for IV drug consumers.[15] The problem was compounded by the inability of the medical personnel adequately to counsel people concerned about their HIV-positive test result. Testing without knowledge or consent is in conflict with the official ethical rules and the law; and an education campaign directed at medical and paramedical personnel has endeavored to limit or eliminate the practice.

Inscribing the test into the list of routine checkups prior to surgery has sometimes been proposed in order to allow hospital personnel to protect themselves more adequately. In response to those concerns, the Ministry of Health published specific guidelines in 1986 that essentially stated that strict obedience to existing hospital rules was deemed sufficient for protection. The legal problem of defining unequivocally whether an unforeseen accident involving needles that resulted in HIV infection could be classified as a work accident was not to be solved by routine testing of all patients under surgery. Once the medical worker concerned had become aware of the possibility of infection through an accident, he or she was to be tested immediately. If the test revealed the presence of HIV, the infection could not be attributed to the accident given the minimum seroconversion period. If the worker tested negative initially, but positive a few months later, then the infection was to be legally treated as a work accident, carrying all related rights and compensations.[16]

Further debate has been raised by the issue of prenatal and premarital tests. The introduction of the HIV antibody test into routine examinations during pregnancy was first proposed by Michèle Barzach in 1986. It provoked criticism, essentially from the AIDS self-help organizations, who feared that this could be but a first step toward wider compulsory testing. In the end the Minister of Health withdrew the proposition but wrote a letter to all concerned doctors asking them to "systematically propose" the test to pregnant women on a voluntary basis. That has remained the official position ever since.[17]

Internationally, too, France has always defended the position of a very strict definition of "informed consent" in the case of HIV antibody testing. This policy position is in harmony with the WHO guidelines and was adopted by the Health Ministers of the European Community, in spite of the existence of divergent regulations in several member countries.

Does this self-imposed limitation on compulsory testing harm public health? With reference to the psychiatric disorders caused by the virus, Michel Boiron, a professor of experimental oncology and hematology, proposed in early 1988 the testing of all "professions with high responsibility for the lives of others." The testing of pilots as well as train and bus drivers was designed to eliminate HIV-positive people from these professions. In arriving at its answer the government waited for WHO expertise and guidance, which was published in March 1988. According to WHO, such disorders had never been proven in the case of asymptomatic HIV carriers. The French government therefore rejected Boiron's call.

Compulsory testing again occupied the newspaper front pages in June 1988. After the reelection of François Mitterrand as President, the Socialists formed a new government. A well-known cancerologist, Leon Schwartzenberg, was named Secretary of State for Health and in his first press conference made a few policy proposals without prior agreement from the cabinet. Among them he suggested systematic testing before marriage and during pregnancy as well as a nationwide methadone program for drug addicts. The AIDES group, consistent with its firm defense of the voluntary nature of all testing, opposed the first proposal, while the press and some professional circles drew on foreign examples to criticize the proposed methadone program as ineffective. Although Schwartzenberg argued that he only wanted to launch a public debate on these issues and that he actually favored a policy of "generalized voluntary testing" rather than compulsory testing, he was fired the same day and had to leave the government for his lack of "government discipline."

Two months later he reiterated his proposals in a popular TV talk show and, seduced by his performance, a majority of over 70 percent in a poll agreed with him. The left-liberal weekly Le Nouvel Observateur then published a manifesto calling on all French citizens to accept an anonymous and voluntary test.[18] It argued that individuals' knowledge about their HIV status would rapidly help to induce behavior changes. In the meantime, however, Schwartzenberg had semantically rearranged his proposals to make them more acceptable. He no longer spoke of compulsory testing, but of "generalized but voluntary testing." These semantic disputes found a resolution in November 1988, when the new Minister of Health, Claude Evin, presented his plan against AIDS, which included the formulation that doctors "should systematically propose the test" to patients who could have been exposed to the virus in specific contexts and situations. Such a formulation obviously aims at the generalization of voluntary testing.

Clearly, consensus is difficult to maintain over long periods on a policy built around the concept of "individual responsibility" and the rejection of coercive and regulatory measures. In such a context expert opinion provides the major guarantee for consensus. In the very first years of the AIDS epidemic only the few researchers and physicians with international reputations in the field and well-known for their treatment of a significant number of AIDS patients were accepted in the public arena as legitimate experts. As described above, they formed a tight network that organized the first French data collection, published popular brochures, and gave conferences for voluntary AIDS associations.[19] Newspapers invited them as guest authors or interviewed them on not only biomedical but also social and health policy problems. In their aim of establishing cooperative relationships with the most exposed communities, they recognized that coercion might have counterproductive effects both on prevention and on early diagnosis and treatment of HIV-infected people. They thus became strong spokesmen for a liberal policy approach.[20] Given the symbolic power of their discourse, hardly any space was left for dissent in the public arena.

The state of impregnable consensus changed only gradually after 1986 in both professional and political communities. Professional dissent first appeared in 1987 when the Southeast regional authorities announced their support for a pilot project in epidemiology. The project was intended as a broad study of the development of the disease from asymptomatic sero-positivity to full-blown AIDS, based on the systematic collection and analysis of data on people treated for an HIV-related infection both in hospitals and by general city practitioners. If carried out, it would have led to the anonymous registration of all HIV-positive people found in the region; and it would therefore have posed problems of data protection and confidentiality. But, since AIDS had been declared a *national* issue, the project also questioned the hierarchical power of central over regional authorities. Defining the issue as a conflict between political and administrative jurisdiction, the central Ministry of Health cut short the region's initiative on the grounds that so major a policy issue as the systematic registration of seropositive cases could not be decided at the local level.

In December 1987 a public statement by Jacques Crozemarie, the administrative director of the French Association for Cancer Research (basically a fund-raising and project-financing organization), again aroused controversy. At a conference then being held in Washington, D.C., he accused the French government of not telling the truth about the dramatic extension of the AIDS epidemic and called for systematic testing of the whole population and everyone entering France. Since he was not a doctor, he was immediately attacked for his lack of medical competence, and his statement was dismissed by the government. Shortly afterward the bulletin of his organization published a whole catalogue of desirable immediate measures against AIDS, which in fact amounted to a watered-down version of Crozemarie's proposals.[21] They clearly reveal a professional strategy around the issue of who should control the new medical field of AIDS. It was proposed that HIV test sites should be integrated into cancer screening centers and that a European epidemiological research institute on cancer and AIDS be created. In the long run, this meant that AIDS research and experimental treatment was to be absorbed into the field of cancerology.

In the early days of AIDS research most experts were doctors in their thirties and forties at a crucial moment of their careers. They perceived a challenging new field that allowed them to combine scientific interests, career considerations, and political and ethical convictions and motivations. They could gain recognition and international reputations much faster than in traditional fields with well-established paradigms and hierarchical structures.[22] But very soon the institutional machinery, which at the beginning was rather reluctant to invest in this new field, moved into the expanding AIDS business. The proposed organizational integration of cancer and HIV testing and the establishment of common epidemiological facilities is but one of the innumerable signs indicating the institutional and disciplinary strategies under way with the goal of structuring and controlling a field in which the need for innovation had allowed a few young scientists and physicians a degree of freedom unusual in the very hierarchical world of medicine. Visibility in the media had been a major source of influence for the young scientists. With the help of spectacular policy statements, the leading figures of traditional institutions are now following the same tactical patterns, and the number of newly established committees and organizations for distributing funds gives additional witness to the scale of competitive interest.[23] Some controversy was provoked by this decision, since two other foundations associated with the Pasteur Institute—the French and American AIDS Foundation and the World AIDS Foundation—had been established only a short time earlier. Almost independent of individual motivations, this strategic cascade produces dissent, damaging the image of a unified field of expert opinion and facilitating political polarization.

It is interesting to note that in a country rather well known for its passionate ideological debates, no significant political controversy over AIDS can be recorded. In 1987 and 1988 the liberal policy line was reaffirmed by Alain Pompidou, the special AIDS counselor of Michèle Barzach, the Minister of Health;[24] and it was confirmed in two parliamentary reports on the AIDS situation in France and Africa. Prepared under the responsibility of two Members of Parliament affiliated to the right-wing RPR, Michel Hannoun and Bernard Debré, these reports were welcomed by socialists and communists.[25] From 1984 to 1986, the declared enemy of the "de-dramatization" policy—irrational fears and ideological exploitation of a sickness—was an anticipated rather than an actually existing phenomenon. Clearly, the media of conservative and right-wing obedience wrote less about AIDS than the left-liberal press.[26] As is well documented in opinion polls, this imbalance corresponds to the expectations of the readership.[27] Not concerned about AIDS in those days, the conservative public showed no interest in the theme. In paying tribute to the internationally known French experts, its members showed that they were not prepared to follow opinion-leaders in developing repressive public health proposals. The left-liberal public, whose members often came out of the generation that had accomplished the "silent revolution," including the sexual liberation trends of the 1970s, soon felt concerned by, if not exposed to, AIDS. They sought medical information and identified themselves with a crusade against irrational reactions that could have threatened their ethical convictions. The editorial line of the Parisian newspaper *Libération*, created in the aftermath of May 1968, is the most typical example of this journalistic presentation.[28]

Only in 1987, when AIDS was declared a national cause and the disease became progressively dissociated in the media from the initial risk groups did the theme become a political issue. That a disease concern everybody and not only a few minority groups is the precondition for a larger politicization. But no major political force would have taken the risk of breaking the prevailing consensus that had kept AIDS out of the political arena.

Denouncing the consensus as a "conspiracy of silence" served the extreme right party Front National as the major theme for its campaign for compulsory testing and for quarantining people with AIDS. In late 1986 a weekly close to the party, *Minute*, published a cover story signed by C. Bachelot, a doctor responsible for health questions for the Front.[29] A few months later the party leader, Jean Marie Le Pen, announced those proposals on a popular TV talk show. He also insisted that the virus could be transmitted in everyday situations and that energetic measures were needed to combat the plague. Associating this health problem with the theme of African immigration, such demagogical language tends to produce AIDS as a metaphor for moral decadence, economic decay, and national decline provoked by a barbarian invasion. But the choice of terms with anti-Semitic connotations such as *sidatoriums* and *sidaïque* to label people with AIDS facilitated an immediate coalition of the whole polity against a Front National accused of using a racist and prejudiced mixture of arguments. Nevertheless, as almost the only candidate during the 1988 presidential campaign to discuss AIDS and to propose coercive measures, Le Pen got no less than 15 percent of the popular vote.

Dissent among professionals and the violent rupture of the prevailing policy consensus forced AIDS onto the political agenda in 1987. At that point gay militancy outside specific AIDS organizations no longer kept its low profile; gays started to campaign on the issue of "AIDS and civil liberties." A gay group closely linked to the Socialist Party, Gais pour les Libertés, started the campaign and enrolled human rights and humanitarian organizations behind their efforts. They not only attacked the extreme right but also criticized the government, in moderate terms, for its inadequate information campaign and its lack of material support for the sick. The mobilization was reinforced by some screening scandals linked to employment. In 1987 the city of Paris had tested some of its job applicants for HIV antibodies without their knowledge during routine medical tests. After months of investigations and public controversy, one HIV-positive person who had been refused a job had to be hired, but no other political or professional sanctions were taken. Rumors about routine testing without consent in prisons and hospitals faced with IV drug consumer patients also appeared in the press.

Another case illustrated the difficulties posed by AIDS as a legally undefined disease. French civil service regulations exclude from employment anyone with an incurable chronic disease as defined in a specific list, which does not include AIDS. When Didier Hutin, a schoolteacher in the Paris suburbs with excellent professional references but under treatment for AIDS, was refused tenure in late 1987, mobilization took place against this measure of exclusion, and Hutin initiated an administrative appeal against the decision not to grant him tenure. At the end of 1988 he won his case, and his nomination was signed by the Minister of Health. It is too early yet to say whether this administrative decision will be considered an isolated one or as constituting a general precedent.

From a general concern, AIDS has been progressively translated into a diversity of concrete and controversial policy problems that are hard to resolve. The policy problems that the government faces today center on the quantitative and qualitative adaptation of the health sector to growing numbers of people with AIDS and a large HIV-positive population that requires, or will require, medical and psychological care. The major expertise on both the shortcomings and their possible remedies has been accumulated in the voluntary sector, which has become a partner that the public authorities can no longer ignore. At the same time, in order to remain faithful to its liberal doctrine, the government has to deal with popular demands for more repressive measures. Economic pressures will be added to the sociopolitical ones. Until 1987 hospital costs in the Paris region were declining because of fewer hospitalizations, with the result that in its early years the increase in costs created by AIDS could be absorbed thanks to these economies. In 1986, however, AIDS was added to the list of chronic illnesses that received full reimbursement by social security. By the end of 1987, for the first time, the hospital costs associated with AIDS could no longer be compensated by economies in other health sectors.

POPULAR OPINION

AIDS is certainly spreading beyond the first exposed groups, which, however, still represent the vast majority of cases. How does social proximity to, or distance from, AIDS victims shape opinions, reactions, fears, and personal involvement in the voluntary sector? Posing these questions reveals, first, that popular perceptions of risk among the majority of the population (who are not personally acquainted with HIV-positive friends or relatives) still feed repressive policy demands; and, second, that the gay constituency continues to shoulder the greatest burden of the struggle against AIDS.

Despite unprecedented media coverage, a government information campaign, and information efforts by voluntary associations, the concern over possible transmission vehicles (insects) and situations (blood donation, swimming pools, public toilets) still persists in the representations of up to 40 percent of the population. The least informed people are over 50 years old, socially located in the traditional downwardly mobile middle classes and in the sectors of the working class that have suffered most from the economic crisis. They tend to project all sorts of fears onto AIDS and favor repressive measures, including quarantine. By the end of 1987, they represented between 10 and 15 percent of the general adult population.[30]

Young, highly educated members of the urban middle classes sharply oppose this demand for state control. Often personally acquainted with HIV carriers, they favor the present liberal policy line. Among them, single persons with several sexual partners have started to use condoms. Among the gay population, which represents a small minority (9 percent) in the general sexually active population, these attitudes and behavior changes are a majority phenomenon. After a slow start in 1985 in making behavioral changes, by 1988, 85 percent of gays had modified their risk activities, and 78 percent were using condoms, 40 percent of them regularly.

But together these two reactions—in their pure, ideal-typical, repressive, and liberal forms—can be found only in a minority (less than 30 percent) of the population. Although rejecting measures of quarantine as useless and inhuman, the majority of the population cannot identify with a completely liberal position based on the concepts of individual responsibility and informed consent. The overwhelming majority (more than 70 percent) favor compulsory testing of the three categories held to be intrinsically "irresponsible": prostitutes, IV drug consumers, and prisoners. Opinions on homosexuals are much more ambivalent, as they are considered to be capable of adapting to the constraints that AIDS imposes on their lives. The most outspoken defenders of a liberal policy line are the voluntary AIDS associations. But they also know that tangible results in the field of prevention are the only long-term guarantee for such a policy.

CONCLUSIONS

AIDS policy in France can be described as liberal insofar as it relies on individual responsibility and consent. This approach precluded the extension and application of existing legislation concerning sexually transmitted disease to AIDS. It also implied the permanent search for political consensus in order to keep the AIDS issue off the political agenda. But this same objective explains the very timid character of the official policies of prevention, which reflect the lowest common denominator between social forces with diverging value commitments. Until the present (early 1989) four phases of AIDS policy can be distinguished:

1. 1981–1984. Before 1984, France occupied a leading role in biomedical research, but AIDS was not yet perceived as a public health issue. Only concerned scientific and professional circles, which were obviously limited in size, started to organize systematic thinking on preventive strategies.

2. 1984–1986. This phase saw alliance-building between the first expert circles and voluntary AIDS associations from the strong gay constituency, which led to the constitution of a tightly knit network that inspired almost all initiatives in the field and was widely publicized in the media. The government persisted in a wait-and-see attitude. No specific measures were taken apart from the systematic

checking of blood and blood products. The decision by the central Ethics Committee on the necessity of informed consent for all testing became the official policy line.

3. 1987–1988. In 1987 AIDS was declared a "national cause." It has since become a growth area in research and in the health sector. Conflict has emerged among professionals eager to gain control over the field—conflicts that have a generational component. At the same time two specific pragmatic measures—liberalizing the sale of condoms and of syringes—have aroused the first, initially small-scale, policy controversies. In public debates AIDS has been progressively dissociated from the initially designated "risk groups." All these elements have converged to create the conditions for the breakup of the prevailing consensus. By doing this with some violence, the extreme right Front National initially provoked a unifying response against itself, apparently reinforcing the liberal consensus among all other political groups. But the consensus is no longer sacred. It is easy to predict that policy debates in the future will concentrate on testing in specific situations (before marriage, during pregnancy) and on the economic ramifications of AIDS that have so far hardly received any discussion.

4. 1989—a new beginning? After commissioning an evaluative report on AIDS policy—which was extremely critical of the inefficiency of present policies—the Minister of Health, Claude Evin, presented a new plan in November 1988 that recognized the urgency of the situation in prevention as well as in hospital care. In 1989 substantial funding of 100 million francs was allocated to information and prevention, which are intended to be better targeted than in the past. Other measures are foreshadowed: an increase in the number of anonymous HIV test sites; the creation of 200 new jobs in AIDS care in the public hospital sector, at a cost of 30 million francs; the allocation of 50 million francs for new hospital equipment and 400 million francs for medication and biological tests. Research, including social science research in the field of prevention, was given 150 million francs. Institutional innovations were also seen as necessary. A national center (Agence National de Lutte contre le SIDA) is now being created in the Ministry of Health, and a National AIDS Council, consisting of an autonomous body of specialists, will advise the Minister of Health in all questions concerning AIDS. It is of course too early to assess the efficiency of the new structures or the effects of the very considerably increased funding for key policies. What is nonetheless plain is that France, as the worst affected European country, and with a predicted 20,000 AIDS cases by the end of 1989, has urgent need of the most effective and rapid policies that the new structures can deliver.

NOTES

1. W. Rozenbaum, D. Seux, and A. Kouchner, *SIDA: Réalités et fantasmes* (Paris: POL, 1984), p. 24.

2. See J. Heilbronn and J. Goudsmit, "A propos de la découverte du virus du SIDA," *Actes de la recherche en sciences sociales* 69 (1987): 99.

3. *Bulletin épidémiologique hebdomadaire* 43 (31 October 1988): 169.

4. M. Pollak, W. Rozenbaum, A. Viallefont, S. Gharakhanian, and F. Aimé,

"Les conséquences psychosociales de l'infection HIV," *Revue d'épidémiologie et de la santé publique* 36 (1988): 202–208.

5. Ibid.

6. *Bulletin épidémiologique hebdomadaire* 43 (31 October 1988): 171, Fig. 1.

7. The two positions are embodied in declarations by the AMG in October 1983 and September 1984.

8. M. Pollak, "AIDS: Risikomanagement unter widersprüchlichen Zwängen," *Journal für Sozialforschung* 27, 3/4, 1987.

9. See M. Pollak, *Les homosexuels et le sida: Sociologie d'une épidémie* (Paris: Anne-Marie Métailié, 1988), p. 149.

10. See the IPSOS survey in *Gai Pied Hebdo* 195 (1985): 16–17.

11. See J. Delumeau, *La peur en Occident* (Paris: Fayard, 1978), p. 147; W. McNeill, *Le temps de la peste* (Paris: Hachette, 1978).

12. M. Pollak and M. A. Schiltz, *Les homosexuels face au sida*, 2 vols. (Paris: CNRS-EHESS, 1987); "Les homosexuels face à l'épidémie du sida," *Revue Française d'épidémiologie et de santé publique* 3 (1986); M. Pollak, M. A. Schiltz, and L. Laurindo, "Ambivalent Reactions to AIDS among French Male Homosexuals," in J. C. Gluckmann and E. Vilmer, eds., *International Conference on AIDS: Paris 1986* (Amsterdam and New York: Elsevier, 1986).

13. A brief account of the major features of the 1987 campaign can be found in Alain Pompidou, "National AIDS Information Programme in France," in WHO, *AIDS Prevention and Control*, papers presented at the World Summit of Ministers of Health on Programs for AIDS Prevention, London, 26–28 January 1988 (Oxford: WHO and Pergamon Press, 1988), pp. 28–31.

14. "De la peur à la solidarité," declaration of the French Bishops' Conference, 23 June 1987.

15. Current anti-AIDS measures in French prisons encourage the voluntary screening of members of risk groups. No special measures are taken for seropositives, but prisoners with AIDS are confined to the prison hospital or transferred to a special center at Fresnes. *The AIDS Letter* 11 (February-March 1989): 5.

16. "Prévention de la transmission de l'infection VIH dans les lieux de soins et laboratoires," *Bulletin épidémiologique hébdomadaire* 40 (1987): 1–2.

17. In mid-1988 a survey of 274, 647 pregnant women in France revealed that two births or abortions per day involved seropositive women. *Nature* 333 (9 June 1988): 486.

18. *Le Nouvel Observateur*, 19–25 September 1988, p. 23.

19. One of the first very widely distributed brochures has the revealing title "Specialists Answer Your Questions": L. Montagnier, ed., "Des spécialistes répondent à vos questions" (Paris: Fondation internationale pour l'information scientifique, 1985).

20. This phenomenon can also be observed internationally; see Denis Altman, *AIDS in the Mind of America: The Social, Political and Psychological Impact of a New Epidemic* (New York: Anchor Press, 1986), p. 129.

21. "Fondamental," *Revue de l'ARC* 37 (January 1988).

22. For these interrelations between career interests, paradigmatic situations, and the strength of social hierarchies in scientific disciplines, see E. Brian and M. Jaisson, "Unités et identités: Notes sur l'accumulation scientifique," *Actes de la recherche*

en sciences sociales 74 (1988): 66ff.; M. Pollak, "From methodological prescription to sociohistorical description," *Fundamenta scientiae* 4, no. 1 (1983): 25.

23. In January 1988 a National Committee for Research on AIDS was announced, under the joint sponsorship of the Pasteur Institute and the Fondation pour la Recherche Médicale.

24. See the introduction by Alain Pompidou to E. Hirsch, ed., *SIDA: Rumeurs et faits* (Paris: Cerf, 1987).

25. M. Hannoun, "Le SIDA: Question de société," *Assemblée Nationale*, no. 1090 (2 February 1988); B. Debré, "La lutte contre le SIDA," *Assemblée Nationale*, no. 1091 (2 February 1988). The only party sharply opposed to this consensual policy has been the extreme right Front National.

26. N. Mauriac, *Le Mal entendu: Dire et savoir le sida* (Bordeaux: IEP, 1988), pp. 68–84.

27. For the relationships between the expectations of the readership and the work of journalists, see P. Champagne, "La manifestation: La production de l'évènement politique," *Actes de la recherche en sciences sociales* 52/53 (1984): 28.

28. Pollak, *Les homosexuels et le sida*, pp. 135ff.

29. C. Bachelot, "On cache la vérité," *Minute* 1288 (December 1986): 14–15.

30. W. Dab, J. P. Moatti, J. Bastide, L. Abenhaïm, and M. Pollak, "La perception sociale du sida en région Ile-de-France," *Bulletin épidémiologique hebdomadaire* 5 (1 February 1988).

AIDS in Belgium: Africa in Microcosm

As of 30 December 1988, a total of 424 cases of AIDS had been reported in Belgium, for a population of some 9.9 million, since the start of the epidemic. Over this same period, 4,013 people were confirmed to be seropositive by reference laboratories accredited to carry out this type of test.[1]

More than half (53.5 percent) of the AIDS cases reported in Belgium since the start of the epidemic concern people who are not residents of the country. They are Belgian nationals or foreigners living for the most part in Central Africa (mainly Zaire, Rwanda, and Burundi) who have come to Belgium for medical care because of the country's historical ties with its former colonies. Even though this trend is currently waning and residents predominate among the new cases of AIDS, this figure still expresses a particularity of AIDS in Belgium.[2] In Belgium more than anywhere else, AIDS is spread by heterosexual contact with people from Central Africa. Besides the fact that the overwhelming majority of the so-called nonresident patients contracted the disease through heterosexual contact, 23.4 percent of the resident patients also contracted the disease in this manner, usually through sex with people who had lived in Central Africa.[3] Homosexual or bisexual transmission is implicated in some 60 percent of the "resident" cases and intravenous transmission (drug addicts) in a mere 5 percent of the cases.

A DOUBLY IMPORTED DISEASE (1983–1985)

Having described the situation, I shall focus on how the AIDS problem has been managed in Belgium until now. To this end, it is useful to distinguish between two periods characterized by particular ways of grasping the problem. The first period extends from the summer of 1983 to the end of

1985, that is, from the time at which AIDS really began making headlines until the first preventive measures were set up (blood screening and public information).

Over this period AIDS can be said to have been a doubly imported disease. The main components of information (type of disease, definitions of risk groups, etc.) came from the United States. At the same time, attention in Belgium had been drawn to the existence of an African focus of infection through patients from Central Africa who began coming to Belgium for treatment rather early. Consequently, the danger was perceived both as an outside threat brought by American homosexuals and Africans and as a relatively remote phenomenon.

In this context, the first preventive measures consisted in instituting systematic testing of all blood and plasma donors and supplies (Belgium is mostly self-supporting in that field). This testing became mandatory as of 1 August 1985 (*Arrêté Royal* of July 18, 1985). Under this law, anti-HIV antibody screening is also required in addition to the taking of a thorough case history for each donor. Furthermore, any specimen that tests positive must be sent to the Institute of Hygiene and Epidemiology (Institut d'Hygiène et d'Epidémiologie) to allow reference centers to confirm the result by further testing. In the event of confirmation of the seropositivity, the donor is to be informed by either the blood transfusion center's physician or his family doctor. To date, not a single case of post-transfusion HIV infection has been reported in Belgium since the measures decided on in August 1985 were implemented.

The first public information measures[4] aimed at calming the fears of the general public (creation of telephone hotlines and dissemination of a brochure) and alerting groups at risk (homosexuals, drug addicts, prostitutes, and foreigners) also took shape at the end of this period (see Table 5.1). This first barrage of information benefited from very modest financial support and was designed rather hastily by the public authorities, which were anxious to meet the steadily increasing demand for information. (The approaching general elections also prompted the government to act quickly, although AIDS has never really been party-politicized in Belgium.)[5] It is clear (here, too, one can speak of an imported phenomenon) that the definitions of the risk groups targeted in this first period were modeled after those developed in the United States (notably by the Centers for Disease Control), where the AIDS epidemic had already reached much larger proportions.

The notion of "groups at risk" is of course central to most of today's preventive strategies. It consists in establishing the relationships among factors that make the appearance of undesirable types of behavior or diseases more or less probable. In other words, factors (statistical correlations of heterogeneous elements), rather than individuals, are treated first. The ob-

Table 5.1
Belgium: Chronology of Major Responses 1983–1988

	Before 1985	1985	1986	1987	1988	Comments
Screening/testing measures		Mandatory screening of all blood & plasma donors and supplies (August 1)		Mandatory testing of foreign students applying for a scholarship (March 3 but unofficially practiced since September 86)		-AIDS has not been included as a notifiable disease (law of 24 January 1845) and this is no longer under discussion. -Many pregnant women, prisoners and patients are being tested without informed consent. -Blood donors who are found seropositive must be informed by the transfusion center of their own family doctor.
Legal innovation				Legalization of advertising of condoms		
General educational campaigns		October: -limited diffusion of an informative leaflet ("AIDS, facts and realities") -creation of telephone hot line		April: National campaign (leaflet + TV spots) "Open your eyes so that AIDS doesn't close them" Informative on AIDS and recommending sexual changes (fidelity or condom)	Summer: National campaign (TV spots) aimed at young people and recommending the use of condoms	
Specific educational actions		Gay community (Appel Homo SIDA): -several leaflets (1985, 1988) -telephone hot line -seropositives counselling		Students: -Multiple talks on AIDS in schools -leaflet in a magazine for young people ("Rock this town")	Travellers: leaflet at the borders (Health Ministry)	
Creation of legitimizing bodies	1983: National AIDS Committee		December Interministerial coordinating committee for AIDS control	January: Permanent cell for AIDS prevention (French-speaking community only)		

jective conditions of the development of the danger are established; new ways of intervening are then deduced from this information.[6]

At the beginning of the AIDS epidemic, epidemiologists, working with a small corpus of information and in the absence of a scientifically validated etiological model, found statistical patterns that enabled them to identify various groups at risk. These were homosexuals first, followed by Haitians and drug addicts, and eventually other groups. Attention should be drawn to the fact that these risk groups were defined on the basis of indicators not all of which were significant for the spreading of AIDS. It is obvious, for example, that classifying individuals on the basis of whether they declared themselves homo- or heterosexual yielded significant correlations with the presence or absence of AIDS. In addition, choosing this criterion (type of sexuality), which corresponds to a perfectly common way of describing sexual practices in our society, almost necessarily focuses the problem on homosexuals, whereas other criteria, including some that are much more relevant in the case of AIDS (e.g., anal penetration, a large number of different partners, etc.), would have produced a different picture of reality and put the emphasis on "risky behaviors" rather than on groups at risk.

As soon as the risk groups are designated, a certain number of social consequences can be and were seen in Belgium, as elsewhere. First of all, group membership, identity, and practices are all equated as one. All of the individuals presumed to belong to a risk group are considered to be aware of such membership, engage in the corresponding practices, and thus be both the vehicles and the victims of the disease involved. Thereupon, the presumed members of these risk groups are readily pointed to as being "responsible" for the epidemic. The fear of contagion among the "healthy" members of society can in such instances be transformed purely and simply into fear of social interaction (avoidance of all interpersonal contact with people from risk groups),[7] while the stigmatized individuals, feeling this attack on their very existence, can react, at least at first, only by counter-denunciations, denials, or paralysis.[8]

At the beginning of the epidemic, these reactions were observed mainly among the Africans living in Belgium, who felt as if they were accused parties and saw in the "charges" brought against them a new form of racism that they denounced. Indeed, many locals identified AIDS with being black. This was particularly noticed by blacks born in Belgium or Africans from countries less affected by the epidemic.

Refusing to accept the grounds for stigmatization, the homosexuals were the only ones to play an active role in tackling the problem of AIDS during this first period. An independent association, Appel Homo SIDA, was set up in the summer of 1985 around the central figure of Professor Michel Vincineau of the Free University of Brussels, a known and acknowledged member of the Belgian homosexual community due in part to the lawsuit brought against him for running homosexual clubs.[9] This association called for the dissemination of information aimed specifically at homosexuals. The initiative was generally well received, including by the public authorities, which found this association to be a reliable interlocutor within an extremely scattered and divided homosexual community.[10] At first, the association's activities were confined to organizing a telephone help line and to disseminating a brochure, but they quickly diversified, notably through work to help seropositives.

AIDS AS A DOMESTIC DISEASE: YOUNG PEOPLE AS A TARGET (1986–1988)

The second periods, from 1986 to 1988, was marked by a sharp turnaround. People began to realize that AIDS might become a genuine domestic disease—a fear confirmed by the fact that the number of new cases involving residents now exceeds that of nonresidents.

The idea that heterosexual transmission of the virus in Belgium was not only possible but proven thrust itself upon society. Thus, N. Clumeck, a Belgian doctor at Saint Peter's Hospital (Brussels), revealed in October 1986 that he had traced a chain of heterosexual transmission of the virus that was linked to the African continent. Here is how *Le Soir* (the leading Belgian French-language daily in Brussels) related the event on the front page of its 22 October 1986 issue, under the title "AIDS: Belgian Doctors Discover Heterosexual Connection":

Everything begins with an engineer and businessman of African origin who is diagnosed as having AIDS. We will probably never know how he contracted the disease. All that is known is that he contracted it before 1982, thus probably not in Europe. Most important, however, is the fact that this man told his doctors that he lived "a bachelor's life," travelled a lot, and granted his sexual favors readily. He was forced to admit that he had unwittingly made his partners run a great risk. He consequently persuaded them to be examined. As a result, ten women, nine of whom were Belgian, were found to be carrying the virus. . . . Here, then, we have ten middle-class women whose only "fault" is to have had an "affair" at some time in their lives. Need it be said that this is the case of several thousand Belgians of both sexes and that not a single epidemiologist would have ever thought of including them in a "risk group?"[11]

The article concludes by asking: "How can one warn and what type of advice must be given to this mass of people who definitely do not believe that their sexuality carries any kind of risk?"

A few days later (30 October) the same newspaper asserted that the danger might be more widespread than formerly believed:

The main revelation of the past few months is that the threat of AIDS is not restricted to male homosexuals with many partners, intravenous drug users, and people who have been in Central Africa. The doctors say that there is a chance that the virus may be spread by heterosexual transmission.

A video produced and unveiled at this time by one of the first AIDS-prevention groups in Belgium, CEDIF, drew the same conclusions, and there are other examples.[12]

It is clear that this "discovery" was twofold, namely, the African origin of the AIDS virus in Belgium and the spread of heterosexual transmission. Consequently, from this time onward the actions and positions taken by all those involved in managing the AIDS problem in Belgium were oriented primarily in these two directions.

The discovery of the African source for the spread of the virus in Belgium resulted in the implementation of some repressive measures against foreigners, especially Africans, by various institutions. One of them, which was particularly ill received by the African community in Belgium, was the institution of compulsory systematic AIDS screening for all foreign students (most of whom are African) who apply for a scholarship from the Belgian Administration of Cooperation for Development. This measure, which went into effect during the 1986/87 academic year and was applied first to grant recipients already living in Belgium, appeared to have been taken by the Secretary of State (Junior Minister) for Cooperation acting on his own initiative. It was subsequently ratified by the entire Council of Ministers (Cabinet) on 3 March 1987, after the press publicized the affair. The universities and various human rights groups managed to pressure the government into agreeing not to send seropositive grant recipients back to their countries of origin. However, such protests did not succeed in abolishing the requirement that all scholarship applicants undergo an AIDS screening test in their countries before the applications can be processed by the Belgian Administration.

Generally speaking, it can nevertheless be asserted that the predominant tendency with respect to the African origin of the spread of AIDS was a definite feeling of uneasiness and a failure to come to grips with the problem, probably in order to avoid any racist drift. The few initiatives taken remained scattered and ambiguous. For example, the Belgian Health Minister took the initiative of publishing "travel recommendations" that were extremely vague about the countries in which the risks were greatest (the brochure claimed only that "no country has been spared").

One may thus well wonder if designating young people as a risk group should not be placed in this context. As soon as the impact of the heterosexual transmission of AIDS became an increasingly real threat, the government was confronted with a duty to intervene. This was less the case when the epidemic was restricted to homosexuals and drug addicts, groups that do not have much political clout in Belgium.[13] Choosing young people as the new targets of prevention campaigns was a simple, inexpensive way to deal with the problem, for an array of health education measures for young people (sex education classes in schools, etc.) that would allow the rapid implementation of AIDS prevention measures already existed. In addition, this was a less conflict-prone way to handle the problem than taking on the African origin of the disease. It was also an approach on which consensus was easy to achieve, for the focus on young people tied in with the concerns of everyone—educators and parents—who feared for the future of coming generations and may not have completely accepted the greater sexual freedom of teenagers. In doing so, however, the policy makers based their efforts on images of teenage sexuality that were not necessarily relevant to the AIDS problem and failed to reach (or reach effectively) the social groups in which the epidemic was really gathering momentum.

What was said about young people? January 1987 marked the start of a burst of texts and pronouncements converging on the same considerations. All of the parties involved in the AIDS problem (see below) who expressed their opinions on this subject insisted on the fact that teenagers go through a period of life marked by instability and experimentation. Due to their emotional and sexual instability, teenagers have much weaker ties to their partners. The hunger for new experiences leads them to switch partners readily but also to experiment with homosexual relationships or drugs. Such behavior leads to serious risks of contamination by the AIDS virus among young people. The situation is all the more alarming as teenagers are becoming sexually active earlier and earlier, are not familiar with condoms, and in any case use them very seldom.

At a later stage, while continuing to insist on the above-mentioned themes, the pronouncements emphasized the fact that young people were not reached as well as other groups by the information campaigns, were not aware enough of the danger that threatened them, and consequently did not take the necessary preventive measures.[14] Here we find a particularly interesting element of *circularity*. If one acknowledges that the entities involved in managing the AIDS problem define the risk itself, it is normal that young people will not be aware of this definition right away. Yet the fact that young people are insufficiently *aware* of the problem becomes the ground for arguing that the means of information aimed at them must be increased urgently. In this way, as one can see, social action creates the conditions of its necessity.

Unlike the other risk groups, the logic behind labeling young people a risk group would thus seem to be based on ideological rather than statistical considerations. This logic, which could be called the *logic of transposition*, consists in deducing from commonly conveyed cognitive schemes about a given category of people (here, young people) consequences for the problem at hand that make it necessary to consider the category as being "at risk." In other words, neither epidemiological nor even sociological data are the initial determinants of the risk group label, even if it will eventually be useful

Figure 5.1
Belgium: AIDS Cases by Age Class 1985–1987

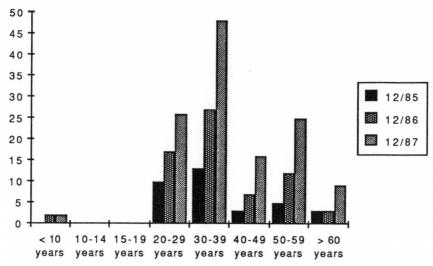

Note: Belgian residents only.

Source: Institut d'Hygiène et d'Epidémiologie, Rapport trimestriel SIDA (AIDS Quarterly
    Report), 31 December 1985, 31 December 1986, and 31 December 1987.

to produce epidemiological and sociological confirmation of the claims concerning this category. The category involved is labeled at risk more because
of an existing set of descriptions of the category, just as the preexisting
structures facilitate the implementation of a solution.

Is such autonomy from epidemiological and sociological data developing
with respect to young people? The National Institute of Health and Epidemiology (Institut d'Hygiène et d'Epidémiologie) provides the epidemiological data on AIDS in Belgium. While, as mentioned above, the proportion
of heterosexuals among the new AIDS cases that are being reported is
tending to rise, the disease cannot be said to prevail among "young people."
As Figure 5.1 shows, the 30–39 year-old age group is the most heavily
affected, accounting for 38 percent of the total on 31 December 1987. In
contrast, there are no AIDS patients in the 10–19 year age class, and the
proportion of AIDS patients between 20 and 29 years of age (20.6 percent
of the total)—the group concerned most directly by the above-mentioned
arguments since, given the virus' average incubation period of about five
years, the individuals in this group would have been infected between the
ages of 15 and 25—is practically the same as for the 50–59 year-olds (as
at 31 December 1987).

Actually, while the number of AIDS patients rose in all three categories
over the three years in question, the rate of increase was not the same

Figure 5.2
Belgium: Changes in Distribution of AIDS by Age Class 1985–1987

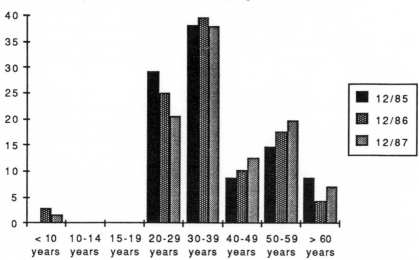

Source: Institut d'Hygiène et d'Epidémiologie, Rapport trimestriel SIDA (AIDS Quarterly
    Report), 31 December 1985, 31 December 1986, and 31 December 1987.

everywhere. The proportion of the 20–29 year-olds in the total number of
AIDS cases dropped between 1985 and 1987, while that of the over–40
group rose (Figure 5.2).[15] An analysis of the age breakdown of the new
cases should only confirm this trend even more clearly, but such figures
have not yet been released by the institute.

One can thus conclude that the emergence of the "youth and AIDS"
theme was diametrically opposed to the trend revealed by the epidemiological data. The theme was developed as the increase in the number of AIDS
patients under 30 was slowing down, whereas the greatest attention should
have been paid to the trend in the population over 40.

Of course, the trends among AIDS patients did not necessarily reflect
those of the seropositives, also known as "healthy carriers" of the virus.
The Institute of Health and Epidemiology has been publishing statistics on
healthy carriers since 31 March 1987, but, given the strict confidentiality
of the screening tests, the epidemiological information related to HIV seropositives is rare and often incomplete.[16]

There is no evidence, however, that a greater proportion of young people
are seropositive than in other age groups. While it is true that the average
age of the seropositive group (33) is lower than that of the AIDS group per
se (39), this is due first and foremost to the virus' incubation period (estimated at about five years).

The flimsiness of the links between the social actors' statements about young people and the epidemiological data is thus confirmed. It also explains both the lack of precise references to epidemiological statistics in talk about "young people and AIDS" and the strong denial of all allegations citing the weakness of such links, as if they were some sort of transgression, or the haste with which any information tending to support such links is exploited. For instance, as soon as a few cases of seropositivity among the 15–19 age group were reported, the Junior Minister for Public Health organized a press conference (March 1988) to stress the importance of the problem.

Still, it might be argued, while young people are not infected by the AIDS virus on a large scale *today*, there is a *potential* for infection due precisely to the instability and experimental nature of their emotional and sexual lives. Even if it appears difficult to base an entire prevention policy at this time on a danger lying in the future, such questions tie in with some of the concerns of research being carried out in the field of the sociology of sexuality. The question that one might then ask is the following: Do the findings of the sociologists of sexuality contain elements supporting the statements about young people made by those involved in the AIDS problem? In other words, do the sociological data confirm the idea that young people engage in more high-risk practices than the other age classes of society?

According to a recent survey of Brussels students between the ages of 16 and 25, a relatively small number of the respondents (16.3 percent) had slept with more than one person in the six months prior to the survey.[17] In addition to the 36.2 percent who had never engaged in sex, 11.3 percent had not had sexual intercourse over the six-month period. More than two-thirds of the remaining 44.4 percent who had sexual relations over this period had had only one partner. Finally, 79.4 percent of those surveyed stated that they personally preferred to know someone better before having sex with him/her (6.3 percent had no opinion; 1.7 percent did not answer this question).

While no one is willing to deny that youth is characterized by a certain sexual vitality, young people (most of whom are single) are distinguished to a great extent from the older age classes (composed of people who are often married or living together) by the reduced *possibility* of having sex. Kinsey had already found that the average frequency of sexual intercourse among bachelors in the United States was half that among married men.[18] Similarly, whereas the *incidence* of sexual intercourse was 100 percent among married couples, it was only 70 percent among 20-year-old bachelors. Likewise, in the case of France, Simon noted that the segment of the population between 30 and 49 years of age contained the highest proportion of individuals engaging regularly in sex.[19] According to his study, 76 percent of the men and 79 percent of the women in this age group had had sex in the month preceding the interview. The proportion of married people was also highest in this age group (84 percent of the men and 86 percent of the women between the ages of 30 and 49 were married as against 40 percent

Figure 5.3
Time Line of Social Actors' Entry onto the "Young People and AIDS" Stage

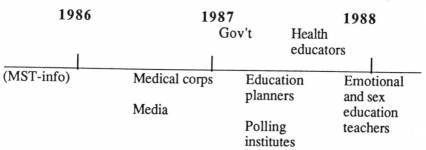

and 59 percent of the men and women, respectively, between 20 and 29), whereas close to 20 percent of the men and women in the 20–29 year age group had never had sexual relations.

SOCIAL ACTORS AND LEGITIMIZING BODIES

All dynamic, living organizations must adapt to market changes if they want to survive. Wherever the services on offer are not marketable (in the area of prevention, for example), the state is the main "buyer," the one who will finance those who dispense the services. The task of the "social actors" is thus to convince the state that there is a public for the services that they offer and, what is more, that the state has a duty to intervene in this area (if it does not intervene, it is liable to popular recrimination).[20] Such a practice tends to increase the *socialization of the state* discussed by Habermas, whereby some areas formerly under government jurisdiction are handled henceforward by private organizations.[21]

Turning to the problem of young people and AIDS, one sees the intervention of a large number of social actors ready to add AIDS prevention to the list of their activities. To date, few organizations have been formed specifically to cope with this new problem.

The recognition of young people as a risk group was not really disputed, as if everyone was convinced right from the start that a public (parents, educators, etc.) anxious about the future of later generations already existed, ready to embrace such a message concerning young people. Rather, the struggle focused on the next step of how to handle the young people and AIDS problem and the promotion of certain individuals or entities to the rank of "privileged social actors."

If the interventions of all of these social actors are plotted on a time line (see Figure 5.3), we find that MST-Info is the only Belgian organization working actively with young people before 1986.[22] In October-November 1986, Clumeck, who is often presented by the media as *the* Belgian expert on AIDS, came to the fore. As we saw, his statements at that time, which were taken up by the press, had important repercussions on the "young people and AIDS" problem, although they did not concern the problem directly. In January 1987, a string of political bodies took positions on various aspects of the AIDS problem, including prevention and young people. The Interministerial Coordinating Committee for AIDS Control, the Council of Ministers itself, the Secretary of State (Junior Minister) for Public Health, and the three linguistic communities' health ministers took action, one after the other.[23] This was followed a few months later by the emergence of social actors concerned primarily with education in their capacities as organizers of education (Ministry of National Education, university chancellors, National Secretariat of Free Education)[24] or teachers and educators (depending on the case, these agents focused on either health education or sex and emotional education). Finally, various polling institutes conducted special surveys of young people or the population at large (with special remarks on young people). Their conclusions were often used by the social actors (especially by those who had the means to commission such surveys and thus secured a monopoly over their use) either to impose a point of view or to justify it retroactively.

How were interactions among all of these social actors organized? The interactions mostly took place between a large group of social actors (whom we can call *claimants*, even if this is an oversimplification)[25] and a few entities who played the role of *legitimizing bodies*. The latter determined which requests were entitled to further hearing and which ones were not and then granted them (or denied them) a certain value.

A number of committees were set up by the government and took on the role of legitimizing bodies. The National AIDS Committee (Commission nationale SIDA) was the first such body to be set up in Belgium. It was created within the Higher Board of Health (Conseil supérieur d'Hygiène) in March 1983 at the instigation of the Secretary of State for Public Health. Composed of doctors only, the committee's role is limited to advice on matters under national jurisdiction, as defined by the laws of 8 August 1980.[26] In practice, the National AIDS Committee has taken stands on such issues as blood testing, information for doctors, and screening at the country's borders. On the other hand, it has played a very limited role in vetting statements and/or information on AIDS prevention for young people. It has, however, served as a trampoline, boosting some of the major social actors in this field to fame.

The use of expert committees (or panels of experts) in fields as new as AIDS (for which at the start there was no "right answer") corresponded to a need of the political decision makers, as any false step (e.g., the institution of discriminatory screening practices) was liable to be judged severely by the public. The backing of an expert committee was a convenient way to create endorsement of the decisions once they were made. The success of such a procedure depends, however, on the credibility of the creation and composition of the committee. The major interest groups involved must be represented or co-opted. Any negative consequences for the group responsible for setting up the committee may be reduced further if the committee uses its acquired independence to occupy center stage by itself more and more often.

One body that has played a more direct—although limited—role in constituting the "young people and AIDS" problem is the Interministerial Coordinating Committee for AIDS Control (Commission interministérielle chargée de la coordination de la lutte contre le SIDA). Created by the Council of Ministers on 12 December 1986, and chaired by the Junior Minister for Public Health, it is composed of a representative of each of the ministries assumed to be concerned about AIDS.[27] In its first report, which was submitted to the Council of Ministers on 23 January 1987, the committee recommended a series of measures, some of which were directed at young people.[28] These recommendations must be seen as a mark of interest by the federal government in the AIDS problem. But most of the effective measures were taken up and developed by the three linguistic communities, which are actually the only authorities in charge of prevention.[29]

In the French-speaking community (i.e., Brussels and the bulk of Wallonia), the Permanent Cell for AIDS Prevention (Cellule permanente pour la prévention du SIDA) is probably the legitimizing body that has played the greatest role in developing AIDS-prevention messages directed at young people. Its main task is to "propose and coordinate all activities aimed at reducing the spread of HIV, especially by proposing and coordinating action aimed at informing the public, schools, and health workers and preventing the transmission of the virus in groups at risk" (Article 2 of the law of 13 January 1987). The AIDS Prevention Cell quickly became a required channel for all entities wishing to participate in AIDS prevention in the French-speaking community. It sorted out requests and arbitrated the various claims, legitimizing certain orientations at the expense of other ones and raising certain actors to privileged positions. I consider this its key function, overriding by far its funding role. Indeed, the AIDS Prevention Cell has a very small budget (about U.S. $500,000 for 1987)[30] that falls short of the needs of the groups that apply to it.

Two ministerial orders (14 July 1987 and 23 October 1987) accredited a total of sixty-three associations that include AIDS prevention among their activities. Those associations cover the target groups that are considered to be at risk of HIV contamination: young people, homosexuals, IV drug users, foreigners, and prostitutes. It is interesting to point out that a large majority of them (fifty-five) are aimed at young people in schools,[31] whereas only one each is aimed at homosexuals, IV drug users, foreigners, or prostitutes, the rest being oriented toward the population at large.

TWO APPROACHES TO PREVENTION

In the absence of a true debate on the reality of the "young people and AIDS" problem (as the state was the one to take the initiative in raising the issue and its role in doing so was not contested), the social actors focused on defining the way to handle the problem. Two approaches to the problem competed with each other at this point: the *educational* model and the *communicational* model.[32]

The *educational* model stemmed above all from the idea that, while there were many ways to reach young people, the school was their "natural environment" and a necessary point of passage for all information campaigns.[33] The educational perspective contains a kind of act of faith in the school's educational mission and its ability to grasp all of the dimensions (intellectual, social, emotional, etc.) of the young person. This being so, the educators entrusted with an AIDS-prevention mission cannot content themselves with simply informing the young people to whom they are speaking. They must take as their point of departure the questions that the pupils ask and see the material to be taught as part of the emotional and sex education that has been aimed for years at helping young people to learn to relate calmly and responsibly to others. Besides the increase in knowledge, the educational model is aimed first and foremost at changing attitudes in directions that may vary somewhat according to the philosophical framework that is adopted.

The learning process must be built around dialogue using discussions (lecture-debates, etc.) and in-depth exchanges backed up by special teaching materials (audiovisual presentations, classroom files, etc.). Guest appearances by outside professionals (e.g., doctors) are encouraged, since they can catalyze discussions that only specialists are in a position to conduct successfully. The teacher, however, is a mainstay, for the learning process requires time.

At the other end of the scale, the *communicational* model works within the context of mass communications. According to this model, each individual is exposed daily to numerous messages urging action. Public service messages have no greater chance of being received by their target audience than any other type of message. "Advertisers" must thus rely on "communication strategies" to reach their objectives, that is to say, to change behavior. This means that a target audience to which a limited behavioral model (for example, using condoms) will be proposed must be defined as precisely as possible on the basis of sociocultural criteria.

As communication is a fleeting phenomenon, it is useful to call on professionals who have mastered all of the techniques of persuasion.[34] Various types of media (personalized mailings, house-to-house distribution of flyers, posters, TV commercials, ads in specialized journals) will be used according to need. After the operation it may be interesting to measure the impact of

Table 5.2
Belgium: Summary of the Educational and Communicational Models

	Educational model	Communicational model
Operating theater	school	media
Target	school children	socio-cultural subgroups
Content	ethical	technical
Change encouraged	attitudes	actual behavior
Principle	dialogue	persuasion
Temporal dimension	long-term	instantaneous
Agents	teaching professionals	communication professionals
Techniques	lecture-debates, AV presentations, etc.	TV commercials flyers, posters, etc.

the campaign on the target population (usually to justify the choices to the client retrospectively) in the same way that one might carry out a prospective study to identify the targets. (See Table 5.2.)

As with all ideal types, it is clear that the educational and communicational models are less clearly distinguished in actual practice than I have described here. A social actor will often use both models at the same time. Such an attitude is exhibited more commonly by those who defend a model that differs from the prevailing one, since it is normal that the proponents of rival models should attempt to clothe their proposals in terms rendering them more plausible to their interlocutors.

The educational model has been favored by the government, school authorities, and sexual guidance, marriage counseling, and family planning centers, whereas the communication model has been adopted by a few private organizations trying to introduce the methods of marketing and advertising in the field of health education.

CONCLUSION

In sum, the perception and management of AIDS in Belgium to date can be divided into two periods. In the first period (until 1985), AIDS was seen primarily as a threat from outside, brought by American homosexuals and Africans. The definitions of the risk groups themselves were basically imported and did not correspond to the epidemiological situation in the country. The generalized screening of blood donations was the main preventive measure instituted during this period. Limited resources were devoted to information or placed at the disposal of a few volunteer organizations, the most active of which was incontestably Appel Homo SIDA, which worked chiefly with the homosexual community of Brussels. In the second period, which ran from 1986 to 1988, AIDS was perceived more and more to be a "domestic threat." Heterosexual transmission appeared not only possible but actually capable of reaching an ever wider range of people. As a result, the management of the problem and definition of the targets for prevention were characterized by a union of ideological considerations on the one hand and an "interventionist" logic of state action on the other. This union resulted in the tendency during this period to focus on young people as the targets of prevention (fifty-five of the sixty-three associations receiving public health funding received this money to spread information in the schools).

As soon as it was realized that the AIDS virus was spreading through the heterosexual population, tackling the problem by starting with young people was a convenient way for officialdom to give the impression that it was doing its job, that is, coping with the problem. Not only was the message about young people one that gained credibility easily because of commonly conveyed cognitive schemes about the sexuality of this category of people, it was also easy to translate into action because a whole array of youth-oriented structures allowing the rapid establishment of a means of confronting the problem already existed. In this way the demonstrated lack of scientific and epidemiological justification for the special targeting of young people was eclipsed by the impression of efficacy.

A much greater effort of social imagination will probably be required to find the "right answer" to the problem of AIDS as regards specific groups, involving both homosexuals and heterosexuals, that are less accessible than young people. However, such a search is not under way yet in Belgium.

NOTES

1. The number of new seropositives did not increase significantly from one quarter to the next (around 300 cases). However, men's cases increased quicker than women's.

2. The ratio of residents to nonresidents among the total number of cases was 0:4 in 1984; it is now 1:7.

3. This percentage is comparable to that found in Greece (21 percent) and, to a lesser extent, Portugal (13 percent), whereas heterosexual transmission accounts for only 4 to 6 percent of the cases in the rest of Western Europe and the United States.

4. Previously, ministerial circulars for physicians were the only type of information to be sent out.

5. Except very recently (1989) when, within the context of the reform of the state, AIDS research and prevention was at the heart of a debate on the degree of decentralization to be reached.

6. This practice led to an increasingly clear distinction between the role of the

technical experts and administrators who define and manage the risk and that of the practitioners, who become simple executors. See R. Castel, "De la dangerosité au risque," *Actes de la recherche en sciences sociales* (1983): no. 47–48: 47–48.

7. Susan Sontag, *La maladie comme métaphore* (Paris: Seuil, 1979), p. 12, described similar attitudes toward other mysterious diseases such as tuberculosis and cancer. In her view, being in contact with a person affected by such a disease is necessarily equated with a transgression.

8. M. Pollak, "Identité sociale et gestion d'un risque de santé: Les homosexuels face au SIDA," *Actes de la recherche en sciences sociales* (1987): no. 68:68.

9. The Vincineau trial, sometimes called "the homosexuality trial," reveals the climate of suspicion that often continues to surround homosexuality in Belgium. Given a suspended sentence of one year in prison in December 1984 for "running a den of iniquity," Vincineau appealed and was acquitted by the Liège Appeals Court in May 1985. The core of his defense is given in the book that he published on this occasion, *La débauche en droit et le droit à la débauche* (Brussels: Brussels University Press, 1985).

10. Aside from the commercial sector, Antenne Rose was the main gay organization already in existence prior to AIDS. Its activities were the publication of a monthly, the organization of meeting places, and a weekly broadcast on an independent Brussels radio. Appel Homo SIDA is an organization close to Antenne Rose that presented itself as independent in order to get the largest audience.

11. This quotation and all subsequent excerpts from French sources have been translated from the French.

12. The CEDIF is a center of documentation and information created in 1980 by the Fédération francophone belge pour le Planning familial et l'Education sexuelle. In 1985 it started its STD and AIDS information efforts by issuing videos and brochures, manning a telephone hotline, etc.

13. Apart from the fact that the rate of IV drug users among the AIDS cases is rather low in Belgium (around 5 percent), another obstacle to general preventive actions for IV drug users is that there is so far no real legal (and thus financial) framework for it. The exact number of IV drug users in Belgium is difficult to assess. In 1987, 4,473 people were convicted on narcotics charges, 32 percent of whom were less than 20 years old. It seems that one of the most alarming aspects of the drug problem in Belgium is that the recruitment of minors is still high in comparison with some other Northern European countries (e.g., the Netherlands, Denmark).

14. These considerations result from a content analysis of various documents (letters, press conference statements, position papers, etc.) produced by all the parties involved in the "young people and AIDS" problem. For a detailed account, see M. Hubert, "La production et la diffusion des problèmes sociaux. Un point de vue constructiviste sur le SIDA," doctoral thesis, Louvain-la-Neuve, Belgium, 1988.

15. The percentage of patients between the ages of 20 and 29 in the total number of AIDS cases fell from 29.4 percent to 20.6 percent between 1985 and 1987.

16. For example, it is not possible to distinguish between residents and nonresidents in this population.

17. M. Hubert, *Les jeunes face au SIDA: Enquête sociologique* (Louvain-la-Neuve: Sociological Research Unit, 1987).

18. A. Kinsey, W. Pomeroy, and C. Martin, *Le comportement sexuel de l'homme* (Paris: Editions du Pavois, 1948), p. 375.

19. P. Simon, *Rapport Simon sur le comportement sexuel des français*, abridged ed. (Paris: Pierre Charron/René Julliard, 1972), p. 193.

20. The term "social actors" will be used throughout the chapter to refer to private organizations and individuals that are involved in managing the AIDS problem in Belgium.

21. J. Habermas, *L'espace public: Archéologie de la publicité comme dimension constitutive de la société bourgeoise* (Paris: Payot, 1978).

22. MST-Info is the former Ligue contre les maladies vénériennes (League Against Venereal Disease). This association's major activity was organizing school information sessions, backed up by slides and films, on the various sexually transmitted diseases. AIDS was simply added to the list of diseases presented within this framework. The association was not a driving force in the management of the "young people and AIDS" problem; see M. Hubert and P. Walraff, *Mesure d'impact des séances d'information de MST-Info dans les écoles de l'agglomération bruxelloise* (Louvain-la-Neuve: Sociological Research Unit, 1987).

23. Belgium is a federation built on two tiers of power—the three linguistic communities (Flemish, French-speaking, and German-speaking communities) and three regions (Flanders, Wallonia, and Brussels)—that overlap geographically but are endowed with very distinct types of powers. Only the communities are empowered to act in the area of preventive health.

24. "Free" as opposed to state-controlled education.

25. A variable degree of interdependence, depending on the case, exists between the partners of a power relationship. Even if it is not always stated explicitly, legitimizing bodies also need claimants to exist.

26. The National AIDS Committee was restructured in April 1988 to include specialists in other fields who would be able to take into account the social, economic, and legal aspects of AIDS.

27. The Prime Minister; Minister of Justice; Budget Minister; the Foreign Minister; the Employment and Labor Minister; the National Education (French-language and Dutch-language), Social Affairs, National Defense, Interior, and Communications (and Transport) Ministers; the Secretary of State of Cooperation for Development, and the Public Health Ministers of the Flemish, French-speaking, and German-speaking communities.

28. The commission recommended:

- general information for the public on the dangers linked to AIDS and ways to avoid contamination (leaflets put in everyone's mailbox, public service announcements, etc.);

- information aimed at specific segments of the population: teenagers, military recruits, hospital staff, prison staff, travelers, and prostitutes;

- allowing advertising for contraceptives.

Teenagers were definitely the prime target for prevention. The other target groups received hardly a leaflet, prostitutes nothing.

29. Cf. note 23.

30. This sum can be compared with the amounts spent on screening: U.S. $3.1 million projected for reference laboratories in 1988; an additional expenditure of U.S. $3.7 million in 1986 alone for the Health and Disability Insurance Institute to

cover the increase in the price of blood resulting from the additional treatment that is required; and U.S. $600,000 to reimburse the cost of screening tests in 1987.

31. They are allowed to give talks on AIDS, provided that such talks fit into the more general framework of sex education and the prevention of STDs.

32. A third model might be the *peer-counseling* model. This consists of training teenagers to relay information on health problems (drugs, sexually transmitted diseases, contraception, etc.) to their peers. These three models each refer back to a "socialization agent" (see R. Rezsohazy, *Les jeunes, leurs parents et leurs professeurs. Valeurs et comportements: continuité et conflit* [Louvain-la-Neuve: UCL, 1979]), namely, the school, peer group, and means of communication. Only the family does not yet seem to have been identified as a specific site for AIDS-prevention work.

33. The following description is based on content analysis of various documents produced by the social actors involved in the "young people and AIDS" problem. For a detailed account, see Hubert, "La production et la diffusion des problèmes sociaux."

34. For a summary, see J. N. Kapferer, *Les chemins de la persuasion* (Paris: Dunod, 1978).

AIDS in West Germany: Coordinating Policy in a Federal System

In the European context, the case of AIDS policy in Germany is of special interest. While a certain lack of coordination between national and local administrative structures may be expected in the management of AIDS, the German Federal Republic (FRG) has seen outright conflict between administrative levels of government. Because one *Land*, Bavaria, has persistently chosen to follow its own path, full harmonization of national policy among all constituent states of the Republic has proven exceedingly difficult. In explicit opposition to the federal government's liberal policy guidelines, Bavaria has opted for a coercive administrative approach. The FRG has thus become almost an experimental testing ground for liberal versus repressive strategies in combatting AIDS. Because the courts have played a significant adjudicative and interpretive role in these political conflicts over measures to combat HIV infection, the legal profession has also entered the public debate in a more direct way than in other European nations. The scope of debate over policies on AIDS has therefore tended to become narrowly focused on one specific—but critical—issue: should existing legislation concerning epidemics and sexually transmitted diseases be extended to cover AIDS or not? Since that question has not aroused such public and legal controversy elsewhere in Europe, this chapter will give it especial weight.

THE EPIDEMIOLOGICAL PROFILE

With 2,580 cumulative AIDS cases registered between 1982 (when the first cases were diagnosed) and December 1988, Germany was then the second European country in absolute numbers. In terms of incidence—with only half the number of cases per million inhabitants recorded for France or Switzerland—it occupied a middle-range position. The distribution of cases among risk groups shows that gays and bisexuals account for three in four cases of AIDS (75 percent) and thus continue to be by far the most affected category. Intravenous drug users provide 9 percent of all cases, but their number is increasing rapidly. Hemophiliacs (5 percent), people having undergone blood transfusions (2 percent), and heterosexuals (3 percent) form the rest of the infected population.[1] As in the United States, AIDS is still a big-city phenomenon. At the end of 1987 four-fifths (81 percent) of all cases were concentrated in a few big cities accounting for only 14 percent of the national population: Frankfurt, Berlin, Munich, Hamburg, and Bremen. In epidemiological terms, the German diffusion model of the disease very much resembles the North American model in respect of the age group primarily infected, since most cases have been concentrated in the 30-to-40-year-old category.[2]

Surveillance data on the diagnosed full AIDS cases are collected by the Federal health service in Berlin (Bundesgesundheitsamt), a technical service of the Federal Ministry of Youth, Family, Women and Health. These data are anonymous and the reporting by physicians, hospitals, and clinics is not compulsory. Consequently accusations of grossly underreporting and of deliberately underestimating the size of the epidemic—perhaps by two to three times the real number of cases—have sometimes been made.[3] However, today experts consider that reporting has become reliable since 1984 and that the federal data are therefore fully comparable to data collected in other European countries such as France, where reporting is mandatory.[4] No doubt, in a country where sensitivity about data abuse is extreme, as shown by a very lengthy dispute over the legality of a population census, to have made the reporting of AIDS cases compulsory would have created controversy and conflict and perhaps even led to a refusal of cooperation by doctors willing to collaborate on a voluntary basis.

In order to gain a more complete picture of the spread of HIV infection, the government introduced, in October 1987, an obligation for laboratories to report anonymously all HIV-positive test results to the federal health service in Berlin. Together with data collected by a network of physicians and clinics working on problems of seroprevalence in the most exposed groups, these data allowed a more sober assessment of the situation than the impression created by media talk about "the plague of the end of our century." In fact, a computerized simulation model calculated for a city of 2.3 million inhabitants projected a total of 107,000 deaths in sixteen years in the worst-case event of no behavior changes, no cure, and no vaccine in the meantime, and a total of 18,000 deaths in the event of rapid changes in behavior, medical therapy after eight years, and a vaccine after ten years.[5]

Based on assumptions of a rapid spread of HIV into the general heterosexual population, this alarming model was contradicted by empirical observations of the progress of infection among the most exposed groups. As the number of people tested increased substantially, the proportion revealed to be HIV-positive declined from 38 percent in 1984 to 21 percent in 1987 among male homosexuals. Over the same period among IV drug consumers, the rate of seropositivity fell from 39 percent (male) and 50 percent (female) in 1985 to 27 percent (male) and 32 percent (female) in 1987. In fact, the first people seeking the test did it for obvious reasons: they felt particularly exposed. As in the United States, a large cohort study of gay men also showed a significant decrease in new infections as a consequence of safer sex behavior.[6] Estimates of the extent of seropositivity and future infection suggested that in early 1987 between 50,000 and 100,000 Germans were already infected and that the figure would approach 500,000 by 1990.[7]

However, although the epidemiological situation in Germany is roughly comparable to that in other European countries, the public debate in Germany grew unusually emotional because of the rapid politicization of AIDS policy.

FEARS OF DISCRIMINATION AND ASSOCIATIVE MOBILIZATION

In all developed countries the concentrated diffusion of AIDS in a few marginalized social groups (male homosexuals, bisexuals, and IV drug consumers) has provoked fears of social stigmatization and legal discrimination. But nowhere were these fears so clearly and explicitly expressed as in Germany where, like other minority groups, gays had experienced the most extreme repression in the Nazi concentration camps. In 1986 a doctor in Frankfurt proposed to tattoo the buttocks of all HIV-positive people in order to mark them visibly for their eventual sex partners.

Although this isolated "public health proposal" was hardly taken seriously, such statements could only reinforce fears about stigmatizing tendencies, especially in the absence of clear directions from the political elite in the early years of the epidemic.[8] In her book on AIDS, Rita Süssmuth, the activist Christian Democrat Federal Minister of Health who took office in September 1985, comments: "One finds such proposals as tattooing the infected and the sick, marking personal identification cards and issuing health passports. All these proposals would create a false feeling of security. And in a country that once visibly and publicly marked people, such proposals remind us of dark and bad times."[9] It must be noted, too, that in 1985 public opinion polls showed that a vast majority of 75 percent of the general public favored official registration of HIV-infected persons and 34 percent agreed with quarantining people with AIDS.[10] Even in the professional medical press the question whether drastic administrative measures were necessary was seriously asked. "Do we soon need AIDS ghettos?" asked the journal *Therapie de Gegenwart* in 1986.

Fears of stigmatization had a contradictory effect on the gay community. Only in 1969 were homosexual relations decriminalized in Germany, after which gay groups, taking their models from the United States, blossomed all over Germany. At the same time a large infrastructure of meeting places— coffeehouses, bars, discos, and bathhouses—emerged in all larger German cities. Militancy has declined, however, since the late 1970s, prior to, and unconnected with, the advent of the then unknown AIDS. Some of it survived in the alternative movement and the Green Party, and some Green candidates and members of parliament are openly gay. In the Social Democratic Party a gay working group also exists, as do its counterparts in the churches. A gay umbrella organization in Cologne coordinates activities and serves as a place for discussion about gay issues. Only slowly did AIDS become recognized as an issue in all these organizations. As long as the importance of the epidemic was not yet fully perceived, mobilization around AIDS and safer sex propaganda was often criticized as the expression of gay guilt feelings.[11]

After 1986 AIDS became clearly perceived as a gay issue and gays played a major role in building up the self-help association network. This network quickly represented some seventy local and regional organizations across Germany, coordinated by an umbrella organization in Berlin. The membership of these AIDS Hilfe organizations reflects local characteristics. Whereas in big cities gays represent the majority of members, the paramedical, social, and medical professions sometimes dominate the organizations in smaller towns. Coordination is sometimes difficult and conflictual since the official liberal policy line—on testing in particular—is not necessarily followed without major discussions by all organizations. The major activities of the AIDS Hilfe concern prevention, the organization of AIDS hotlines, and the provision of individual support for people with AIDS.

THE INSTITUTIONAL FRAMEWORK OF AIDS POLICY

In 1984 a national advisory council on AIDS was created in order to concentrate the necessary policy expertise in the Federal Ministry of Health. This council is composed of medical doctors, social scientists, psychologists, and the representatives of major social organizations. It discusses all problems whether or not they have legal implications.

Regional policies are coordinated and harmonized by the Conference of State Health Ministers, at which the health ministers of all ten German states participate in the discussions. The conference published its first report on AIDS on 27 March 1987, shortly before a national information campaign. Its position is in line with the liberal guidelines developed by the national advisory council, which from 1984 onwards had rejected the idea of applying the existing legislation on sexually transmitted diseases and epidemics to AIDS. In particular, the council warned that contact tracing and administrative registration might have counterproductive effects; and it also rejected all routine obligatory testing of the general population and of so-called risk groups. It underlined more particularly that routine testing in hospitals was "unnecessary" and that the test should only be done with the explicit consent of the patient. As an advisory body to the minister, the council's statements have no legal force, but they have a decisive moral and symbolic influence.

On most issues, in fact, the Conference of Health Ministers followed the council's arguments and gave them more concrete meaning, particularly in financial terms. In 1987, for example, it announced a special allocation of 135 million DM for continuing research and information efforts. At the same time it rejected any measures for compulsory testing. But it encouraged all those "who had knowingly been in a risk situation as well as all couples wishing to have children, to undergo a voluntary test." The same report stipulates which agencies are permitted to add the HIV antibody test to their routine pregnancy tests.[12] A few months later a second report was issued, agreed to by all states except Bavaria, which had in the meantime formulated its own, rather repressive, policy.

Coordination has also taken place between the Federal Republic and the health authorities of the German Democratic Republic. In fact, the two Germanies have obvious interests in cooperating in this area of policy. Circulation of people between the two countries is intense, television programs can be seen on both sides of the border, and information policy in the German Democratic Republic has to take into account these basic facts. The first meeting between politicians responsible for health in the two countries took place in Cologne in late 1988, where it was decided to intensify the exchanges of data and research results and to examine the possibility of clinical exchanges.

CONFLICT AND COOPERATION BETWEEN THE PUBLIC SECTOR AND THE ASSOCIATIONS

For the implementation of its policies the Federal Ministry of Health relies on its technical services (Bundesgesundheitsamt) and the Central Administration for Health Education, or CAHE (Bundeszentrale für gesundheitliche Aufklärung). The latter body devises and manages information and education efforts in cooperation with social groups. In the case of AIDS, collaboration has been established with the associative network of AIDS Hilfen, whose umbrella organization receives some 90 percent of its funds from government, mostly from the CAHE. Between 1986 and 1988 the budget of the federal umbrella organization grew by four times, from 2 million DM in 1986 to 5 million DM in 1987 to more than 8 million DM in 1988.[13] Over the same period its salaried personnel increased from 8 to 35, while local and regional organizations provided some 250–300 full-time positions.

The relation of financial dependence on the CAHE can sometimes generate conflict, since the funds are made available on a negotiated project basis. In 1987, for example, the AIDS Hilfe published a leaflet on the HIV antibody test, advocating the use of the test for diagnostic reasons only and rejecting its employment as an instrument of prevention and education. Particular insistence was also given to the still-existing possibilities of a lack of confidentiality, which might in turn lead to discrimination and "social quarantining" of HIV-positive people in their work environment. On the grounds of the leaflet's critical overtones and disagreement with its contents, the Central Administration of Health Education refused to finance its production and distribution.

Other conflicts have occurred in relation to work with IV drug consumers and prisoners. In 1988 a project volume of only 200,000 DM was financed out of a total of 2 million DM. In the state of Rhineland Pfalz the Health Minister threatened the AIDS Hilfe with suspension of its funds because of political differences. In addition, the AIDS Hilfe insists on the shared responsibility of both sexual partners to protect themselves irrespective of their HIV antibody status, whereas the minister insists on the particular responsibility of the HIV-positive person for informing his or her partners and for taking the necessary precautions.

A further example highlights the difficult position of the AIDS Hilfen between the public administration and their own constituents. In 1987, with specific public funding, the organization launched a survey among the gay population to assess the extent of changes in behavior and, indirectly, the viability of a strategy of "individual responsibility." The survey showed very encouraging results, as a majority of gays had already converted to safe sex practices, using condoms and/or reducing the number of their partners.[14] A year later the same questionnaire was distributed to measure the evolution of behavior changes. But when the federal court confirmed the punishment of a young HIV-positive man for having had insufficiently protected sex, the general assembly of the AIDS Hilfen in Hamburg decided that the survey results should not be analyzed because the organization would not assist the state in spying on the sexual behavior of minority groups.

The Hamburg meeting of all regional AIDS Hilfen on 12–13 November 1988 also showed clearly the divisive internal conflicts between those organizations, for example from Frankfurt, which defined themselves in the terms "we are ourselves all prostitutes, gays, junkies," and the organizations from provincial towns such as Pforzheim, where the AIDS Hilfe is composed of the local medical establishment. A gay newspaper, commenting on the crisis, wrote of the lack of imagination and innovative thinking in the AIDS Hilfen.[15]

The work of the AIDS Hilfe nonetheless has been generally described in rather laudatory terms. Indeed, the quality of its counseling work has been confirmed by a study comparing different counseling services in the public health sector, private hospitals, and the AIDS Hilfe. Having tested the eleven offices of the AIDS Hilfe, nine public health agencies, and eleven hospital services, the survey concluded that the best welcome and the best guarantee for the respecting of anonymity were provided by the AIDS Hilfen.[16] The Hamburg meeting blurred this overly positive image. But it did highlight the contradictions and tensions inherent in a situation in which associations with the double task of promoting public health and protecting minority groups depend almost exclusively on financial support from public bodies.

In the eyes of public authorities, the close cooperation with the associations is justified to the extent that the latter are better prepared for targeted information and education efforts in the most exposed groups, which are rarely within easy reach of the official structures. Nevertheless, the public authorities simultaneously mobilized their traditional services (general practitioners, medical organizations at school and work, social workers) for information and education. Before 1988 everybody recognized the competence and efficiency of the voluntary associations. Now their qualities are increasingly questioned, and the public authorities have clearly been trying to multiply their partners, including commercial communication and marketing agencies, and to rely more heavily on the actors they are used to working with. Most of the project support given to the Deutsche AIDS Hilfe expires in 1991. At present the respective weight of the different actors engaged in the fight against AIDS is being renegotiated and the eventual outcome is very open.

THE LIBERAL LINE OF THE FEDERAL GOVERNMENT

The various debates in the national AIDS advisory council and the reports published by the Conference of State Health Ministers confirmed the liberal policy line developed from the beginning. Defined as a strategy of "individual responsibility," the AIDS policy gives especial weight to the two tasks of information and education. At the same time obligatory testing is refused, except in the case of pregnant women.

As far as the policy toward IV drug consumers is concerned, the various reports advocate the use of substitution drugs (methadone) in individual cases, under strict medical surveillance, in case therapeutic efforts and detoxification programs do not work. A street worker program with social workers specifically trained for AIDS education has been proposed as a means of reaching the IV drug population.

In their report the Health Ministers ask all people with multiple partners to use condoms. But they also insist on "fidelity in the couple as the safest protection against an infection." This statement has often been attacked as a concession to the Roman Catholic Church, which has condemned the use of condoms as "dehumanizing love." The Protestant Church, by contrast, has agreed with the necessity for public campaigns in favor of condom use.

The different documents that have emerged from the Conference of State Health Ministers reflect the majority position of nine states, with the tenth—Bavaria—often voting against the adoption of these liberal texts. But such documents hardly allow one to understand the differences of implementation that often cut across political party lines. In particular, the approaches to the categories of IV drug consumers and prostitutes differ significantly from one state to another. The political color of regional governments can account only in part for these differences.

Berlin, for example, which has a conservative Christian Democratic government, must also take into consideration the existence of a well-organized gay community and a wide network of "alternative" organizations with a strong mobilizing capacity. It is therefore no surprise that AIDS policy in Berlin can be described as very liberal: indeed, in 1985 Ulf Fink, the city's Health Minister, financed the entire cost of printing a special issue of the gay magazine *Siegessäule* devoted to AIDS. In addition the Ministry of Health collaborates actively with Hydra, a self-help organization of prostitutes, which helps members of the category who want to change their careers.

Methadone programs are a highly controversial issue. When the Social Democratic administration of North Rhine Westphalia introduced methadone programs in large cities, very critical reactions came not only from Christian Democratic governments but also from Social Democratic Bremen. At the level of concrete policy discussions AIDS reveals contradictions and taboos and fuels controversy. The dividing lines then become much too complex for any simple opposition between the repressive Bavarian government and the rest of the country.

Party political differences and cleavages in approaches to AIDS can best be observed in the reports published by the Parliamentary Commission on AIDS. Although the general text is in line with the official federal policies, the different minority votes show how political convictions shape the approach to AIDS. Consensus generally prevails among the Christian Democrat, Liberal, and Social Democrat members of this commission. Minority votes by the Christian Social Union (CSU) members are usually consistent with the repressive policy guidelines adopted in the state, Bavaria, where their party has its stronghold. They also insist on the possibility of yet unknown modes of HIV transmission in daily-life situations and ask for special measures against "the minorities that participated in the import of AIDS."[17] The Greens always adopt the perspective of the most directly concerned categories (seropositives and people with AIDS) as well as the interests of gays and IV drug consumers; and they also refuse all cost-benefit analysis of different treatments and hospitalization models: "Such analysis is of no help to the people concerned. Financial thinking should never be used against the best possible treatment of HIV-positives or people with

AIDS." Furthermore, the Greens are against research into sexual behavior on the grounds that it could constitute an invasion of privacy.[18]

That same parliamentary report includes some proposals for legislative action concerning the most exposed groups. In order to strengthen trust and to increase the willingness to behave responsibly, a suggestion is made to abolish the last remaining discriminatory articles in German law against gays; and a clear position is taken in favor of methadone programs and schemes for the free exchange of syringes. In those recommendations the report demonstrates once again how isolated the Bavarian government is. Witness too the rejection of the compulsory testing of foreigners and candidates for civil service employment in terms that can already be found in a report from the Conference of the State Health Ministers: "The public sector should not become the first employer to exclude seropositive individuals."

THE BAVARIAN MODEL

When it became clear that there would be no majority backing for repressive measures at the federal level, the Bavarian government decided to follow its own policy within the state territory. Having tried and failed to get a federal law enacted, it proceeded by way of administrative orders—a way of circumventing the fact that state governments have no legislative power in this matter. Publication of these orders in May 1987 introduced AIDS into the existing state legislation covering epidemics, immigration, and police powers. The health administration was thus empowered to administer a test for HIV to all persons who could be infectious, in particular male and female prostitutes and IV drug consumers. Even in the case of a negative test result, the test can be repeated every three months. By the same orders prostitutes are obliged to use condoms in their work, irrespective of their serological status. In the case of a positive test result, prostitutes are not allowed to continue in their profession. All people who test positive for HIV antibodies are obliged to inform their sexual partners, doctors, and dentists. Failure to respect these obligations can lead to a court decision to isolate HIV carriers from society. In addition, the Bavarian government compels all of its candidates for civil service and judicial positions to take an HIV antibody test.

The introduction of AIDS into the legislation concerning immigration means that the HIV antibody test becomes part of the routine medical examinations that all foreigners who wish to live in Bavaria and who need a residence permit have to undergo. In case of foreigners already living in Bavaria with regular residence papers who turn out to be HIV-positive, termination of their residence permit should be considered. Foreign IV drug consumers and prostitutes should not be eligible for residence permits for

Bavaria even if they are seronegative. Shortly before Bavaria decided on these measures, the then Federal Minister of the Interior, Friedrich Zimmermann, who represented Bavaria's governing Christian Social Union Party, ordered the federal border police to refuse entry into the Federal Republic to all seropositives. Asked by his officers how this should be decided, the minister answered that people falling under suspicion could be subjected to a test. This suggestion provoked an immediate protest by the Minister of Health and the order was finally annulled. The measure was assuredly proposed in order to test public reaction shortly before the Bavarian government published its own orders. The dispute showed not only that almost all political forces except the CSU were against such actions but also that the practical application of such measures ran into grave difficulties.

The difficulties were further compounded by legal issues of discrimination applying to member states of the European Community. Because of their incompatibility with legal norms of a higher order, the Bavarian rules had therefore to make an exception for all residents of the European Community.

The third dimension of the catalogue of the state government's repressive measures concerns police surveillance of meeting places. Institutions that encourage the dissemination of the virus (bordellos, meeting places for prostitutes, saunas) should be permanently controlled and can be closed by a simple police order. In such places the police are allowed to carry out identity checks of the prostitutes and their customers. Prostitutes have to possess a certificate stating that they are seronegative. Finally, the Bavarian rules explicitly punish the transmission of the virus and, in cases where transmission cannot be proven, even the sexual activities that could transmit it.

One year after the introduction of the various rules, what can be concluded about the range of consequences that these forms of repression have had? First, some rules could not be implemented at all or could be implemented only in part. The liberal city of Nuremberg, for example, refused to impose the test on its candidates for civil service employment, resulting in legal action pitting it against the Bavarian government. When the administrative court in Ansbach had to declare in favor of the state or the city government, its judgment in fact established no clear rules. It accepted that the state of Bavaria was no doubt entitled to subject the candidates for its civil service posts to the test, but at the same time the city of Nuremberg, like the other autonomous administrative units in the state, could refuse to follow suit with its own employees. As the Bavarian rules are only administrative orders and not laws, they are, according to the same court decision, binding for the state administration only. This ruling has in fact considerably limited the scope of their application.

A further court challenge was initiated by an IV drug user who had been asked to present himself to the health administration in order to undergo an HIV antibody test. On the grounds that many legal problems were still unresolved, the court decided, in this specific case, that "private interests should have precedence over the public interest of an immediate systematic test." At the same time the press reported that the Bavarian orders had immediately motivated prostitutes to leave the state for other German states with no such repressive measures. It was also often said that the orders created social fears as well as the unforeseen consequence that people who wanted to know their serological status but who were skeptical about the confidentiality of test results preferred not to get tested. But the actual number of prostitutes or IV drug consumers reported as "fleeing" to other German states was small; and only a few seropositives or people with AIDS who were resident in Bavaria sought treatment elsewhere in order to avoid administrative registration.

In all respects, therefore, the Bavarian administrative rules had quite limited effects, as suggested by the statistics on their role in HIV detection. Out of the state's more than 11 million inhabitants, 1,047 people suspected of being infected and all civil service candidates were subjected to the compulsory test during its first year of application: only eight (six IV drug consumers, one male and one female prostitute) turned out to be seropositive.

The very limited results of such cost-intensive administrative measures have naturally increased skepticism about their necessity and utility. Following the death of Bavarian Prime Minister Franz Joseph Strauss in the fall of 1988, the State Secretary of the Interior responsible for its AIDS policy, Peter Gauweiler, was replaced. It is not yet clear if this change of personnel can be interpreted as the sign of a gradual redirection of Bavarian policies toward convergence with general federal AIDS policy. Such a resolution, if it comes, lies in the future. For the time being, the Bavarian example continues to serve as the negative model of repressive AIDS policies for the whole of Europe, since it revives images of coercion and of a lack of respect for human rights characteristic of an earlier period.

"INDIVIDUAL RESPONSIBILITY" AS DEFINED BY COURTS

If it can be said that Bavaria's measures had only limited effects, the criminal charges brought against people on the grounds of having knowingly transmitted the virus will have much longer-lasting consequences on the general social climate and on the very conception of "individual responsibility" in the case of AIDS. Several cases have been brought to the courts, one of them concluded in front of the federal court in Karlsruhe on 4 November 1988. A U.S. Army cook had been sentenced by the state court in Nuremberg-Fürth to two years in prison for causing "grievous bodily harm" to three sexual partners by not informing them that he had AIDS: the verdict was upheld by the federal court. Although the federal court considered that the length of the jail term was too harsh with regard to the crime committed and requested that the state court revise it, the higher court set out a clear definition of the responsibilities of seropositive people in their sexual lives. According to its sentence, anyone diagnosed as seropositive bears sole responsibility for informing his eventual sex partners of his infection and for implementing safe sexual practices. In the commentaries on the judgment it is clearly stated that the proven transmission of the virus is of lesser importance than the simple possibility of transmission. All sexual behavior not completely safe must be considered criminal if engaged in by someone who is HIV-positive. In the case in question the accused had practiced coitus interruptus and had used condoms in order to prevent sperm entering his partner. These precautions were considered insufficient by the federal judges, despite the further fact that none of the three "victims" could be proved to have contracted AIDS.[19]

That verdict clearly puts the burden of proof in exculpating themselves on seropositives and people with AIDS; and it leaves them with the exclusive responsibility for not spreading the disease. The legal definition of responsibility interferes with the major arguments for prevention that have been developed by the AIDS Hilfen and by the health ministers; and it goes against the stress on the sharing of responsibility for taking sexual precautions and for using condoms. Both groups voiced immediate criticism of the judgment for its potentially negative effects on prevention inasmuch as it would be likely to create a quite false climate of security in the supposedly uninfected population. But irrespective of the validity of the different arguments for and against the judgment, the fact of the determination of individual responsibility in the courtroom shows how the legal professions may enter the arena of the formation of AIDS policy. While acting in accordance with their own rationality, its members of course also contribute to the shaping of substantive policies and of the wider social climate in which the issues surrounding AIDS are managed.

NOTES

1. The figures for the distribution among risk groups were calculated at 31 December 1987. WHO, *Weekly Epidemiological Record* 15 (8 April 1988): 107, Table 2.

2. M. Koch, "Kein Massiver Einbruch der Infektion in die Normalbevölkerung," *Weltgesundheit* 4 (April 1988): 20ff.

3. *Der Spiegel* 18 (1986): 209.

4. Koch, "Kein Massiver Einbruch."

5. *Der Spiegel*, 18 (1986).

6. Koch, "Kein Massiver Einbruch."

7. *Nature* 325 (19 February 1987): 650. The estimate is attributed to the Federal Minister of Health.

8. The Health Committee of the Bundestag appears to have been first briefed

on AIDS in the fall of 1985; and the first plenary Parliament debate, which lasted only half an hour, took place in 1986. *Nature* 325 (19 February 1987): 650.

9. R. Süssmuth, *Wege aus der Angst* (Hamburg: Hoffmann and Campe, 1987), p. 15.

10. *Der Stern* 43 (1985).

11. See the discussion between the social scientist Martin Dannecker and the filmmaker Rosa von Praunheim, "Das finde ich kriminell," *Konkret* (1986): "Sexualitä": 15–21.

12. Resolution of State Ministers and Senators Responsible for Health Affairs, Bonn, 27 March 1987.

13. Deutsche AIDS Hilfe, *Jahresbericht 1987/1988* (Berlin, May 1988).

14. M. Bochow, *AIDS: Wie leben schwule Männer heute? Berichte über eine Befragung der deutschen AIDS Hilfe* (Berlin: mimeo, September 1988).

15. A. Salmen, "Tief in der Krise," *Siegessäule* 12 (1988): 11–12.

16. See the consumer research newspaper *Test* 3 (1987): 257–262.

17. CSU politicians have recommended compulsory tests and registration, initially for the high-risk groups and later for the entire population, as well as segregation at school and work for seropositives.

18. *Zur Sache. Themen parlamentarischer Beratung. AIDS. Fakten und Konsequenzen* 3 (1988): 205ff.

19. *Vor-sicht. Die AIDS Zeitschrift* (December 1988): 11–14. A brief English-language commentary can be found in *Nature* 330 (26 November 1987): 304.

AIDS in Italy: Emergency in Slow Motion

In December 1984 Italy showed the lowest reported numbers both of absolute cases (fourteen) and of rates of AIDS per million population (0.3) in Western Europe. By the end of 1988, a bare four years later, Italy had become second only to France in the absolute numbers of AIDS cases in Europe (3,235), its rate per million population had increased by more than one hundred times (36.5), and it had entered the list of the ten most affected nations in the world.[1] At that point an official forecast suggested that after a further four years, by the end of 1992, there would be 142,000 people who had developed, or had already died of, AIDS; and the Minister of Health finally acknowledged the position as "a true state of emergency."[2] Professional and press commentators have, not surprisingly, agreed both that the recognition of the threat posed by the lethal virus, which entered Italy at more or less the same time that it entered the United States, was extremely belated and that the prolonged failure to acknowledge openly the scale of the health risk was not only a likely contributory factor to its rapid expansion but also a revealing exemplification of the unreasonably slow, and apparently ineffective, responses to AIDS by the public authorities.

Emergencies, viewed as occasions for urgent institutional and individual response, are of course not made merely by ministerial pronouncement. Nor do emergencies simply emerge. They are created by variously authored and heterogeneous measures serving to extract the specific focus of intervention from its surrounding foliage of routine misfortune: ill health, criminal activity, unexpected environmental change, or the many banal passages to untimely death. Invariably, public claims that particular issues are accurately characterized as "emergencies" assert or imply allocations of responsibility to act, recipes for successful prophylaxis, efforts to enroll and mobilize allies in the combat, demands for exceptional procedures, and rigorous account-ability. Contemporary Italy is well acquainted with the notion of an emergency and with exhortations to treat many natural and social events with appropriate urgency. Earthquakes, dam collapses, floods, political violence, Mafia and camorra slaughter—all punctuated, and in some cases helped to characterize, the decade prior to the first AIDS diagnosis in 1982. In all cases the government, and its civilian and armed public servants, were accused of failing to prevent avoidable death and guarantee public safety, the accusations coming not merely from political opponents but, in the case of the 1980 earthquake in the South, from the President of the Republic. Necessarily, in fragmented political systems such as Italy, managed by fragile coalition governments and marked by substantial ideological disputes, the polemical implications of acknowledging emergencies and the means actually employed to resolve them generate conflicts of a potentially paralyzing and publicly confusing kind. Pressures toward unambiguous, consensual portrayal of the nature of a particular emergency and the formulation of consistent policy are notoriously weak.

In four major respects, however, by comparison with those previous emergencies, the problems generated by HIV infection have been raised in an exceptionally benign environment for coherent responses. First, the years 1983–1987 were uniquely stable in postwar Italian politics. A single continuing government throughout the entire period effectively eliminated the characteristic regular disruption of policies and personnel.[3] In particular the Ministry of Health has had only two incumbents since 1983, both from the same party, compared to the succession of four ministers from three different parties between 1977 and 1982. Moreover, the steady electoral decline and oppositional forcefulness of the Italian Communist Party (PCI) has removed a substantial restraint on the government's freedom to formulate whatever controversial or unpopular policies it might deem necessary in the public interest without much fear of electoral punishment. Second, each above-mentioned emergency precipitated immediate allegations of the criminal and moral responsibility of individuals and groups from the country's politico-administrative elites. AIDS of course has morally accountable actors, but they are not found among the groups whose strategies for public defense are usually inimical to rapid policy formation. Third, the years between the introduction of divorce in 1970 and the referenda on abortion in 1981 had seen mass mobilization on controversial biopolitical issues. Such extended activity might have been expected to provide experience and organizational platforms for action on AIDS, both among the relevant social movements and the political parties that had translated their demands into parliamentary decisions. Finally, whereas responses in other societies have been fettered by restrictive laws on homosexuality, drug-taking, and personal privacy, the absence of similar laws in Italy has excluded the accompanying delays specifically attributable to disputes whether tacitly to condone illegal acts in the effort to control the spread of HIV infection.

Given the apparently abnormally favorable circumstances for effective and rapid intervention, some explanation of the factors hampering response needs to be provided. I shall argue, first, that the particular profile of HIV infection in Italy aggravates the difficulty of effective intervention; second, that the delay in response from the central authorities in particular is due less to any such cultural feature as homophobia, as Shilts has argued in the case of the United States,[4] than to fragmented and ambiguous institutional responsibilities resulting, most notably, in the tardy acquisition of knowledge about the exact profile of HIV infection and incidence of AIDS in Italy; and, third, that the legally liminal—and politically insignificant—positions occupied by the major risk groups have weakened pressures for more rapid action.

THE DEVELOPING SOCIAL PROFILE OF AIDS AND ITS IMPLICATIONS

The initial form taken by AIDS proved to be deceptive. The first case was diagnosed in June 1982, not long after the appearance of the first mass-circulation article in Italian on AIDS. The article's title ("For Gays Only"), the identity of the first sufferer (a gay man from Rome with regular contacts with the United States), and the implications of the fact that twelve of the first fifteen people with AIDS to be reported to the central health authorities were gay or bisexual suggested a straightforward delayed replication of the early United States profile.[5] However, the figures in Table 7.1 show that within three years a very different pattern of infection had imposed itself.

By the end of 1985 the cumulative number of intravenous drug users (ivdus) with AIDS had overtaken the total of gays and has progressively increased its dominance. New ivdu cases, already double the number of new gay cases by 1986, were five times as numerous by 1988 so that by December of that year ivdus accounted for two-thirds of AIDS cases, gays for only one in six. The transmission route of HIV infection through drug users has further implications for the contours of the problem and the responses.

First, it leads to a more variegated infected population than elsewhere. Women now represent nearly one in five AIDS cases (19 percent), as compared to the much smaller proportions in the United States (6 percent in 1987) and in Britain (3 percent).[6] In consequence the numbers (ninety-two), and proportional significance (3 percent), of children infected at birth remains the highest in Europe. Furthermore, the possibility of transmission to the heterosexual population is higher where the numbers of ivdus infected are greater: AIDS acquired through heterosexual contact now accounts for

Table 7.1
Italy: Cummulative AIDS Cases by Transmission Group 1982–1988

Year	Gay/bisexual	Ivdu	Gay & Ivdu	Haemophiliac	Transfusion	Pediatric	Heterosexual	Unknown	Total
1982	-	-	-	-	-	-	-	1	1
1983	3	-	-	-	-	-	1	1	5
1984	15	11	-	1	-	3	1	1	32
1985	70	98	12	4	4	15	4	6	213
1986	158	364	32	26	14	32	18	13	657
1987	321	1027	57	44	32	56	73	42	1652
1988	531	2123	93	67	54	94	182	91	3235

Notes: At 31 December 1988. According to COA the delay in reporting AIDS is such that less than half (43%) of new cases are in fact notified in the trimester of diagnosis: it takes two years for all cases to be reported. COA estimates the real figure of diagnosed cases at the end of 1988 to be approximately 4,000.

Source: Centro Operativo AIDS, *Aggiornamento dei casi di AIDS conclamato notificati in Italia al 31 dicembre 1988*, Rome, 1989, Table 7, n.p.

only 5 percent of all cases, but since 1986 the proportion of new cases through heterosexual contact has risen from 2 percent to 7 percent.[7] Drug-using prostitutes, male and female, represent a clear passage point for infection, especially since ivdu prostitutes have double the number of partners, twice as much anal intercourse, and a vastly greater indifference to condom use than their non-ivdu colleagues.[8] The very diversity of the populations at risk, which is a consequence of the centrality of drug users as the primary infected category, is itself of course a major factor rendering prevention more difficult. Moreover, the socially heterogeneous nature of the ivdu groups in Italy implies a reduced impact for informal social barriers to the transmission of HIV to wider social groups, such as appears to be favoring a disproportionate volume of AIDS cases in New York to (the poorer segments of) black and Hispanic groups.[9]

Second, because introduction to drug use begins young, the average age of AIDS cases is lower in Italy than in countries where gays are the principal sufferers. One-half of persons with AIDS in 1987 were aged between 20 and 29, in contrast with one-fifth in the United States: in Lombardy, for example, the average age of ivdus with AIDS is 27, that of gays 39.[10] The relative youthfulness of the Italian AIDS and seropositive population has clear implications for the nature and direction of educational campaigns. Moreover, the likelihood that the young infected will survive longer than the older entails a greater call on hospital and health services, especially when taken together with the fact that the prevalence of opportunistic infections is twelve times higher than Kaposi's sarcoma among Italian AIDS cases, requiring a much greater amount of regular medical attention that cannot be provided at home.[11] The probability that many ivdus with AIDS have in any case broken off relations with their families and have little household support from uninfected partners or friends reinforces the scale of the need for public services.

The third significant aspect of the distribution of AIDS is its geographical spread. The retrospective natural history of HIV infection in Italy attributes its earliest appearance to Milan in 1979, from which the virus spread to the other major cities, reaching even relatively remote outposts such as the island of Sardinia within two years.[12] However, reported progression to full-blown AIDS remained geographically restricted. As Table 7.2 shows, as late as 1985 three in every four new cases were still confined to the four regions of Lombardy, Veneto, Emilia Romagna, and Lazio.

By 1988, however, those four regions accounted for rather nearer to one-half (61 percent) of all cases; and, with the single exception of Val d'Aosta, AIDS had become a direct concern for every region. Indeed, the incidence of AIDS in peripheral regions such as Sardinia (6.3 cases per million inhabitants) had rapidly overtaken the national figure (4.8).[13] The dominance of ivdus is everywhere apparent, indicating not merely the national spread of HIV infection itself but also of the drug use through which the virus is

Table 7.2
Italy: AIDS Cases by Region and Year of Diagnosis 1982–1988

REGION	1982	1983	1984	1985	1986	1987	1988	TOTAL
Piedmont	-	-	2	9	37	68	124	240
Val d'Aosta	-	-	-	-	-	-	-	-
Liguria	-	-	-	9	25	65	93	192
Lombardy	-	1	11	72	160	335	509	1088
Trentino	-	-	-	1	3	9	13	26
Veneto	-	-	3	10	25	55	86	179
Friuli	-	-	-	2	4	10	10	26
Emilia	-	-	4	22	33	114	158	331
Marche	-	-	1	1	7	13	32	54
Tuscany	-	-	-	10	31	53	82	176
Umbria	-	-	-	2	1	1	8	12
Lazio	1	2	3	21	50	112	206	395
Campania	-	-	1	5	15	27	63	111
Abruzzi	-	-	-	-	3	8	6	17
Molise	-	-	-	-	-	1	1	2
Apulia	-	-	-	3	8	32	45	88
Basilicata	-	-	-	-	2	1	2	5
Calabria	-	-	-	1	5	14	11	31
Sicily	-	-	-	3	21	41	60	125
Sardinia	-	-	-	8	12	33	66	119
Non-Italians	-	1	3	1	3	4	9	21
TOTAL	1	4	28	180	445	996	1584	3238

Notes: 1. At 31 December 1988; 2. Cases classified by region of residence.

Source: Centro Operativo AIDS, *Aggiornamento dei casi di AIDS conclamato notificati in Italia al 31 dicembre 1988,* Rome, Table 2, n.p.

transmitted. Gays with AIDS constitute no more than one-third, and ivdus no less than two-fifths, of any region's total number of cases. Geographically and administratively speaking, HIV infection and its supportive networks of drug dissemination and abuse are by no means simply a limited metro-politan predicament. Given the distinctive profile of AIDS in Italy, therefore, within what kind of institutional framework do the primary relevant actors have to frame their responses?

FIVE CHARACTERS IN SEARCH OF THEIR RESPONSIBILITIES

So variegated and diffuse a spread of HIV infection calls for action from a wide range of institutions to cover the tasks of acquiring epidemiological knowledge, organizing prevention campaigns, and managing all degrees of infection between the asymptomatic carriers and the terminally ill. Five principal (sets of) actors can be identified: the central government, the regional governments, organizations of members of the principal risk groups, voluntary organizations established specifically to combat AIDS, and Catholic groups. In contrast particularly with actions in the United States, but in keeping with the generally restricted role of self-help groups among the sick in Italy, no formal associations of AIDS patients or people diagnosed as seropositive have been established, nor have there been any consciousness-raising public mobilizations by those most directly affected. Responses are organized through the formal and informal linkages among the five largely institutionalized actors; they are obstructed by the relative autonomy of institutions and by the concentrations of relevant powers to intervene at different, and therefore not easily coordinated, levels in particular institutions between the center and the periphery.

At the central level the state institutions dealing with the varied populations exposed to AIDS have maintained their formal distance from one another. An especially significant fissure divides the centralized education and radio-television services—which, given the youth of drug addicts and the HIV-infected, are especially crucial—from the decentralized health services. Despite demands to establish a body to coordinate the health services with the most obvious channels of education (as well as the ministries responsible for the prison system, armed forces, and scientific research), no such organ has been created.[14] Moreover, no representatives of the education bureaucracy or the state television services (RAI) sit on the committee to advise the Minister of Health on AIDS. As a result the major agencies of mass prevention and management remain separated from each other, so that not only are practical initiatives harder to put in place but the sense of urgency that a single organized set of responses might successfully communicate to the widest public is also diminished.[15]

Furthermore, while the educational and mass media systems are highly centralized, the health services are characterized by dispersal of powers to local levels. Following the health reform of 1978 substantial responsibilities, including the management and prevention of infectious diseases, were transferred to the twenty effectively autonomous regional governments and to the grass-roots agencies for the delivery of services, the Local Health Units (USL).[16] The state retains overall financial responsibility—which falls some way short of control, since the health budget has been overspent by progressively larger amounts each year, while nonetheless constituting a smaller proportion of GNP (5.3 percent) than in other advanced industrial societies. The Minister of Health also retains the power to issue emergency decrees binding on all regions and to order forms of compulsory treatment (sc. quarantine or isolation) for the infected. In responding to the spread of HIV infection, however, neither the financial power to allocate extra resources for directed regional spending nor the administrative power to isolate known

HIV carriers has been used. Up until the end of 1988 no special funds had been granted to any region to combat AIDS, a failure eliciting strong protests from the worst-affected areas.[17] The 38 billion lire (U.S. $29.4 million) that had been allocated in 1988, for example, were divided among scientific research (16 percent), the training of medical and paramedical personnel (32 percent), and the first national educational campaign (52 percent). Moreover, as I shall show below, not only had the state not used its most extensive powers against infection, but it preferred generally to make recommendations rather than issue orders. These policies, reinforcing rather than overcoming the fissures in an institutional framework characterized by central coordination rather than control, permit substantial variation between the management of AIDS in different parts of the country. Regional governments have been left to make their own decisions at their own pace for their own territories. The positive consequence has been the encouragement of extreme flexibility in responding to a disease of uneven incidence, unequal costs, and uncertain direction. Nevertheless, because HIV infection is also marked by asymptomatic and mobile carriers, a long latency period, and a demand for accurate and consistent public information, use of the existing health system also makes it much harder to prevent contradictory public messages, to ensure complementary rigor in prevention measures, and to compensate for the gross existing regional imbalances in the provision of services to the sick.[18]

Analogous disjunctures of various kinds characterize the activities of the other actors in search of clear roles in the campaign to halt the spread of AIDS. As far as the organizations directly associated with the risk groups are concerned, the shift in health responsibilities toward regional and local levels has encouraged more territorially circumscribed and fragmented mobilization on biopolitical issues and has therefore not favored the formation or survival of national pressure groups to stimulate central government policy. One clearly related casualty of this process has been the women's movement—the major actor in the preceding biopolitical issues—whose national-level mobilization has virtually disappeared since 1978.[19] Significantly, despite the considerably higher proportion of women among HIV-infected cases in Italy than elsewhere, caused by the salience of the ivdu transmission route, no public initiatives have been taken by women's organizations. The gay movement, politically far weaker than the women's movement and with little access to political parties or state authorities in the years before AIDS, has not achieved the status of legitimate interlocutor in the formation of national AIDS policies; nor have its leaders been visibly incorporated in the public policy process. Finally, the other major risk group, drug users, lacks any direct first-person public representation. While of course that lack is equally common elsewhere, in Italy the scale of HIV infection among drug users makes the failure to achieve regular access and self-organization for prevention much more costly. The specific problems of mobilization and response among both gays and ivdus will be discussed separately below.

In so state-centered and religiously saturated a society as Italy, the role of secular voluntary organizations has traditionally been small. While they have enjoyed a very considerable recent expansion in numbers, they possess few resources and must therefore be clearly limited in the practical contributions that they can offer to the control and management of HIV infection. At the center two national associations have been established to address aspects of AIDS: ANLAIDS (National Association for the Struggle Against AIDS) in July 1985 and LILA (League for the Struggle Against AIDS) in July 1987. ANLAIDS was the creation of the then Under-Secretary of Health from the Liberal Party, in criticism of the inactivity of his Christian Democrat minister, and has been largely concerned both with organizing and funding scientific research and with public education, in particular advice to seropositives.[20] As the stimulus for its creation suggests, ANLAIDS has been in some tension with the Ministry of Health: its president has publicly described ANLAIDS' work as necessary compensation for the ministry's failures, while its senior scientific adviser and vice-president was excluded from the official ministerial committee on AIDS in early 1988.[21] The other national creation, LILA, is an umbrella organization for a wide range of existing professional, trade union, and voluntary groups from the left, with a particular concern for the civil rights aspects of AIDS prevention and treatment. While the organization has not been a formal interlocutor in government policy, it has promoted micro-campaigns in several cities to distribute condoms and syringes carrying warnings of infection.

The remaining significant set of actors is composed of Catholic organizations. The pronouncements of the Church hierarchy can be presumed to have some, but hard to determine, influence on policies devised by Catholic politicians and health professionals. The Church has opposed any narrowly pragmatic prevention campaign in favor of a drastic reform in sexual mores. Not only did it sharply criticize the government's national education campaign in 1988, but the repeated, and allegedly confusing, public emphasis on the unreliability of condoms by the Ministry of Health and the Minister of Health himself can be attributed to pressure by the Church for at least tacit acknowledgment of the need to encourage more rigorous forms of prevention.[22] At the grass-roots level religious organizations have always played an important role in emergency, hospital, and caring services; and interventions by single organizations and priests in favor of both seropositives and the terminally ill have been noted from all major cities. A particular area of attention is represented by the numerous private therapeutic communities for drug addicts, many of religious inspiration, which of course contain members infected with HIV. But the very diversity of inspiration, organization, and practice of such communities has prevented any unified "representation" of their infected members to public authorities.[23]

Responses to AIDS have been organized through the formal and informal linkages among these sets of actors, in a framework that is institutionally fragmented and traditionally hostile to intervention by secular, nonpolitical party groups in policy formation or execution. How, then, have the tasks of accumulating knowledge about the actual spread of AIDS, managing general prevention campaigns, and controlling the spread of HIV infection among the categories most at risk been taken on and performed?

ACCUMULATING KNOWLEDGE

Knowledge of the national profile of AIDS cases and HIV infection has been created slowly and unevenly, partly because of the delay in creating a formal unit to provide advice on AIDS and partly because of the powers at the disposal of the Ministry of Health to create knowledge. The first official notice taken of AIDS appeared in a Ministry of Health circular in August 1983, providing information for local use, establishing an ad hoc study group for the surveillance of AIDS in the National Health Institute (Istituto Superiore di Sanità), and encouraging the notification of all diagnosed and suspected cases to the group. Not until January 1987, however, was the group given formal institutional status as the Centro Operativo AIDS (COA), in tandem with the creation of a twenty-two member National Committee for the Campaign Against AIDS (CNLA), composed overwhelmingly of medical researchers and administrators (the two exceptions were a philosopher of law and a journalist). The CNLA's mandate was to provide advice and coordination for the initiatives against HIV infection; the COA, whose role was not formally defined until February 1988, had the primary tasks of surveillance and the monitoring of scientific research. Somewhat belatedly, therefore, with regard to the rapid increase in AIDS cases and the measures already taken by some regional governments, the central government provided itself with an authoritative organ of exclusively medical expertise to propose and evaluate possible initiatives to contain the spread of HIV infection.

Following the establishment of the two new bodies, as of February 1987 notification of all AIDS cases to the central authorities was first made compulsory, then expanded to include the actual name of the patient.[24] This decision was both tardy with respect to initiatives by the most-affected regions and risked breaching their guarantees for the absolute privacy of all AIDS cases. Thus the two most affected regions, Lazio and Lombardy, had already made AIDS a notifiable disease, respectively in June 1985 and January 1986, and had taken pains to create unequivocal guarantees of confidentiality precisely to ensure the maximum effectiveness of regional surveillance. Both regions initially resisted the introduction of new rules for the indication of patients' names but were eventually persuaded that the registration procedures at COA were both secure and useful.[25]

The uneven attention given to AIDS both among the regions themselves and between regions and central authorities has had two results. First, it has raised doubt whether the natural history of AIDS represented by the reported figures is more an artifact of the different pressures to report the disease than an accurate indication of the exact path HIV infection, and progression to diagnosed AIDS, has followed. Second, it has led to considerable disparities in the statistical patterns presented at regional and national levels. Thus, in September 1988 the official figures of the Lombardy region showed a cumulative regional total of 932 cases; the cases counted by the COA for Lombardy amounted to only 866, some 7 percent fewer.[26] If similar divergences exist elsewhere, then the smaller and recently affected regions may have had their contributions both understated and underweighted in the portrayal of the incidence of AIDS at the national level. To the extent that the disparities are long-standing, then the statistically and territorially reduced profile of AIDS obtainable in Rome may help to account for the prolonged failure of the government to recognize the extent of the spread of AIDS.

Since the invention of reliable tests in 1985 the second major technique for generating official knowledge about the dissemination of HIV infection has been through screening. This issue has been confronted in two stages, both characterized by extreme caution: in 1985, when the government took its first explicit actions to combat AIDS, and in 1987, when the CNLA reviewed the potential advantages, disadvantages, and costs of screening a wide range of specific populations. In the course of 1985 the government recommended screening in three cases. The first population for whom testing was made available, but only encouraged rather than enforced, was prison inmates, among whom infection was believed to be extensive. According to official figures as of 31 December 1986, roughly half the 42,000 prisoners had opted to be tested, with one in seven resulting seropositive.[27] Although local surveys show considerable variation around this figure (approximately one in two prisoners in Lombardy were revealed to be seropositive, but only one in ten in Umbria's major jail), overall, Italy appears to have one of the highest rates in Europe of infection in prison.[28] However, unlike in some other, less affected, European countries (notably West Germany, Ireland, and the UK), seropositive prisoners have not been made the subject of any special measures.[29] Nor, despite reiterated suggestions—notably by the Minister of Health in November 1986, the CNLA in April 1987, and the director of prison services in the Ministry of Justice in May 1988—has the mandatory testing of prisoners been imposed.

The second instance of government recommendation of screening concerned not people but blood donations and blood products. Italy's estimated 2,800 hemophiliacs rely in particular on blood products from the United States (80 percent) and Austria (20 percent), while blood itself is mainly imported from less developed countries. In July 1985, not long after the first reported deaths of a hemophiliac in November 1984 and a transfusion patient in June 1985, the government recommended that all regions advise donors that blood from persons at risk of HIV infection would not be used and that in any case all units of blood would be tested.[30] At this time the government was explicitly concerned not to designate formally any particular entire group as prohibited from donating blood, preferring the strategy of encouraging self-exclusion rather than publicly indicating polluted social categories.[31] By the time that the government made the screening of all blood mandatory in January 1988 and explicitly forbade donations from specified categories at risk (all ivdus since 1977, male homosexuals, sexual partners of HIV antibody positives, sexual partners of all categories at risk of AIDS, and all transfusion recipients since 1978), not only had many regions imposed compulsory testing of all blood but some of the blood banks had also taken their own initiatives. Lombardy, for example, required the testing of all blood from early 1987; and the principal association of blood donors (AVIS) had, controversially, announced in the Veneto in 1984 that it would refuse all blood donations from gays and prostitutes. Regions and blood banks favored confining blood donations to a known local circle of regular donors whose habits were more easily maintained under surveillance and whose sexual lives appeared more transparent. The result of the initially relaxed policy was to ensure that by the end of 1986 the proportion of donors revealed to be seropositive was higher in Italy than elsewhere: 2.5 per 10,000 as compared with 2 per 10,000 in the United States and 1 per 50,000 in the UK.[32] But, over a longer period and notwithstanding the fact that Italy's list of excluded blood-donor categories was shorter than that in, say, the UK, by the end of 1988 Italy had one of the lowest rates in Europe of hemophiliac and transfusion-related AIDS: compare its joint 4 percent (89 cases) with France's 8 percent (349) or the 9 percent (139) reported in the UK which, by including prostitutes, men participating in even a single homosexual act since 1977, and the sexual partners of Africans in its list of excluded categories, had a more restrictive policy than Italy.[33]

The third case in which the government advised screening in 1985 was for drug abusers who attended the drug treatment centers of the local health units (USL). However, because regional governments acted slowly to make testing mandatory and treatment centers reached only a minority even of intravenous drug users, the response rate was poor. Only 6,483 tests had been carried out by the end of 1986, equivalent to one-quarter of the total number of addicts registered at such centers and probably no more than 4 percent of all addicts.[34] Apart from the obvious consequences of leaving the overwhelming majority of the major risk category in ignorance of its HIV status, such small and probably unrepresentative samples were scarcely an adequate base for formulating public policy. In reviewing the value of screening specific and general populations in April 1987, the CNLA calculated that its overall cost would amount to 1450 miliard lire (U.S. $1.1 billion) and produce no fewer than 3.5 million false positives. Because of the serious personal and social consequences of such figures, notably for the potentially large category of pregnant women who might be tempted into unnecessary and traumatic abortions, the CNLA advised unequivocally against imposing screening on any category. It further argued against the provision of generalized test facilities for members of categories not believed to be at any risk.[35]

Exclusion of such sources of policy-informing data compelled the central authorities to rely on relevant information gathered as a by-product of biomedical investigations of the virus and its carriers. Despite the absence of a national research plan on AIDS, which was not launched until August 1988, a considerable volume of local research had nonetheless been undertaken, sponsored by a range of public bodies, universities, and groups such as the Association for Cancer Research. The national AIDS conference in Rome in May 1987 attracted 246 papers by Italian researchers, who also provided 101 contributions to the Fourth International Congress on AIDS in Stockholm in June 1988; and no fewer than 535 proposals were elicited by the funding opportunities of the national project a few months later.[36] Until 1988, however, there had been no central coordination of research priorities or directions. Dependent on small-scale and not easily generalizable results, progress toward any reliable overall profile of the distribution and future of HIV infection was inevitably slow, haphazard, and unreliable, with the result that until 1988 all predictions from the center on the development of AIDS fell far short of the reality. In March 1985, for example, a leading immunologist spoke—as he then claimed, pessimistically—of the likelihood of 1,000 AIDS cases in Italy by 1990, a figure that had already been surpassed by mid–1987. Likewise the forecast made in April 1987 by the CNLA that there would be 1,900 AIDS cases by the end of 1988 underestimated the eventual total by more than 40 percent.[37] It was of course on the basis of such underestimates that the CNLA advised the minister of the likely resources required to combat the disease.

A principal stimulus to a major revision of predictions was the first national enquiry into the extent of seropositivity promoted in 1985 by the then recently constituted ANLAIDS. When its results were finally made known in autumn 1987, the first serious quasi-official prospect of the future of AIDS in Italy became available. For they indicated, on the basis of tests by a sample of 52,880 volunteers, an estimated national total of some 200,000 seropositives, with levels of HIV infection in specific populations ranging from 47 percent among ivdus to 25 percent among gays.[38] Less than a year later, in August 1988, the implications of so large a pool of infection were drawn out in a forecast of 27,000 cases of full-blown AIDS by 1990 and 61,050 by 1991, nearly nineteen times the reported total for 1988.[39] Such predictions suggested a problem of hitherto unimagined dimensions, requiring a major revision of likely costs. The scale of recalculation can be illustrated by the estimated demands for hospital beds. In April 1987 the CNLA reckoned that 1,362 new beds would be required by the end of the following year; in December 1988 it indicated that 10,000 would be required within one year.[40] Finally, the dissemination of HIV infection could clearly be proclaimed an emergency—ironically, just two months before the COA reported that the increase in new cases had slowed for the first time and that the forecasts for cumulative AIDS cases in 1990 and 1992 had been dramatically revised downwards to the (still very considerable) figures of 5,864 and 15,000, respectively.[41]

DISSEMINATING KNOWLEDGE

Not surprisingly, the tortuous and error-prone process of accumulating reliable knowledge about the distribution and transmission routes of AIDS entailed some diffidence toward the need for, and content of, supposedly reliable messages to educate the public about the disease. In fact, not until the early summer of 1987 did the Minister of Health call for proposals for a three-pronged media campaign on AIDS, directed at the general public; at doctors and health personnel; and at specific populations in schools, prisons, and military establishments and among drug users. Budget conflicts forced further delays, and the national media campaign finally got under way only in July 1988, more than six years after the first AIDS diagnosis in Italy. The subsequent dissemination of a brochure and a controversial letter on AIDS by the Minister of Health himself to every Italian household had to wait until December 1988.[42]

Despite exposure to information initially circulated widely in 1987 by regional authorities, local health units, private organizations such as AN-LAIDS, and gay groups, it seems likely that the absence of a clear national information campaign was a factor in maintaining fairly high levels of ignorance about AIDS among at least the general public. As late as December 1986, 33 percent in one national opinion survey had either not heard of AIDS at all or had learned about it only in the previous few months; as many as 44 percent believed that the disease was serious but curable; and 67 percent claimed not to know its symptoms. According to the agency responsible for the content of the national campaign, only 45 percent of Italians considered AIDS a serious disease and 40 percent had very confused ideas about its transmission prior to the campaign's launch.[43] It must, however, be said that the scarcity of officially validated information did not appear to make Italians less tolerant toward HIV carriers than other better-informed populations: in an eleven-nation survey of attitudes to people with AIDS carried out in early 1988 the Italian sample was more tolerant and readier to accept close contact with AIDS patients than all other European societies.[44]

It is unlikely that the content of the campaign itself has altered such tolerant attitudes. Its messages have consciously eschewed both the generalized alarm intended by, say, Australia's Grim Reaper symbol and the specification of any otherwise identifiable social category as the primary vehicle of infection. Central policy can thus be seen either as a refusal to provide authoritative state sanction for existing prejudice or, given the delay in launching the campaign, as a willingness to educate only when the heterosexual population is clearly threatened. Before 1988 the RAI had refused to transmit a privately produced sequence of information on the grounds that it was too explicit; and it had also rejected a set of film clips produced by, and directed toward, the gay population.[45] The texts of the television and newspaper information and of the minister's letter to all households emphasize how difficult it is to be infected, the ways in which the virus is not transmitted, and "the advisability of conducting a normal life as a couple." Nowhere are the categories at risk picked out for public attention: gay relations are merely embedded in the warning against casual sexual partners, explicitly recognized as either heterosexual or homosexual, and the dangers of infection through syringes are not specifically tied to intravenous drug abuse but appear along with a general warning against the promiscuous use of all personal toilet instruments. Condoms are mentioned only once, without emphasis, and designated by the remote and poorly understood term *profilattico* rather than the widely comprehensible but "vulgar" *preservativo*. It is explicitly stated that they do not provide absolute protection against infection and that their use is an option essentially for those of feeble moral character who cannot avoid "nonnormal" sexual behavior.[46]

The generic nature of the term "normal" as applied to sexual practices or partnerships—a characterization dominating the Minister of Health's letter to all households, where it is tied to family life—is the counterpart of the refusal to draw clear boundaries between the pure and the polluted. Specific types of risky behavior are not mentioned, leaving it entirely unclear what actual forms of "nonnormal" sexual activity might be intended in this context. In effect the information campaign evades defining particular social categories in terms of specific risky practices, although at the same time it does not specify what such practices, which by implication might enter anyone's repertoire of sexual activities but ought to be eliminated, might be. One effect of declining to identify any category of victims as especially significant is to refuse both to legitimate its members as deserving of special treatment and to acknowledge their representatives as institutionalized interlocutors in a joint campaign to contain HIV infection. The message of the central authorities has been framed in terms that withhold formal recognition of special status for any particular category of HIV-infected persons. For the gay movement in particular, therefore, the spread of AIDS has not been an occasion on which it has been able to transform its image or status in the wider society. It has not been "legitimated through disaster."[47]

THE ROLE OF THE GAY MOVEMENT

Homosexual acts, between men or women, have not been a crime in Italy since the promulgation of the first national penal code in 1889. Although attempts have occasionally been made to declare them, and any public approval for them, illegal, none has succeeded, despite an apparently widespread disapproval of homosexuality.[48] In the most recent case, in 1963, the draft bill did not even reach the discussion stage in Parliament. Some activists have suggested that the gay movement in Italy is weaker than elsewhere precisely because there have been no specifically discriminatory laws to contest and thus provoke an active gay solidarity in the face of a common threat to its community existence.[49] In that respect gays in Italy have been faced with more severe mobilizational difficulties than women, for whom the contests over the laws (and referenda) on divorce, abortion, and sexual violence have provided significant national issues for feminist debate and political intervention almost continuously since 1970. Conversely, freedom from obvious legal constraints has not enabled the gay movement to impel the government into rapid national action or to transform itself into a quasi-institutionalized contributor to the formation of public policy. The reasons are epidemiological, social, and political.

An important consideration may simply be the diminishing extent of gay vulnerability to AIDS and to HIV infection. Gays represented the majority of cases only in the very earliest days of the epidemic, before the need for comprehensive action, directly incorporating members of risk groups, was clear. Since 1985 the proportion of AIDS cases by gay transmission has fallen from just under one-half of all cases (46 percent) to less than one-sixth (16 percent). While evidence on seropositivity trends is mostly local and hard to interpret, reports from Milan, Rome, and Bologna suggest a clear rise in HIV infection among gays between 1983 and 1986 but a decline thereafter.[50] All studies, retrospective and prospective, indicate that from the first appearance of HIV the levels of seropositivity among gays have been substantially lower than among ivdus; and it is therefore likely that simply because the gay population appeared to be at lower risk and was in any case able to change its behavior rapidly, direct involvement by its representatives in more general decision making on public health measures was unjustified.

One alleged feature of Italian gay life is regularly invoked to explain the apparently low proportion of gays among the victims of AIDS and seropositives both with respect to other Italian risk groups and to gays elsewhere: a low level of promiscuity by contrast with other advanced societies.[51]

Whether or not such a feature, if it were clearly defined and proved to be true, would account for the level of incidence of HIV infection among Italian gays (a level that might in fact be no lower in regard to the unascertainable total gay population than in other societies where gays are relatively more prominent in the AIDS statistics, as they may well be in those societies' general populations), it might at least indicate a less dense and extensive network of gay social relations in Italy and thus help to explain the difficulty of mobilizing gays.

Certainly community life among Italian gays is less visible as well as more exclusive and self-sufficient than in, say, some major cities of the United States. Accepted sites for transient sexual and social encounters are relatively few. In Milan, for example, only five small and recently opened gay saunas existed in 1988, so that there has been a very restricted "bathhouse culture" for anonymous sex: fewer or no opportunities exist in other cities.[52] However, the infrequence of public and exclusively gay meeting points should not be taken to mean that Italian gays are necessarily markedly more restrained in the number and choices of their sexual partners than gays in other societies. A study in the Naples region found that one-quarter of the sample of 86 sexually active gay men had more than 200 partners annually.[53] More precise data are available from a sample of 123 gay men attending a clinic for sexually transmitted diseases in Milan.[54] Sixteen percent had more than ten partners each month and a further 24 percent had between six and ten partners. Rather more than one-third (38 percent) declared that they had a fixed partner (i.e., a relationship of at least six months' standing), although that stability does not entail a reduced range of sexual relationships: roughly half (47 percent) of those with fixed partners recorded six or more (other) partners monthly, as against only slightly more than one-third (36 percent) of those without fixed partners. Even if Italian gays are indeed more "monogamous" than elsewhere in the sense of favoring the creation of one relatively enduring relationship, that preference by no means excludes a network of other sexual partners.[55] As the ARCI Gay movement in Bologna has observed, social prejudices and informal discrimination lead rather to "a virtually non-existent community life, an extreme difficulty in establishing stable relationships."[56]

Furthermore, sexual encounters are far from being confined to the gay community. Thirty-eight percent of the Milan sample claimed to have "occasional" heterosexual relations and 7 percent to be fully bisexual, leaving the exclusively gay in only a bare majority. Again, even those with fixed partners were only slightly less involved in such relations than their apparently freer fellows. Approximately one-third (29 percent) of those with fixed partners maintained such heterosexual relations, as against a rather larger proportion (44 percent) of those without fixed partners. The extent of involvement in both gay and heterosexual sex, while it follows patterns observed among gays in other societies, appears nevertheless to be rather more extensive in Italy than elsewhere. If the pattern of relationships in the Milan sample is characteristic of other gay networks, then there is clearly a greater risk in Italy than in societies with more strongly bounded gay communities that HIV will pass into the heterosexual community not only through drug-taking but also through gay links to heterosexual partners. The level of this risk is unknown, although recent research in Rome and Sicily suggests that the risks of infection for both gays and heterosexuals is directly correlated with the numbers of sexual partners and encounters.[57] Moreover, the high proportion of gays who regularly or occasionally enjoy heterosexual activities suggests why an exclusive gay identity and its public recognition might be less widely sought, or indeed acceptable, within the gay population: the incentive for active involvement in highly visible pressure-group politics to influence the response to AIDS is correspondingly reduced.

Reinforcement for relative public inactivity has come from the structure and policies of organized gay representation. The major national gay organization, ARCI Gay, established itself with a formal statute and representative structures only in 1985 and now claims some 9,000 members, who are more or less actively affiliated with its twenty-eight sections, mainly concentrated in central and northern Italy. Its sections in southern Italy, where AIDS is becoming increasingly salient, are few and generally inactive—a fact that bodes ill for the institutional support for self-management on the part of the HIV-infected. ARCI Gay's political association is with the left—a more institutionalized left than represented by the earlier-established (1972) but now dissolved group FUORI, whose activities have been primarily confined to Turin. At the national political level, however, where the balance of power favors the parties of the center, the gay movement is not strong, either in terms of its influence on political party policy or in interaction with the government. Indeed, the political weight of the gay movement is not sufficiently great for the parties to seek their own advantage by cultivating it. In the 1987 national elections, for example, the explicitly gay candidates, standing as independents in various left-wing parties, secured only 20,000 preference votes, of which one-quarter alone went to the national secretary in the movement's leading stronghold, Bologna; no gay candidates were elected.[58]

Until the early 1980s this weakness was partly a matter of choice since, like some segments of the women's movement, the gay world favored a policy of separatism and "diversity." Recently, however—no doubt partly in response to the need to collaborate with state agencies and politicians in combatting AIDS and partly in consequence of the new visibility and scrutability of the gay world that AIDS has provoked—the emphasis of the movement's leadership has been to achieve a legally defined position within Italian society as a recognized rights-bearing minority. Thus, since 1987 it has proposed legislation extending a series of rights and opportunities to gay couples that hitherto have applied only to heterosexuals (principally inheritance, public housing, and adoption of children). In an effort to appeal to a broader constituency it has also advanced general libertarian objectives for all ethnic, linguistic, religious, and sexual minorities, to be embodied in a Charter of Rights and in legally recognized opportunities to defend members and sue for damage from discrimination. While perhaps ensuring some wider support, so broad a policy—epitomized by the claim of ARCI Gay's secretary that the word "homosexual" did not even appear in the organization's legislative proposals[59]—necessarily reduced the potential for recognition of specifically gay concerns and any formal institutional incorporation.

As far as the response to AIDS is concerned, the combined effects of the epidemiological, social, and political factors have reduced any national-level impact of the gay movement. Meetings demanded with the Minister of Health have not been realized, the national broadcasting corporation (RAI) has refused to transmit information prepared by, and directed toward, the gay population, and the CNLA suggested that all preventive activities should be organized in tandem not with the central authorities, whose primary task was information, but with the regions.[60] The content of the major educational leaflet ("Against AIDS, New Love Practices") produced in 1988 by ARCI Gay in collaboration with the CNLA in fact reflects the policies of both contributors to aim at the broadest audience: the text makes a single, unobtrusive reference to gays. Thus, although the gay movement began its own educational campaign in the autumn of 1984, its success in mobilizing the national authorities to indicate the gay community as in especial need of defense has not been great. Protection of gays has not been acknowledged as a valid trigger for a public health emergency; the acceptance of an emergency itself has been rendered more difficult without the public acknowledgment of a clear set of victims.

The primary contributions by the gay movement to the struggle against AIDS have been informal and local. In the area of epidemiological research a gay club in Rome has been collaborating with the surveillance group in the National Health Institute since 1983, and informal association with local hospital services, especially to guarantee the anonymity of testing for gay men, is common. Given ARCI Gay's affiliation with the political left, its AIDS initiatives could be expected to receive the most sympathetic institutional responses in cities with left-wing administrations, notably in the region of Emilia Romagna and its capital Bologna, which has gone first and furthest in integrating the gay movement into the formation of AIDS policy and prevention. Educational activities, often simply the translation of German materials, began in 1984. Meetings were held with the regional health authorities and political leaders from 1985 onwards; and ARCI Gay endorsed their Program Against AIDS, which was approved in May 1988. The only aspects of which the movement was critical were the domination of the AIDS advisory committee by medical experts and the absence of any particularized recognition and ensuing funding for the role of voluntary groups such as ARCI Gay itself.

In Milan, where HIV infection appeared earlier and has been most widespread, the less organized gay community began its work against AIDS much later—an illustration of the relative independence of epidemiology and response. In late 1986 local gays established the Associazione Solidarietà AIDS (ASA), which has organized the distribution of educational materials, managed three professionally oriented courses on safe sex, staffed a daily telephone information service (and, since 1987, has contributed to the staff of the line run by the city council), and sponsored a conference in mid–1988 on gays and health. ASA has also concerned itself directly with the management of seropositives and people with AIDS: first, by establishing self-help groups for seropositives (the first group consisting entirely of seropositive women), which now contain some fifty members; and, second, by providing domiciliary care for up to fifteen people with AIDS. The group has plans (1988) to collaborate with the city council in creating and staffing a group of flats for people with AIDS. ASA has received funding from the region and the concession of premises from the city council; but its professional expertise is provided by volunteers, who also guarantee a network of informal collaboration with local medical centers.

Rome, Milan, and Bologna represent the most extensive initiatives and institutional collaboration by the gay movement. Elsewhere resources are lower and even a minimal local organization may be lacking. As I shall suggest in the conclusion, this bodes ill for the South in particular since an important stimulus to official action will be lacking. Nevertheless, whatever difficulties exist for gays, they are overwhelmed by the problems associated with Italy's major category of AIDS cases: the intravenous drug users.

MANAGING AIDS AMONG DRUG USERS

Intravenous drug abuse as a publicly visible problem entered Italy in the mid–1970s, with the first official death from overdose recorded in 1973. The annual death toll has continued to rise, slowly until 1979 and—with the exception of a sharp fall in 1985—very rapidly thereafter.[61] Heroin consumers were estimated at 65,000 in 1980; by 1987 the figure had nearly tripled to at least 150,000.[62] The appearance of HIV infection has therefore been coterminous with an increasingly serious drug problem, signaled between 1979 and 1988 by a sixfold increase in annual deaths from overdoses (126 to 785), a tenfold rise in the number of arrests for trafficking (2,714 to 28,629), and a sevenfold increase in the quantity of heroin sequestered by police (79 kg to 572 kg). That escalation signifies also the spread of drug abuse from metropolitan centers to provincial towns, a movement reflected in the wide regional dissemination of AIDS cases.

Undoubtedly this rapid expansion was facilitated by the passage of law

No. 685 in 1975, which legalized the possession of "a moderate quantity" of drugs for personal use. To sell drugs (including heroin) was a serious crime: to buy them was not.[63] A second facilitating factor is also important: the ready availability of syringes in Italy, since no doctor's prescription is needed, at the accessible price of 300 lire each in 1987. It is reasonable to suppose that, despite the obligations on police and doctors to inform either the magistrature or the regional drug treatment centers of anyone caught in possession of drugs, the removal of the threat of direct criminal sanctions reduced the perceived need for surveillance and knowledge of the drug-abusing world, with obvious implications for the ability to track and combat HIV infection. Moreover, although local magistrates could order attendance at treatment centers, few pressures could be brought to bear on recalcitrant nonattenders. In one study of rural Lombardy between 1984 and 1987, only 47 percent of identified drug addicts had actually made contact with the local drug abuse unit, even though in their catchment area of twenty-two villages visibility would be higher, and pressure to conform much greater, than in the metropolitan centers.[64] In fact, the overall number of drug addicts in attendance at (public) treatment centers or resident in (private) therapeutic communities amounted to 24,947 in 1986, representing no more than 16 percent of the total estimated regular drug-abusing population.[65] Moreover, in some areas of concentration in drug abuse, the services themselves are not established or are unable adequately to manage drug addiction itself, let alone the further problems of HIV infection. The lack of effective contact between drug users and the state makes any efficacious information campaign on AIDS to change both injecting and sexual practices extremely difficult.

Ensured by the simple scale of intravenous drug use, the difficulties are aggravated by three characteristics of the drug-using world itself. First, the international network of provision of drugs into which Italy is firmly inserted ensures that any attempt to combat AIDS by reducing the availability of injectable drugs requires coordinated action far beyond national frontiers. International collaboration on such a scale is hardly easy. Second, regular consumption of both hard and soft drugs from an early age encourages the continuing reproduction of the category. In the sample from rural Lombardy one in four of the sample had begun regular use of drugs before the age of 20: two-fifths of the men and one-quarter of the women had actually begun their drug careers directly with heroin.[66] A broader investigation of drug use in central and northern Italy showed that 6 percent of 11- to 16-year-olds had at least experimented with drugs (mostly cannabis), rising to a maximum of 26 percent among 21-year-olds.[67] Third, drug abusers in Italy have no formal organizations of self-help outside the mostly religious framework of therapeutic communities. Unlike the Dutch and, more modest, New York examples, Italian drug users have not mobilized into groups with formal leadership through which information can be effectively spread and safer practices encouraged.[68] No defensive, self-created network has been, or looks likely to be, created. Indeed, the therapeutic communities, which represent the nearest equivalent to an organizational structure for potential mobilization, account for only one-fifth (22 percent) of addicts in treatment and are too diverse for any coordinated action. In some cases, as noted below (p. 161, n.23), such communities have attempted to avoid the problem by demanding a certificate of seronegativity as a condition of residence. In the face of such apparently comprehensive difficulties, what responses have been made?

Partly because of the initial preoccupation with the risks to gays both in Italy and in the United States, which acted then as the image of all Western European societies' futures, attention to the ivdu transmission route was relatively slow in emerging at national and local levels. The government's first specific initiative on AIDS among drug users was to recommend to all regional authorities in November 1985 the mandatory testing of all ivdus who attended drug treatment centers. Very slow compliance (by the end of 1986 only 26 percent of the approximately 25,000 attenders had in fact been tested) ensured that even among the minority of ivdus who attended clinics, only a small proportion were made aware of their HIV-antibody status. In Lombardy, with one of the highest proportions of ivdus among people with AIDS and the highest absolute number of sufferers, the problem was especially acute. All drug users attending treatment centers were regularly tested from the beginning of 1986; the results suggested that in 1987 there were between 17,500 and 21,000 seropositives in the region. However, the structures to permit adequate surveillance and management of drug users at the local level were not always present. For example, in 1987 some seventeen Local Health Units of the Milan hinterland—where the drug problems were especially intense—had still not created specialized sections to offer medical and psychosocial services to drug users. Likewise the Italian South, where the health services have long been inferior to the North's, accounted for only 17 percent of treatment centers and 16 percent of residential therapeutic communities in Italy. The structures of HIV management are therefore very uneven in Italy. While most local authorities had organized information campaigns, more radical initiatives adopted elsewhere, such as the exchange of syringes or mobile clinics for information and assistance, have not been introduced.

The consequences of the problems as just described ought to be disastrous and without remedy. But, surprisingly, the fragmentary evidence available by late 1988 gives slight but necessarily uncertain cause for optimism, based on small-scale studies of trends in HIV positivity and in other diseases associated with the same risky behaviors that facilitate HIV infection. First, analyses of seropositive rates suggest that no behavior changes were taking place among ivdus in the period before 1985, that is, before AIDS was widely portrayed as a serious risk for that population. From 1986, however, a fall in seropositivity rates among both recent and long-standing ivdus in an early-affected region has been observed. Second, a sharp decline in the incidence of viral hepatitis in Lombardy, especially in 1985–1986, and in smaller northern cities over the same period has been suggested as evidence of behavioral change following educational campaigns. A third possible indicator may be found in the decline in the numbers of births to HIV-positive women in 1987, again arguably a response to the reception of information about the risks of pregnancy to both mother and child.[69] It seems likely that at least in the North changes in both needle-sharing and sexual activities are taking place, which jointly must lead to a long-term decline in HIV transmission.[70] A study in Padua, for example, found that after an intensive local campaign beginning in 1986 the proportion of ivdus who shared needles had fallen from 64 percent to 20 percent and users of condoms had increased from 6 percent to 22 percent.[71] One reason for these changes may lie in an increasing "normalization" of (mostly the inveterate) users: the majority of attenders at treatment centers are employed, either full or part-time, and most are living at home, that is, in environments reachable through ordinary channels of education and no longer dominated by a simple countercultural attraction to drug addiction.[72] At present, however, little more can be said than to note the presently scarce data and to add that any reduction in the vulnerability of the ivdu category is being achieved in the absence of an extensive national campaign or of innovative methods for dealing with the most intractable transmission route for HIV.

CONCLUSION

Seven years have passed since the first AIDS diagnosis in Italy without clarifying the local future of the epidemic. In their responses the national and regional governments have refused all drastic forms of intervention through innovations or more rigorous applications of existing public health law. No attempt to vary the general legal definition of criminal responsibility in order to control the behavior of seropositives or AIDS sufferers has been made; and the existence or extent of liability for transmitting the virus is assessed in the ordinary courts. In the most significant such case a doctor and a manufacturer of defective medical equipment were brought to court in Turin for their responsibilities in the accidental infection of a nurse in 1987. In March 1989 both were convicted and sentenced to six months in prison: the victim was awarded interim compensation of $101,450 while awaiting the decision on her claim for the full sum of about $500,000.[73] The severity of the sentence—and the clear indication of the personal responsibility of senior doctors to ensure absolute conformity with infection-control guidelines—did not elicit immediate responses from professional medical associations. Their public role has continued to be a limited one in the debates on AIDS policy, and they have not developed an independent or critical line on issues such as testing or risk reduction for medical staff.

In some respects the dominance of ivdus makes the Italian case an anticipation of what is described as the second manifestation of the disease in countries such as the United States where gays have hitherto been the largest category of victims but are now steadily reducing their future vulnerability. Some figures suggest, too, that Italy is producing its own version of a trend visible in the United States toward a concentration of infection among poorer social groups. For an increasing number of new AIDS cases are located in the South, where income, employment rates, and the provision of welfare services have been consistently (and perhaps recently increasingly) inferior to those in the North. In 1985, 22.6 percent of newly diagnosed cases were from Rome and the regions to its south; in 1988 the figure was 30.4 percent. Over the same period the proportion of the total number of cases in the South increased from 22.5 percent to 26.7 percent.[74] Moreover, local studies have found a seropositivity rate in southern towns at least equal to the North, particularly among ivdus.[75] If those figures for progression to AIDS accurately indicate a continuing trend, then the presence of AIDS will constitute merely the health dimension of the long-standing "Southern Question" and become as endemic as the previously epidemic cholera bacterium.

It will also call for far more active responses, since the South is precisely the area where services for infectious diseases are generally agreed to be less effective and where the limited organizations of gays and their institutional connections, if they exist at all, are less active vehicles for education and local pressure than in the North. The same consideration, of course, applies, only more strongly, to ivdus. Because both market and community organization is least effective in the South, the state is likely to have not merely to coordinate regional and local initiatives more attentively but to stimulate responses by active intervention. It will not be the first time or the only dimension of social life in which that kind of remedy has been prescribed for the social problems of the South. But until a cure is found for AIDS itself, it may be necessary to underline its urgency.

NOTES

I would like to acknowledge the help I have received from Drs. V. Carreri, M. Morretta, D. Greco, and E. Rossi, and in particular from Drs. Marcello Innocenti and Hartmut Sasse. None, of course, can be held responsible for the interpretations I have made of the information that they very generously made available.

1. *Weekly Epidemiological Record*, no. 12 (22 March 1985): 86, Table 1; ibid., no. 45 (4 November 1988): 342. By comparison, in December 1984 France had reported ninety-four cases and a rate of 4.8 per million, West Germany forty-two cases and a rate of 2.2 per million.

2. Centro Operativo AIDS (COA) document, as reported in *La Repubblica*, 5 August 1988, p. 7.

3. A specific case in point: two days after the Sondrio flood disaster of July 1987 the outcome of factional deals for the composition of the new government forced the replacement of the long-serving Minister of Civil Protection who was organizing the response by a party colleague with no previous experience in that portfolio.

4. Randy Shilts, *And the Band Played On* (Harmondsworth: Penguin, 1988).

5. The article, "Per soli gay," appeared in the weekly *Panorama*, 11 January 1982. The figures on the early AIDS cases are taken from R. Ferracini, ed., *AIDS* (Turin: Edizioni Gruppo Abele, 1985), p. 30, Table 12.

6. *The Lancet*, 17 September 1988, 697. Figures for the three countries include female children.

7. Centro Operativo AIDS (Istituto Superiore di Sanità), *Aggiornamento dei casi di AIDS conclamato notificati in Italia al 31 ottobre 1988*, Table 7.

8. U. Tirelli et al., "HTLV-III Infection among 315 Intravenous Drug Abusers: Seroepidemiological, Clinical and Pathological Findings," *AIDS Research* 2, no. 4 (1986): 330. Male prostitutes, including transvestites, show significant levels of seropositivity and constitute a further linkage between populations at higher and lower risk. U. Tirelli et al., "HIV–1 Seroprevalence in Male Prostitutes in Northeast Italy," *Journal of Acquired Immunodeficiency Syndromes* 1, no. 4 (1988): 414.

9. See S. Friedman, J. Sotheran, A. Abdul-Quader, B. Primm, D. Des Jarlais, P. Kleinman, C. Maugé, D. Goldsmith, W. El-Sadr, and R. Maslansky, "The AIDS Epidemic among Blacks and Hispanics," *Milbank Quarterly* 65, Suppl. 2 (1987): 455–499.

10. *L'Espresso* 22 November 1987, p. 223; Regione Lombardia, Settore Sanità e Igiene, *Andamento epidemiologico dell'AIDS in Lombardia e relativi confronti con i dati nazionali*, October 1988, p. 2.

11. Commissione Nazionale per la Lotta all'AIDS (CNLA), "VII Documento: Proposte per la Programmazione degli Interventi Sanitari da Effettuare contro le Infezioni da HIV e le Sindromi ad Esse Conseguenti," February 1987, reprinted in Istituto Superiore di Sanità (ISS), *Relazioni: Documenti della Commissione Nazionale per la Lotta all'AIDS dal 9/1/1987 al 14/5/87* (Rome, 1987), p. 173, Table 6. See also M. Moroni, A. Pagano, A. Lazzarin, G. Privitera, and C. L. Parravicini, "Opportunistic Infections in AIDS Patients in Milan," *Antibiotics and Chemotherapy* 38 (1987): 174–179. While the youth of patients may prolong their survival in the absence of a cure, a countervailing factor is the higher mortality rate for opportunistic infection cases than for Kaposi's sarcoma. Moroni et al.'s study further indicates that the opportunistic infections of Italian AIDS patients are more diversified than in the United States, with *P. carinii pneumonia* playing a much less dominant role (p. 176), thus requiring a wider range of medical treatments and expertise.

12. See F. Titti et al., "Human Immunodeficiency Virus (HIV) Seropositivity in Intravenous (IV) Drug Abusers in Three Cities of Italy: Possible Natural History of HIV Infection in IV Drug Addicts in Italy," *Journal of Medical Virology* 23 (1987): 241–248; P. Farci et al., "Introduction of Human Immunodeficiency Virus Infection among Parenteral Drug Abusers in Sardinia: A Seroepidemiological Study," *American Journal of Epidemiology* 127, no. 6 (1988): 1312–1314. Rates of HIV infection could, however, vary markedly between adjacent areas; for the eightfold difference between the adjoining provinces of Udine and Pordenone in Northeast Italy see S.

Franceschi et al., "Increased Prevalence of HTLV-III Antibody among Drug Addicts from Italian Province with US Military Base," *The Lancet*, 5 April 1986, p. 804.

13. G. B. Cherchi, M. S. Mura, M. G. Calia, C. Gakis, R. Ginanneschi, G. M. Zara, A. Flumene, and G. Andreoni, "L'infezione da HIV nella Sardegna Nord-Occidentale," *Bollettino del Istituto sieroterapico milanese* 66, no. 6 (1987): 449. The figures on incidence refer to 31 March 1986.

14. The demand for an interministerial committee to close this institutional gap was made by, *inter alia*, a former Under-Secretary of Health in August 1987. *L'Espresso*, 9 August 1987, p. 19.

15. On World AIDS Day 1988 the Minister of Health was quoted for the first time as favoring the creation of a single center to combat AIDS, incorporating in particular an advertising agency to devise and disseminate programs in harmony with his own health service advisers. *La Repubblica*, 2 December 1988, p. 19.

16. The Ministry of Health has retained the purse-strings, the power to issue emergency decrees applicable to all regions, and the role of coordinator of initiatives in line with a still to be formulated national health plan. For English-language summaries of the 1978 reform, see J. H. Robb, "The Italian Health Services: Slow Revolution or Permanent Crisis?" *Social Science and Medicine* 22, no. 6 (1986): 619– 627; and M. Ferrera, "The Politics of Health Reform: Origins and Performance of the Italian Health Service in Comparative Perspective," in G. Freddi and J. W. Bjorkman, eds., *Controlling Medical Professionals* (London: Sage, 1989).

17. See the comments by the Lombardy region's health department in its manual on AIDS produced in 1987 for health personnel, section 5.4. V. Carreri and C. Porro de' Somenzi, "Piano Regionale degli Interventi per Contrastare e Prevenire l'AIDS in Lombardia—Linee Guida (Anno 1987)."

18. The scale of Italy's internal migration since 1945 has made the population highly mobile, resulting in the easy spread of infection to outlying areas. Travel not only abroad but within Italy increases the risk of infection; a study of ivdus in Northeast Italy indicates that addicts who had traveled out of their region were three times as likely to be infected with HIV as those who had not left it. See S. Franceschi, U. Tirelli, E. Vaccher, D. Serraino, M. Crovatto, P. De Paoli, S. Diodato, C. La Vecchia, A. De Carli, and S. Monfardini, "Risk Factors for HIV Infection in Drug Addicts from the Northeast of Italy," *International Journal of Epidemiology* 17, no. 1 (1988): 162–167. Under these circumstances it is obviously preferable to have consistent policies on prevention, testing, and treatment throughout the country.

19. For a brief summary of the trajectory of the women's movement in Italy, emphasizing the decline since the late 1970s, see E. Eckmann Pisciotta, "Challenging the Establishment: The Case of Abortion," in D. Dahlerup, ed., *The New Women's Movement* (London: Sage, 1986). There were of course other reasons for this disappearance than the pressures exerted by the new health system.

20. ANLAIDS (funded by voluntary contributions) is managed by a twenty-member National Council, dominated by biomedical experts. It offers sixteen annual scholarships for young researchers and organizes press conferences, scientific congresses, and the publication of brochures for specific populations. Also among its tasks is the recruitment of volunteers to assist the infected, but this aspect has remained subordinate in practice.

21. For remarks on the role of ANLAIDS by its president, Francesco De Lorenzo,

see *Panorama*, 14 February 1988, p. 70. The removal of ANLAIDS' vice-president, Ferdinando Aiuti, from the ministerial committee caused some press comment in February 1988; in addition his candidature for the Radical Party in the elections of 1987 cannot have improved his acceptability to the Christian Democrat minister. Whereas the ministerial committee had initially shared three members with the ANLAIDS advisory council, by 1988 this was reduced to one. The tensions have not prevented some collaboration, however (see note 38 below). Indeed, in July 1989 De Lorenzo himself became Minister of Health, quickly restoring Aiuti to his ministerial committee: it is too early to assess the likelihood of changes to AIDS policy.

22. The Church's opposition to the state's educational campaign is summarized in *La Repubblica*, 27 July 1988, p. 6, and *Panorama*, 7 August 1988, pp. 124–127.

23. On occasion therapeutic communities have refused to admit seropositive patients, and the Ministry of Health has requested the USL to intervene to discourage this practice; see the note of 6 July 1985 circulated by the Ministry, "Problemi collegati con presenza movimento anticorpale contro retrovirus HTLV-III," reprinted in the Lombardy region's *Notizie Sanità*, no. 8 (1985): 103.

24. COA was established by ministerial decree on 9 January 1987, but its functions (primarily the surveillance of AIDS and HIV) were not formally defined until a further decree was issued more than one year later on 1 February 1988. AIDS was made a notifiable disease by ministerial decree on 28 November 1986 (to come into operation on 11 February 1987), its details specified by Circular No. 5 of 13 February 1987. The circular is reprinted in ISS, *Relazioni*, pp. 305–317.

25. The controversy was recognized in a ministerial note to all regional health authorities (Health Ministry D.G.S.I.P. Div. II, Nota 400.2/30.35), reprinted in ISS, *Relazioni*, pp. 318–319. On 26 July 1988 the Chamber of Deputies approved a document committing the government to ensuring the confidentiality of people infected by HIV and to preventing discrimination; if acted upon, this resolution would abrogate the reporting of any case by name.

26. Both sets of figures are included without comment in Regione Lombardia, Settore Sanità e Igiene, *L'andamento epidemiologico dell'AIDS*, appendices 2 and 5. The disparity shrinks to only 3 percent if the numbers of cases resident (rather than diagnosed) in the region (859 and 832) are considered.

27. Commissione Nazionale per la Lotta all'AIDS (CNLA), "VIII Documento. Gli screenings per anti-corpi anti-HIV," 9 April 1987, in ISS, *Relazioni*, p. 261.

28. For some comparative European data see T. W. Harding, "AIDS in Prison," *The Lancet*, 28 November 1987, pp. 1260–1263; and A. McMillan, "HIV in Prisons," *British Medical Journal* 297 (8 October 1988): 873–874. For the rate of infection in prisons in Italy I have used V. Carreri, personal communication; G. Stagni, D. Francisci, R. Pegiati, and F. Baldelli, "Prevalence of anti-HTLV III Antibodies in Detainees at the Jail in Perugia," *Bollettino Istituto sieroterapico milanese* 66, no. 6 (1987): 453–455.

29. For a comparison of screening policies toward prisoners in seventeen European countries as of early 1987, see Harding, "AIDS in Prison," pp. 1260–1263.

30. Ministerial Circular No. 28, July 1985. The descriptions of the first hemophiliac and transfusion-associated deaths are in R. Dal Bo Zanon et al., "First Case in Italy of Fatal AIDS in a Hemophiliac," *Acta Haematologica* 75 (1986): 34–37; A. Lazzarin et al., "First Case of Transfusion-Associated AIDS in Italy," *Vox Sang*

52 (1987): 155–156. Interestingly, the prevalence of AIDS and HIV-seropositivity among hemophiliacs is markedly lower in Italy than in the United States, France and West Germany (A. Gringeri et al., "National Survey of HIV Infection in Italian Hemophiliacs: 1983–1987,"*Ricerca Clinica in Laboratorio* 18, no. 4 (1988): 275–280.

31. A. Ferrari-Sacco, "AIDS e trasfusioni di sangue," *Minerva Chirurgica* 40, no. 20 (1985): 1439.

32. CNLA, "VIII Documento," p. 254.

33. *Weekly Epidemiological Review* 42 (14 October 1988): 321, Table 2. The categories excluded in the UK are listed in *The AIDS Letter*, no. 8 (August 1988): 2. The presence of substantial numbers of Africans among Italy's roughly 800,000 clandestine immigrants has not fueled demands for any particular racial surveillance.

34. For the numbers of ivdus tested by 31 December 1986, see F. Tarentini Trojani, "I rapporti sulla sorveglianza dell'AIDS in Italia al 18 gennaio 1987," *Clinica Terapeutica* 121 (15 April 1987): 80. The size of the ivdu community and its relations with the state are examined below.

35. CNLA, "VIII Documento," pp. 281–283. The specific categories examined were blood donors, the general population, hospital patients, pregnant women, military personnel, prisoners, health service personnel, ivdus, the partners of sero-positives, gays, and transfusion and blood-product recipients. The screening of 510 pregnant women in Padua, begun in 1985, revealed seropositives only among ivdu women; the authors of the study estimate the cost of actually identifying each true HIV-positive woman at $340,000, and they support the CNLA's rejection of generalized screening at pregnancy. A. De Rossi et al., *The Lancet*, 26 March 1988, p. 714.

36. *La Repubblica*, 2 December 1988, p. 19. The papers at the 1987 conference, of which only twelve (5 percent) specifically concerned epidemiology, have been published in F. Aiuti, M. Moroni, and F. Pocchiari, eds., *AIDS e Sindromi Correlate* (Bologna: Monduzzi, 1988).

37. For the two forecasts see the interview with F. Aiuti in Ferracini, *AIDS*, p. 126; CNLA, "VII Documento," p. 154.

38. See *L'Espresso*, 22 November 1987, pp. 222–227, as well as an anticipation of other conclusions from the research in *Nature* 328 (30 July 1987): 385–386. I characterize the report as quasi-official since, although promoted by ANLAIDS, it was also authored by staff at the proto-COA in the National Health Institute.

39. Figures released in a press conference by the Minister of Health reported in *La Repubblica*, 5 August 1988, p. 7. A slightly higher figure for 1990 (27,438) was given later that month by a prominent member of the CNLA; see *Epoca*, 4 September 1988, p. 71.

40. ISS, *Relazioni*, p. 205; *La Repubblica*, 2 December 1988, p. 19.

41. See the figures quoted from the National Health Plan, *La Repubblica*, 24 February 1989, p. 7. The same plan acknowledged a need to increase qualified doctors from 891 to 3,400, and nurses from 2,470 to 11,200, between 1988 and 1992 to care for the growing number of persons with AIDS. A total expenditure of 4,500 milliard lire on AIDS-related hospital beds, professional training, and research was called for, along with the acquisition of 3,000 apartments for the terminally ill.

42. In June 1987 a centralized information hotline was activated for the first time

at the COA. In the first three days 1,863 calls were made, falling away to fewer than 100 per day within one year. The largest proportion of calls came from people not at risk (34 percent), while only one call in eight came from gays (9 percent) and ivdus (3 percent); and by far the largest number of calls (29 percent) concerned the modes of transmission of the virus.

43. For the various survey details see *L'Espresso*, 18 January 1987, pp. 30–33; *La Repubblica*, 2 December 1988, p. 19; and *The AIDS Letter*, no. 9 (October/November 1988): 5.

44. *La Repubblica*, 12 March 1988, p. 21. Italy had the highest percentage of respondents (13 percent) who declared that AIDS was a self-inflicted disease but the lowest percentages in favor of isolation for gays (12 percent) or ivdus (17 percent) with AIDS.

45. Some of the clips privately produced by the not-for-profit agency Pubblicità Progresso in 1987 were transmitted by private television channels. The clips made by a gay organization, the Associazione Solidarietà AIDS, were refused by the RAI.

46. "Those who do not have sufficient will power to avoid the risks of sexual relations [with casual partners, prostitutes, or ivdus] should at least try to protect themselves with a condom."

47. D. Altman, "Legitimation Through Disaster," in D. Fox and E. Fee, eds., *AIDS: The Burdens of History* (Berkeley: University of California Press, 1988).

48. Surveys (e.g., *Epoca*, 6 December 1987, p. 90) regularly report a widespread antipathy to gays, with significant proportions of men from all classes, political parties, and professions declaring their hostility to the homosexual world. Even in environments directly linked to the management of AIDS surprising comments can be heard: the rapporteur for a conference on AIDS and blood transfusion in 1985 referred to homosexuality and drug abuse as "these two social plagues." Ferrari-Sacco, "AIDS e trasfusioni di sangue," p. 1438.

49. See Giovanni dall'Orto, "La tolleranza repressiva dell'omosessualità," *Omosessuali e Stato* (Bologna: Quaderni di Critica Omosessuale no. 3, 1987), p. 50.

50. E. Alessi, "Sexually Transmitted Diseases in Italy," *Annali Sclavo*, no. 1–2 (1986): 371, Table III, shows an increase from 5 percent to 23.5 percent among gay clients at the major screening center in Milan between 1983 and 1986; F. Titti et al., "Epidemiology of HIV in a Cohort of Italian Homosexual Men, 1983–1987," Fourth International Congress on AIDS, Stockholm, June 1988, abstract no. 4104, shows a seropositivity increase among gay men in Rome from 10.9 percent in 1983 to 19.8 percent in 1986, followed by a fall to 14.5 percent in 1987; and an analogous decline has been claimed for Bologna since 1985 (*La Repubblica*, 27/28 November 1988, p. 21). The national study referred to in note 38 above found a seropositive rate of 25.5 percent among gays.

51. See, for example, Aiuti (quoted in Ferracini, *AIDS*, p. 126), comparing Italy not only with the United States but also with France, Germany, Denmark, and England; Margaret Owen, "Italy Seeks a Strategy," *AIDS Watch* 3 (1988): 5; and, for the particular region of the Veneto, L. Maiori et al., "Seroepidemiology of HIV Infection in a Group of Homosexuals in the Venetian Region," paper presented at the Fourth International Conference on AIDS, Stockholm, June 1988. Other social factors that have been proposed to explain the allegedly low risks for gays in Italy are, first, a supposedly distinctive preference for a single active or passive identity among gays, which reduces risks for the active, and, second, a general absence of

drug-taking among Italian gays, which eliminates the second source of infection often found among gays elsewhere. Although discussion of those suggestions is out of place here, neither is strongly supported by the (admittedly slim) evidence.

52. See *Italia Gay 1987–8* (Milan: Babilonia Editions, 1988), listing all gay organizations and meeting places. In Rome, for example, only one exclusively gay meeting place or sauna is listed, although—by contast with other European societies—more emphasis is probably placed on open-air contacts in Italy.

53. G. Castello et al., "Relationship Between Immunodeficiency Conditions and AIDS-Associated Retrovirus (ARV) Infection in Homosexual Men and I.V. Drug Abusers in the Campania Region," *Haematologica* 71 (1986): 454. The study also indicated that 16.3 percent of gays in the sample were seropositive.

54. I am very grateful to Marcello Innocenti for providing me with the data from the Centro Malattie Trasmesse Sessualmente of the First Dermatology Clinic of the University of Milan. The sample covers all first-time attenders of the clinic's Centro antivenereo section in November-December 1984 and July-August 1985, consisting of Milan residents and probably biased somewhat toward middle-class gays.

55. There was no significant difference in the average ages of those with (27.7 years) and without (29.2 years) fixed partners.

56. *Piano Regionale di Prevenzione contro l'AIDS tra la Popolazione Omosessuale elaborato dall'ARCI Gay Regionale* (Bologna, November 1987), p. 2.

57. N. Romano et al., "Main Routes of Transmission of Human Immunodeficiency Virus (HIV) Infection in a Family Setting in Palermo, Italy," *American Journal of Epidemiology* 128 (1988) 2: 259. One reason for uncertainty is straightforward ignorance about gay sexual practices, what acts respondents count as "experiences with heterosexuals," what activities "partners" engage in, and so on. Romano's conclusions seem to go against research elsewhere that suggests that the nature of sexual acts is a much more significant variable than the simple number of acts/partners in transmitting the virus.

58. *Omosessuali e Stato*, Appendix p. 69.

59. *Epoca*, 6 December 1987, p. 88.

60. *Piano Regionale*, p. 7.

61. Ferracini, *AIDS*, p. 136; *Vita Italiana* 36, no. 1 (1986): *La Repubblica*, 13 March 1988, p. 21.

62. *World Health Statistics Quarterly* 36, no. 4 (1983): 460; CNLA, "VI Documento. Prevenzione della Transmissione Materno Infantile dell'HIV," in ISS, Relazioni, p. 137. The CNLA figure appears to use an estimate from 1982; more recent calculations have reckoned the numbers of regular heroin users at between 250,000 and 300,000 (according to a survey on behalf of the Higher Judicial Council, reported in *La Repubblica*, 31 January 1989, p. 5).

63. At the time of writing (December 1988) the government, to general approval, had just submitted to Parliament a revised bill abolishing the right to legal possession. It seems certain that the right will indeed be eliminated, much less certain what penalties will be introduced for offenders. Surveys show that a substantial majority of Italians favor prohibition of all drugs; see, for example, the poll published in *Epoca*, 16 April 1989, p. 16, which indicates that 62 percent were in favor of punishing casual users of soft drugs, 71 percent of hard drugs.

64. Eugenio Rossi, *Indagine e riflessioni su aspetti biografici e di trattamento terapeutico relativi ad utenti del Nucleo Operativo Tossicodipendenza dell'USSL*

25 *della Regione Lombardia* (report presented at the seminar "Adolescenza, Droga e Identità," Clusone, 26 November 1988), pp. 1–2.

65. *Annuario Statistico Italiano 1986* (Rome: Istat, 1987), Tables 3.26, 3.27, pp. 116–117.

66. Rossi, *Indagine e riflessioni*, p. 6, 8. The later the age of encounter with drugs, the more rapid the passage to regular use.

67. Study by the Pharmacology Institute of the University of Ancona, summarized in *L'Espresso*, 24 May 1987, pp. 207–208.

68. For summaries of the Dutch case and the role of the so-called Junkies Unions, see E. C. Buning et al., "Preventing AIDS in Drug Addicts in Amsterdam," *The Lancet*, 21 June 1986, p. 1435; for New York and the attempt to create a self-help group under extremely unpromising legal and other conditions, see S. Friedman, D. Des Jarlais, J. Sotheran, J. Garber, H. Cohen, and D. Smith, "AIDS and Self-Organisation among Intravenous Drug Users," *International Journal of the Addictions* 22, no. 3 (1987): 201–219.

69. For the studies containing the basis for optimism, see Aiuti et al., p. 386; De Rossi et al., *The Lancet*, 26 March 1988, p. 279; Regione Lombardia, Settore Sanità e Igiene, *Andamento epidemiologico dell'AIDS*, p. 4, appendix 13; R. Pristerà et al., "Drug Addiction and Fear of AIDS," *The Lancet*, 17 January 1987, p. 160; Italian Multicenter Study, "Epidemiology, Clinical Features, and Diagnostic Factors of Pediatric HIV Infection," *The Lancet*, 5 November 1988, p. 1045.

70. For evidence that a positive HIV test convinces ivdu carriers to limit needle-sharing, use condoms, and restrict their sexual promiscuity, see H. Sasse et al., "Significance of HIV Antibody Testing as a Preventive Measure in Intravenous Drug Users," *AIDS* 2, no. 5 (1988): 402–403. Ivdus who tested antibody-negative or who were not tested at all showed far fewer changes toward safe sex and safe injection practices. A study of the behavior of seropositive ivdus by the Institute of Social Health Research of Salerno indicated that 90 percent of the sample in the northern cities of Verona and Brescia used condoms. *La Repubblica*, 1 December 1988, p. 19.

71. F. Bortolotti et al., "AIDS Information Campaign Has Significantly Reduced Risk Factors for HIV Infection in Italian Drug Abusers," *Journal of Acquired Immune Deficiency Syndromes* 1, no. 4 (1988): 412–413. The study also indicates a fall in seropositivity rates among local ivdus after 1985 and a significant decline in the incidence of acute viral hepatitis.

72. Rossi, *Indagine e riflessioni*, pp. 12, 38. A study in Bologna confirms this pattern of integration among 383 attenders at local drug clinics; P. Faccioli and S. Simoni, "Identità e droga nelle società complesse," *Dei Delitti e delle Pene*, no. 3 (1984): 578. How far this picture can be extended to regular drug abusers who do not attend treatment centers is unknown.

73. See *La Repubblica*, 23 March 1989, p. 18. AIDS has not been included in the list of formally recognized occupational diseases in Italy.

74. Centro Operativo AIDS, *Aggiornamento dei casi*, Table 2. The South includes the regions of Lazio, Campania, Abruzzi, Molise, Puglie, Basilicata, Calabria, Sicilia, and Sardegna.

75. For some recent results: 45 percent in Bari in 1985 (G. Angarano et al., "Rapid Spread of HTLV-III Infection among Drug Addicts in Italy," *The Lancet*, 7 December 1985, p. 1302); 57 percent in Sardinia in 1986 (Farci et al., "Intro-

duction of Human Immunodeficiency Virus," p. 1313); and 64 percent in Palermo in 1986 (F. Vitale et al., "AIDS in Sicily: Prevalence of Antibodies to Human Immunodeficiency Virus (HIV) in Low and High Risk Groups," *European Journal of Epidemiology* 3, no. 3 (1987): 281).

AIDS in Poland: The Fear of Unmasking Intolerance

Compared with Western Europe and the United States, the impact of AIDS in Poland, and in Eastern Europe generally, has so far been much less dramatic. In the first place, the number of reported cases from the region in late 1989 is relatively low, ranging nationally between the fifty-eight cases notified from Yugoslavia in 1988 to the three cases in Bulgaria (see Table 8.1).[1] Second, infection by HIV was first detected in Eastern Europe when knowledge concerning the disease was well advanced. Not only had the specific virus been identified, but the HIV antibody test had already been invented. Theoretically, therefore, Eastern European countries were in the fortunate position of being able to learn from Western experiences. However, since the health structures that determine the efficacy of responses are in many ways inferior to their counterparts in the Western world, taking advantage of the opportunities for second-comers has been very difficult. Moreover, the estimates of present seropositive rates and future progression to AIDS suggest that taking comfort from the present low incidence of actual cases would be to ignore the likelihood of an epidemic of proportions somewhat similar to that in the West only a few years away.

Shortage of even the most basic equipment has already had an impact on the development of the AIDS epidemic throughout the region. In a remote city in the south of the USSR, for example, unsterilized needles caused an outbreak of HIV infection. The discovery that twenty-seven children had been infected with HIV in a hospital in "what might have seemed the most AIDS-immune part of the world—a provincial town in deepest Russia where few foreigners ever set foot—underscores the Soviet Union's health problems."[2] If theirs is a system where the supply of needles and syringes does not meet even 10 percent of national needs, where hot water and main

Table 8.1
East Europe: AIDS Cases Notified 1986–1988

Country	1986	1987	1988
Albania	-	-	-
Bulgaria	-	3	3
Czechoslovakia	5	7	12
German Democratic Republic	-	4	6
Hungary	-	6	15
Poland	1	3	4
Rumania	2	2	9
USSR	-	4	4
Yugoslavia	3	21	58
Totals	11	50	111

Note: Cases notified at different times in each year.

Sources: WHO, Weekly Epidemiological Record 47 (21 November 1986): 362, Table 2; WHO, Weekly Epidemiological Record 3 (15 January 1988): 14; WHO, Weekly Epidemiological Record 1 (6 January 1989): 2.

drainage are not connected to even half the country's medical establishments, their ability to manage the estimated 15 million seropositive cases by the year 2000 is in serious doubt.[3]

The effect of the underdeveloped medical infrastructures of Eastern European countries is exacerbated by the low health status of their respective national populations. Again, in the Soviet Union, mortality in some parts of the country stands at more than 30 in 1,000 births; in other countries life expectancy has recently been falling—in Hungary, for example, average male life expectancy has declined from 67 to 63 over the last eight years.[4] This state of affairs is further eroded by the low morale of medical and paramedical staff: "There is the injustice; not just the formal injustice of separate, better-supplied hospitals for the Nomenklatura [the party privileged] and the police, but the informal injustice of corruption and graft, when in practice you have to pay illicitly (preferably in hard currency) for the surgeon to perform an operation, for the nurses to look after you in hospital."[5]

Many of these problems have already been brought to public attention by the mass media. Although the Eastern European media are controlled by the state, their role has recently been changing. Today they are increasingly the forums for discussion of previously unacknowledged problems, although, unlike the Western mass media, there is still a taboo on discussion of sexuality. While low-key rational reporting based on the opinions of medical researchers avoids the hysteria and sensation frequently found in the Western press and thus minimizes prejudice and discrimination against AIDS victims, the low degree of trust in the content of the official media and the absence of a widely circulating alternative press make the results of any educational effort unpredictable.

What makes the context for responses to AIDS in Eastern European countries interesting is that most are in the process of liberalization. Political life is being democratized, and features of market economies are being adopted, albeit at varying speeds and to different degrees. Observations on the hitherto rigid constraints determining the responses to HIV infection are likely to be rapidly overtaken by events, making generalization on the basis of a single case such as Poland especially hazardous. In any case, political, legal, and cultural differences between Eastern European countries signify very varied conditions for intervention. The legal status and public acceptance of homosexuality varies widely. Hungary—alone in the region— allows the open organization of the gay community. In East Germany gays have obtained a measure of toleration and some meeting places, thanks to support from the Protestant Church. In Poland, although homosexual activity is not a criminal offense, participants have had to lead a largely underground existence. In the Soviet Union, however, gay activities can lead to prison sentences of up to eight years.[6]

Another set of contrasts concerns the conditions of testing and the consequences of diagnosis as seropositive, where the differences between countries largely reproduce the degrees of liberal treatment of homosexuality. Eastern European societies have been consistently ready to impose mandatory testing on a wide set of specific populations. In Bulgaria the entire population aged 16–65 is being tested,[7] while in the Soviet Union testing is compulsory for all foreigners who stay for more than three months, Soviet citizens returning after more than twenty-eight days abroad, and members of high-risk groups.[8] Hungary shows a still wider catchment area: people suffering or suspected of suffering from sexually transmitted diseases, sexual partners of AIDS patients, prostitutes, prisoners, juvenile delinquents, and drug users.[9] Czechoslovakia has instituted mandatory HIV tests for anyone with a record of venereal disease: those who test positive must sign a statement agreeing to limit their circle of sexual partners and use condoms in all sexual encounters. Where voluntary testing has been made available, it is not anonymous except in Hungary and East Germany. In most countries of East Europe serious consequences follow for seropositives who infect their partners. In the Soviet Union, for example, anyone who tests positive and then infects another can expect to receive a five-to-eight-year prison sentence;[10] in late 1988, for example, a court in the southern Ukrainian town of Kakhovka sentenced a woman to four years' imprisonment for knowingly infecting her sexual partners. As a result of mass tests hundreds of foreign students are reported as having been expelled from the country.[11] Punitive jail sentences have also been imposed elsewhere: in October 1988, a Prague court sentenced a homosexual to three years in jail for having several sexual partners while aware that he was suffering from AIDS. These brief and selective examples show that in Eastern European societies there have been no common response to the disease, despite the fact that its countries share the Pattern 3 transmission route for infection (see Table 8.2).

This chapter examines the situation in Poland. Poland has experienced the most severe economic crisis in Eastern Europe, yet its economic and political liberalization is relatively advanced. While the country's economic conditions have been the most significant factor limiting state responses to the problems posed by the new disease, other factors initially made any cooperation between the state and society problematic. Despair in civil society has been generated by the impossibility of influencing the political process, and the loss of legitimacy suffered by the government has inhibited any capacity for centralized direction of responses. However, very recent developments such as the legalization of Solidarity and the general mood of "national reconciliation," combined with actions such as registration by the Polish authorities of an independent health fund set up by Solidarity to administer a U.S. $1 million grant from the United States government, provide some encouragement for future policies. Despite those changes, however, the health authorities will continue at best to muddle through many problems, among which AIDS is likely to play an increasingly significant role. But for the first time, the state bureaucracy is not alone on the stage. Social movements involving gays and drug addicts are also becoming important supporting players.

MANIFESTATIONS OF THE DISEASE

At first, AIDS was treated as merely interesting news from the United States. Being so distant, it posed no threat to any Pole. Gradually, with more alarming information reaching Poland from abroad, AIDS attracted the attention of a small group of scientists who began to try to establish the hitherto invisible rate of HIV infection in the country. Between June 1985 and March 1986, the first test found 14 out of 8,262 samples to be HIV-positive. These included 4 homosexuals (2 percent of the 199 tested), 6 hemophiliacs (1.5 percent of 482), 3 prostitutes (0.3 percent of 1,000),

Table 8.2
East Europe: AIDS Cases by Transmission Category 1987–1988

Country	Homosexual/ Bisexual		Intravenous Drug User		Homosexual IVdu		Hemophilia/ Coagulation disorder		Transfusion		Heterosexual		Other		Total	
	1987	1988	1987	1988	1987	1988	1987	1988	1987	1988	1987	1988	1987	1988	1987	1988
Albania	-	-	-	-	-	-	-	-	-	-	-	-	-	-	-	-
Bulgaria	-	-	-	-	-	-	-	-	-	-	-	-	1	3	1	3
Czechoslovakia	6	10	-	-	-	-	-	-	-	-	-	-	2	1	8	11
German Democratic Republic	2	2	-	-	-	-	2	2	-	-	-	-	2	2	6	6
Hungary	5	9	-	-	-	-	-	-	2	3	1	1	-	-	8	13
Poland	2	2	-	-	-	-	-	-	-	-	1	1	-	-	3	3
Rumania	1	1	-	-	-	-	-	-	-	-	2	7	-	-	3	8
USSR	-	1	-	-	-	-	-	-	-	-	-	-	3	3	3	4
Yugoslavia	10	13	7	13	1	-	3	6	-	1	2	3	2	4	25	40
TOTAL	26	38	7	13	1	-	5	8	2	4	6	12	10	13	57	88

Note: Cases notified at different times each year.

Sources: 1987: WHO, *Weekly Epidemiological Record* 15 (8 April 1988): 107, Table 2; 1988: WHO, *Weekly Epidemiological Record* 42 (14 October 1988): 321, Table 2.

and 1 baby. A later survey in August 1986 revealed that 15 out of 30,000 individuals (0.05 percent), including many from high-risk groups, were HIV-positive.[12] Shortly after that survey the first victim died in October 1986, followed by two others in early 1987. All three men had lived some years abroad. Two were infected in the United States and returned home only to die. The third was infected in West Germany. By December 1988 Poland had reported a total of five AIDS cases to WHO. All had already died.

The slow but inexorable spread of infection through existing and new transmission routes has been progressively recorded. By November 1986, nineteen seropositive cases had been notified, comprising eight homosexuals, nine hemophiliacs, and two prostitutes, the total increasing by March 1987 to twenty-four and by the end of the year to fifty-eight. Mass testing of 1.7 million people in mid–1988 revealed that eighty-eight were HIV-positive: about 60 percent of these were homosexual or bisexual men, 10 percent foreigners, 12 percent hemophiliacs, 5 percent prostitutes, several persons infected through blood transfusions, and—for the first time—four drug users.[13] Although no drug users are reported to have developed AIDS, the number infected stood at twenty-two at the end of 1988.[14] All infected hemophiliacs received blood products from overseas. Although all early victims of AIDS had traveled abroad or had significant contacts with foreigners, the most recent pattern of infection points to domestic routes of transmission. At a rough estimate, there are approximately 25,000 seropositive cases out of a total population of 37.5 million.

OFFICIAL RESPONSES TO THE AIDS PROBLEM

Until the mid-1980s medical experts interested in AIDS saw no immediate need for a widespread campaign aimed at the general public, believing that the risk of the disease spreading was low and that the country had time to prepare itself. In an address to the Polish Parliament in October 1985, Mikolaj Kozakiewicz, a Member of Parliament, sociologist, and chairman of the Association for Family Development, demanded a more active response. As a result, in 1985 the Minister of Health and Social Welfare appointed an AIDS Council of forty-five members, consisting of eight subcommittees staffed mainly by medical experts, journalists, and lawyers. The council was charged with the responsibility for instituting an education campaign and prevention programs and for mobilizing the health system against the disease.

In 1988 the AIDS Council prepared a battle plan for the period 1988–1990. Under its guidelines, AIDS was added as item 46 to the list of communicable diseases in October 1988, and, as item 10, to the list of diseases where victims are subject to compulsory treatment at an outpatient care establishment. According to these regulations, persons diagnosed as HIV-positive are required to take special measures for prevention and treatment of the disease and to provide information about their sexual contacts. Doctors are required to notify the central medical authorities of any suspected cases. The medical test for detection of infection is not anonymous but is voluntary; only foreign students are compulsorily tested. In addition, a new provision was added to Article 160 of the Criminal Code, stating that anyone who tests positive and then infects another is liable to three years' imprisonment.[15]

Since those regulations represent a significant intrusion into the private lives of AIDS sufferers, they caused considerable controversy at a conference devoted to legal aspects of AIDS in June 1988. As a result, they are presently being reanalyzed by the Legal Commission of the AIDS Council.[16]

According to the official assessment, Poland is "one of seven countries that have already planned action against AIDS to the year 2000."[17] The plan itself reflects a central feature of the Polish government's response: utilization of the established health bureaucracy rather than the creation of new structures. Prevention and treatment of the disease are centered around existing health institutions (hospitals, clinics) no new testing centers have been inaugurated; and programs are centrally organized and there are no local AIDS committees. Diagnosis and treatment have been allocated to venereologists and dermatologists, for two reasons. First, a network of outpatient care centers already exists; and, second, since prostitutes and homosexuals frequently use these establishments, doctors have experience in exercising discretion and are able to make contact and gain their confidence easily. Training programs for doctors have been introduced into medical school curricula and courses made available for those already in practice (an official agreement between Poland and Sweden makes it possible for some Polish doctors to undertake this training in Sweden).

Public education too is recognized as an important aspect of the AIDS prevention campaign. In this regard, the AIDS Council approach, according to the *New Scientist*, "is exemplary by East European standards."[18] Up to 40 million copies of various information-carrying publications have been printed, and 10 million leaflets explaining what AIDS is and how the spread of the virus can be prevented were produced for distribution to every home in Poland.

Systematic testing of donated blood for HIV infection did not begin until October 1987. Until recently, the test kits had to be imported, which meant that valuable hard currency was being used in their purchase. While the kits are now being manufactured under license following an agreement with the American firm Abbot, "it has taken Poland more than a year to catch up with Bulgaria, Hungary and Czechoslovakia in providing enough tests."[19]

The official acknowledgment of AIDS as a social problem was largely the result of the growing flow of international information. This enabled the AIDS Council to formulate a program incorporating the experiences of other countries as well as the World Health Organization's suggestions for the

Polish case. Its features and implementation, however, were deeply influenced by Poland's economic difficulties and by the competition posed by the growing number of vastly more significant social problems. A particular account of "the AIDS problem" was developed, designed to present the disease in a nondramatic, nonhysterical way and as a comparatively unimportant issue. But the progressive revelations of the spread of infection and the publicizing efforts of grass-roots movements together ensured that the official perspective did not come to dominate public discourse as completely as its authors had hoped.

ACTIONS ON AIDS: THE REALITY

Lack of Funding

Without doubt the single most important factor undermining efforts against the spread of AIDS has been the lack of resources. Evidence of Poland's economic crisis is everywhere. The standard of living is falling dramatically; services of all kinds are increasingly inadequate; industrial pollution of the environment is among the highest in the world; successive attempts at reform have faltered because of the government's loss of legitimacy; government actions are paralyzed by the enormous foreign debt; and the absence of economic and political decentralization eliminates the opportunities for compensatory initiatives at local levels. Those constraints ensure that nonproductive sectors such as education, health care, culture, and welfare are chronically under-resourced. The competition for the limited resources available, especially in the form of hard currency, is intense.

In 1988 the AIDS Council operated on a combined budget of 400 million zloty and U.S. $7 million. For 1989 a total of U.S. $9 million was promised for use in testing, information campaigns, and training programs. According to official statements by General Jerzy Bonczak, the Deputy Minister for Health and Social Welfare who then commanded the AIDS Council, this sum would suffice; but other members of the council disagreed, insisting that it would leave no funds for the acquisition of essential medical and scientific literature from the West, let alone permit support for essential social or medical research. Moreover, the centralized bureaucratic response to AIDS makes it practically impossible to estimate actual allocations and expenditures. Judging by the AIDS Council members' comments, this fund seems to resemble the Loch Ness monster: everybody talks about it, but nobody has seen it. In reality, spending has been offset against the regular operating budgets of various health institutions involved in the battle against AIDS, thereby stretching financial resources more thinly across a service which is already one of the most devastated areas of Polish society. It took four years of bureaucratic battles to set up the first AIDS ward in a Warsaw hospital in early 1989. However, in protest against the appalling conditions of the ward, all four doctors employed there resigned within a few months. In their joint statement of resignation denouncing the government's lack of action on AIDS, they described the conditions in the AIDS ward: blood was tested in the corridors, the patients did not have their own toilet or bathroom and there was no hot water. Prompted by the doctors' report, in August 1989 Solidarity staff in the hospital demanded that the Minister of Health dissolve the AIDS Council and establish a Parliamentary Commission of Inquiry to scrutinize its operations and expenditures.[20]

The Status of the Health Sector

Since the health system is part of the social, political and economic system, many of its problems and inefficiencies are derived from its broader context. Generally speaking, the Polish health service is scarcely in any shape to confront the AIDS epidemic adequately. It suffers from "grave systematic pathologies which are reflected in petrified, rigid structures, continuous underfinancing and underinvestment, and a lack of adequate investment."[21]

Expenditure for health and social welfare in the national budget decreased from 4.3 percent in 1970 to 3.7 percent in 1978. Despite recent increases (by 1987, spending had increased to 5.3 percent of GDP), Poland has one of the lowest levels of expenditure on health in Eastern Europe. Consequently, hospitals and hospital beds are in short supply, and the hospitals themselves are poorly equipped. In Warsaw alone, for example, there is a shortfall of 5,000 beds, and in some cities such as Gdansk, the ratio of general hospital beds to population has declined to the level in 1945.[22]

Furthermore, because medical facilities are inadequate for the needs of the population, infectious diseases contribute substantially to morbidity and mortality rates, which are disproportionately high for an urbanized country.[23] The incidence of viral infections is alarming. Rubella is widespread because of insufficient hard currency to purchase vaccine. The incidence of hepatitis-B is the highest in Europe, mostly as a result of unhygienic conditions in hospitals, and viral hepatitis appears more frequently than in other European countries, with health workers themselves representing 13 percent of all acute cases.[24] Among twenty-seven European countries, Poland recorded the highest incidence of tuberculosis, and there are frequent epidemics of poisoning due to salmonella.

Since even basic needs are barely met, there is vigorous competition for scarce resources. For example, hospitals can obtain only 40 percent of their requirements for disposable syringes, needles, and rubber gloves, and there are insufficient gloves even for analytical laboratories. An immunologist from the AIDS Council commented, "In my laboratory, people do not have gloves, nor do all dentists. . . . In most outpatient clinics they have signs saying: "Patients wanting to use disposable syringes must bring their own."[25]

Given the inadequate supply of the most basic instruments and protective devices and the shortage of nurses and medical doctors willing to treat AIDS patients, nonsexual transmission of the HIV virus is a serious threat for health workers—something of which they are well aware and for which they want to be financially compensated. Taking a different kind of advantage of this opportunity, many medical experts are exploiting "the AIDS fashion" in an attempt to convince the government that health services need to be improved,[26] hoping thereby to compete more effectively with the spokespersons for other social problems for both public attention and funding.

The state of family planning highlights another inefficiency of the health system, suggesting that the virus might well enjoy considerable freedom of movement among the population not in contact with health institutions. This service is underdeveloped and underfunded, notably for the provision of contraceptives, where demand has always exceeded supply. While the AIDS leaflet distributed to Polish homes recommends the use of condoms, the domestic industry produces only 15 to 20 million annually for a population of 37.5 million, and the volume of imports has recently been reduced.[27] Furthermore, the quality of those that are available leaves much to be desired. Most youths are sexually active before reaching 18 years of age, yet are ignorant about methods of birth control and safe sex, and generally do not accept condoms.[28] The inadequacy of advice and provision is further aggravated by the negative stance of the Catholic Church toward all forms of contraception and public discussion. That attitude may, however, now be softening to some extent: an anonymous priest was recently reported as saying that "on ethical grounds it is now hard to condemn the use of contraceptives if they are helping to save lives."[29] Nonetheless, without the active support of the Church hierarchy in a country where at least half of the population attends church weekly, such individual voices are unlikely to be heard.

Risk Groups

One factor reducing the effectiveness of the struggle to control AIDS is the long-standing failure to recognize openly controversial issues or real social problems because their existence contradicts the official vision of a socialist society which is supposed to be free of such problems. This attitude has made prevention difficult. Although the emergence of Solidarity from the beginning of the 1980s has improved the situation somewhat by allowing debate on unacknowledged social problems to be brought out into the open, the lack of experience in how to deal with them handicaps efforts at public presentation and pragmatic management. Members of the three currently most significant risk groups—homosexuals, intravenous drug users, and prostitutes—are in any case unable to identify themselves as part of distinct communities due to a characteristic mix of legal prohibitions and deep social disapproval. In contrast with Western societies, in which those groups have at least some direct or indirect organized representation, their social invisibility in Poland, and generally in Eastern Europe, makes any attempt to target them directly especially difficult.

Homosexuals are the major group at risk from AIDS since they constitute 60 percent of all diagnosed seropositives. The results of a recent opinion survey show that Poles generally perceive them as abnormal, even criminal, and deny that gays have a right fully to participate in social life.[30] Among respondents, 65.2 percent stated that Polish society has hostile attitudes toward homosexuals, and 45.6 percent declared that the state should take steps actively to combat the practice. These traditionally rigid attitudes owe much to long-standing Catholic prescriptions for sexual activity. As a result, homosexuals are forced to mask their preferences or isolate themselves silently from the rest of society.

Coupled with Catholic intolerance has been the puritanism of the Communist Party. Although the establishment of a gay club was one product of the 1917 Revolution in Petersburg, the rapid and rigid closure of political and cultural experimentation forced the redefinition of homosexuality as an example of bourgeois decadence. While in Poland, unlike the Soviet Union, homosexual acts were not made criminal offenses, the level of police harassment of known or suspected gays has always been high.

The difference between East and West in this respect is very considerable. In many Western countries today gays enjoy a measure of protection against overt discrimination; such a development is still unheard of in Poland. Altman argues correctly that to speak of homosexuality is to use

a concept that ceases to have much meaning outside the affluent developed countries of the First World (North America, Western Europe, Australasia, and perhaps Japan) and that seems dependent on a certain level of both economic development and political liberalism to flourish. It must be galling for those fundamentalist defenders of "the American way" to reflect that it is only their "way" that allows for the creation of a homosexual minority, and that the so-called socialist states of Eastern Europe are much more successfully repressive of public homosexuality than are those of the "free world." Cities like Warsaw and Budapest have homosexual worlds rather akin to those of North America in the fifties.[31]

It appears, nevertheless, that the situation as described by Altman only a few years ago is showing some signs of change. AIDS has been a catalyst, leading not only to the formulation of a case for legal rights by members of this minority and to their increasing mobilization but also helping to shape a new gay consciousness. The development of an active gay solidarity was the result both of a common threat to life and of the reaction to the government's prevention campaign—a response that was perceived by Polish gays as providing a further weapon against them. Public reporting has

consistently linked AIDS exclusively to homosexuals, offering powerful support for existing intolerance. Police have used the disease as an excuse to
raid homosexuals' homes and interrogate them and their friends. "In small
towns," says a homosexual, "we are sometimes more afraid of police than
AIDS. In this way we differentiate between the real danger and the potential
one."[32] Anticipating both discrimination and the growing need to establish
support structures for the HIV-infected, homosexuals have attempted to
establish associations that are legally recognized by the state and thus achieve
a public voice. However, the Warsaw Homosexual Movement, set up in
late 1987, has so far been refused registration by the authorities and has
therefore been allowed only a semi-clandestine existence. The refusal reflects
the view of the general public: only 24 percent of 1,493 people polled in a
1988 survey agreed that the government should allow these organizations
to be registered. For homosexuals themselves, however, the battle for registration is tantamount to a fight for the right to public recognition as a
distinct social category. In its absence, the interests of homosexuals, insofar
as they are recognized at all, have to be incorporated in existing structures.
In contributing to responses to AIDS, their opportunities to be heard are
largely confined to participation in the work of the special AIDS section
established in the Association for Family Development.[33] That work consists
primarily of grass-roots pragmatic interventions such as the distribution of
educational leaflets. The chairman of the association, Kozakiewicz, has
nevertheless sent a memorandum to the state authorities signed by thirteen
prominent people in science, art, and medicine, calling for recognition of
the rights of association for homosexuals and arguing that such organizations could play an important mediatory role between gays and the state
health authorities in preventing the spread of AIDS.

Perhaps the most significant support for gays in Poland has come from
their contacts outside the country. Among thousands of Poles who left the
country after 1980 were a large number of homosexuals, mostly well-ed-
ucated young people. Using the informational resources and the self-confidence gained from living abroad, they have been trying to help raise the
consciousness of their friends who remain in Poland: the first article on gay
issues to appear in a Polish newspaper, for example, was written by a Pole
living in Vienna. Gays from Hamburg, The Hague, West Berlin, and elsewhere send gay publications carrying the general message that they need to
fight for their legal rights and make the discrimination they suffer known
to the public.

The still overwhelmingly hostile environment has obvious consequences
for prevention. Although gays constitute the major risk group and are a
target of the AIDS screening program, few homosexuals come forward to
be tested. According to many gay men, the interview that precedes the test
resembles an interrogation, which, when combined with the prevailing social
climate, the lack of counseling before or after the test, and the refusal of

anonymity to testees, makes a substantial contribution to the failure of the screening program. Moreover, those who test positive cannot expect much help, since no organization provides nonmedical forms of assistance such as counseling, housing, and services, nor is there any defense against discrimination and the abrogation of their ordinary rights. On the contrary, they are required to list their sexual contacts and sign a statement saying that they will stop having sex.

As has been observed for other societies, the impact on the gay community in Poland has provoked a wide variety of immediate threats to basing their identity publicly on sexual preference. But, as some of the category's representatives have also observed, the appearance of HIV has simultaneously had the consequence at least of forcing the issue of sexual identity into the public domain for the first time.

The second high-risk group consists of drug users, estimated to number up to 100,000 regular users and up to 700,000 casual users, mostly young, unemployed men who live in large cities.[34] Fortunately, thanks to the dominant practices of drug consumption in Poland, drugs do not pose as great a threat in the spread of AIDS as they do in the West. Heroin is simply too expensive and syringes are not easily available, so the possibility of contamination through sharing needles is more limited. Most drugs are illegally cultivated and manufactured inside Poland. The majority of drug addicts drink the juice domestically manufactured from poppies, use opium-based derivatives, inhale volatile substances, or produce synthetic or semisynthetic drugs from legally available chemicals. It is estimated that around 100,000 people regularly sniff or take drugs orally.[35] The 26,000 drug users who do inject their drugs, however, face a higher risk than their Western counterparts because they are forced to reuse and share probably contaminated equipment. In 1988 the drug consultation centers warned that they expected 20 percent of injecting drug-users to be HIV-positive and that unless immediate measures were taken, 70 percent of the drug-using population were at risk of contracting the virus.[36]

After the official mass media began reporting this new social problem in the early 1980s, state agencies, parastate agencies (the Society for the Prevention of Drug Abuse), social organizations (MONAR, the Youth Movement Against Drug Addiction) and Church groups have combined to combat drug abuse. Even given some initially positive results (since 1985, for example, the number of hospitalized cases has declined) and despite the barriers mentioned above, AIDS may become a serious threat for the drug community. Realization of this possibility has promoted new social initiatives, among which the actions initiated by MONAR—collecting money to make HIV testing available in Poland, organizing counseling services—have been the most visible. The major achievement, however, is a needle exchange scheme, set up by the Ministry of Health and Social Welfare in close collaboration with eighteen drug consultation centers. This scheme, launched on 15 March 1989, is the first Eastern European project to provide clean needles in exchange for used ones without requiring any registration. The MONAR drug consultation center in Warsaw, where the experiment was initiated, has already attracted about 1,000 drug users.

The third major risk group comprises prostitutes. Although prostitution is not illegal, the women practicing this profession—about 16,000 in 1982— are under police control and are regularly examined by health workers.[37] But the economic and social crisis has also made it an attractive option for nonprofessionals. Young boys and girls work as prostitutes during their vacations but make themselves available only to foreigners in order to obtain highly valued foreign currency. Unlike the professionals, this group evades police control and avoids contact with the health service, and is therefore held to represent a significant problem in controlling the spread of AIDS into the general population.[38]

Only the fourth high-risk group has received systematic care and help: the hemophiliacs. Studies of HIV infection among Polish hemophiliacs show them at lower risk than their Western counterparts, largely because their treatment with imported blood products has been less intensive.[39] As patients are generally very attentive to their health, they have considerable medical knowledge and have dealt with the threat of infection by early testing for antibodies. In any case, from October 1987 onwards, all blood and blood products available through the health system have been guaranteed as safe.

The Role of Mass Media and Education

Before AIDS reached Poland, it was presented in the Polish mass media as a Western disease, the price paid by the West for its affluence and promiscuity. After the first national cases were registered, however, emphasis was placed on the fact that HIV is one of the least contagious viral infections, and that there was therefore a need to avoid hysteria. Nevertheless, the Polish media, "the most unfettered in East Europe," have been accused by members of the AIDS Council of having been "guilty of shocking sensationalism."[40] Such impressions were an unintended consequence of the combined reporting of two facts: the emergence of AIDS in Poland, and the shortage of means of protection. The message was strong enough to trigger actions on the part of the government and social groups. Without press involvement, Poland would have waited much longer for state reactions and social initiatives. Although not always scientifically reliable, the mass media campaign has had an important impact on the organization of the battle against AIDS.

Rather less successful have been the media education campaigns to inform the general public about prevention against HIV infection. According to members of the AIDS Council, for example, the education campaign of late 1987, directing general information about the disease to a mass audience through a leaflet distributed to their homes, was a failure. Several factors were regarded as having contributed to the lack of success. First, the leaflet intended to spread the message around the country did not in fact reach every household. It was evidently easier to publish than to distribute. Second, its contents were insufficiently clear. It did not provide simple, straightforward answers to uncertainties about the transmission of HIV. In the determination to avoid a hysterical approach, the leaflet suggests at one point that "AIDS does not come by itself. You need to try to get it. You can avoid the infection." Presentation of the disease as avoidable through the exercise of self-control and individual responsibility contradicted earlier public statements about its contagiousness. The leaflet's credibility was further undermined by the incorrect claim that all health care institutions used only disposable syringes. Third, the general public was simply not prepared to discuss the issue of sexuality. As mentioned earlier, the attitudes of Poles toward sex have been influenced by a dominant Catholic culture and by the puritanism of the Communist Party to the extent that, in 1987, public opposition forced educational authorities to remove from schools a book which for the first time directly addressed the topic of sexuality. Until recently, discussion of sexual matters had been entirely absent from official publications. The message contained in the AIDS leaflet about safe sex confused people and made many of them angry. Their response was unexpected. In numerous telephone calls, newspaper articles, and letters to the AIDS Council, self-described "honest" citizens protested at being the recipients of this "dirty" pamphlet and complained of its language—asserting, for example, that they had "wives," not "partners." In sum, because the public lacked the motivation to absorb information, perceived the risk of the spread of AIDS to be low, and were generally loathe to discuss the issue, the educational effort was not particularly successful.

The recent thrust of media reporting has been to emphasize the need for tolerance and to attempt to convince the public both that the danger is avoidable and that Polish society, at least in this dimension, should conform to what are seen as "civilized standards." The press is now leading the campaign against homophobia in particular and deploring the social isolation that AIDS victims suffer. Indeed, gays are for the first time a topic of public discussion, and the mass media are playing an important role both in trying to change people's attitudes and in preventing the mass hysteria they say is characteristic of the West. De-dramatization of the disease, coupled with the relatively low rate of infection, has moderated attitudes toward AIDS, especially among health workers, and has encouraged at least a superficial attitude of indifference.

Social Reactions

Indifference has not always marked social attitudes to the disease, however. A survey carried out at the end of 1987 asking respondents to state the greatest threats facing the contemporary world revealed that, of the thirteen current problems indicated, Polish teenagers regarded AIDS as the most significant.[41] Such attitudes, however, do not necessarily translate into behavioral changes to restrict the spread of infection or produce rational attitudes toward victims of the disease. In fact, there is little public sympathy for AIDS sufferers. The level of intolerance, prejudice, and discrimination directed against them suggests a frustrated and intolerant society. Raised on the myth of generalized tolerance and the supremacy of their culture— an image that, reinforced by the election of a Polish pope, has been a very important factor in their survival in times of deep economic crisis—it is difficult for Poles to admit to the unmasking of their intolerance. The effect of news items about how a 14-year-old seropositive hemophiliac was forced to leave her school, about the total isolation of an AIDS victim in his village, and the cruel and hostile treatment of AIDS sufferers in hospitals has been to force Poles to reexamine their preferred self-image.

Information about HIV carriers and AIDS patients percolates through institutions without any respect for issues of personal confidentiality and privacy. An interesting illustration can be seen in Szczecin in early 1988 when a local newspaper carried the information that four foreign students at the local polytechnic were HIV-positive. The director of the dormitory where they were living immediately asked her superiors for their names, which, after initial hesitation, she was (illegally) given. The reaction of the university rector was even more puzzling: he ordered that every student, Polish and foreign, take the HIV test on pain of dismissal. Unfortunately there were no medical facilities through which his order could be implemented. The decision flew in the face of the reality of the lack of medical resources, illustrating the purely rhetorical "solution" to many social problems. New administrative rules are promulgated with the sole intention of convincing the general public that authorities are actually doing everything they can.[42]

Yet preserving all sources of motivation is vital for a society that feels unable to act independently in public life and blames the state authorities for its own performance. This "learned helplessness" is a result of "nationalization of the initiative of action in collective life"[43] and is associated with an attitude "which may be described as shortening of the temporal perspective of the actions undertaken and planned, and adopting temporary solutions without considering their long-term effects."[44] In the light of this, it is perhaps surprising that there were any groups at all trying to organize action in connection with the AIDS issue.

One initiative came from an unusual source. The guru of a circle for drug addicts, Marek Kotanski, who had previously organized social initiatives such as a campaign against alcoholism, pushed effectively for HIV testing by starting the Bank of Hope, the aim of which was to raise funds to import HIV test kits. With his followers he attempted to raise money (namely, foreign currency) by collecting on the streets of Polish cities. In early 1987 these actions were publicized on radio and television and drew the first contributions from prominent people in the arts and sciences. Thanks to the Bank of Hope, Poland was able to purchase test kits from the American manufacturer, Abbot. In fact, in recognition of Kotanski's work, Abbot provided free of charge the Quantum apparatus that was necessary for testing. However, the funds collected (U.S. $4,000) remain in the Bank of Hope account, their fate illustrating the impact of bureaucratization on social initiatives. Their use requires approval by an office of the Ministry of Finance and Foreign Trade and the state export bank, but as of early 1989 neither has given its consent.

CONCLUSION

For the present, AIDS is not a serious problem in Poland. It is only one among many problems competing for public attention and money. It is, however, destroying the sense of certainty granted to society by an omnipotent state and will continue to do so as the (predicted) epidemic in Eastern Europe spreads.[45] For almost forty years the socialist state was based on the myth of security (state provision of employment, housing, free health care, and education), protection from social problems, and a commitment to provide for the needs of its people. These illusions are now gone. The democratization process started by the Solidarity movement, reinforced by the introduction of glasnost, has revealed many problems that have been further deepened and dramatized by the economic crisis.

In this context AIDS appears as the type of threat that can return Poland to a New Dark Age. Something of this threat is conveyed by a recent article in the journal *Konfrontacje* describing a possible scenario for the spread of AIDS.[46] Its major premise was that as confirmed cases increased, so would a generalized panic. The prices of needles, syringes, and condoms on the black market would skyrocket, fueling intolerance and even the lynching of homosexuals. Draconian regulations would be only one of the state's responses. The health system would simply succumb to unmanageable demands. In the end, when a vaccine against AIDS invented in the United States eventually came to Poland, the society would already have been destroyed less by HIV itself than by the social and political consequences of obscurantism and ignorance. This representation, neatly illustrating Mann's distinction between the three types of epidemics associated with AIDS, not only offers the disease as a symbol of the fight against the unknown forces of nature but also uses it to signal the consequences of ignorance and intolerance concerning the existence of social problems.[47]

One characteristic of the Polish response to the AIDS problem is that the whole task of tracking, controlling, and preventing infection has been thrown onto the AIDS Council without giving it the necessary power and resources effectively to carry out its task. It has no mechanisms, for example, to demand that the rubber industry produce more condoms or the pharmaceutical industry test and introduce new drugs. The purely nominal allocation of responsibility in this way functions only to shore up the image of state competence in a period when in both practical and ideological terms that competence is being challenged.

A second feature has been the way in which, under the formal responsibility of government organizations, individual initiatives have been allowed to direct the workings of existing agencies. Both Kozakiewicz and Kotanski, as individual players, have used the space provided by their official co-optation to initiate new types of intervention. In the absence of organized pressure groups to force the government into action, positive actions emerging within the institutional structure are valuable. To some degree this "privatization of institutions" has been possible because of the prestige and visibility of the two individuals mentioned, helped by the fact that their proposals did not require new investments. Lack of resources in fact necessitated the centralization and incorporation of AIDS care and prevention programs within the framework offered by the existing health system. The resulting possibility of the spread of the AIDS virus within the health system itself needs to be faced. Equally, because of the low visibility of risk groups, and since social intolerance prevents members of risk groups from openly identifying themselves, controlling the spread of AIDS will be quite difficult. The refusal to provide the gay movement with official legal recognition and the lack of legitimacy enjoyed by the state limit the effectiveness of the battle against AIDS by obstructing popular participation in initiatives for wider education and behavior change.

It is quite clear now that unless more money becomes available, success in curbing the spread of HIV will be strictly limited. Since the government's efficacy in launching initiatives has been poor, the power publicly to define and address the problem has been taken over principally by medical experts. But this shift in the balance of definitional power is conditional and will be reversed should the political leadership choose to define the AIDS crisis in terms of strategic-political considerations rather than public health indicators. At present the history of AIDS in Poland has revealed the urgent need for a new "culture of crisis solving" similar to that displayed by the continuing Soviet attempts to eliminate alcoholism. As Feher suggests, those campaigns show a concern with the specific substantive problem but at a deeper level reveal much more general aspirations of the Soviet state. The official steps against alcoholism serve "a symbolic-cultural function which is closely related to crisis solving: alcoholism is a metaphor for the politics of modernisation."[48] Similarly, the effort to combat AIDS in Poland is seen by many as a condensed symbol for the national ability to behave collectively in a responsible way, for the preservation of national and personal dignity, and for the extent of the determination not to allow the world to leave the country behind.

It is clear, however, that the international determinants of the AIDS problem and the measures to combat it are very significant. The need for foreign currency to obtain medical resources, the continuing significance of Catholic morality reinforced by a conservative Polish Pope in Rome, the vital support given to the gay community by its members outside Poland and the early infections imported from abroad and associated with the presence of foreign students in Poland itself, the transmission of HIV among prostitutes working with foreign clients—all those factors demonstrate the ways in which both the spread of the disease and the reaction to it has been deeply embedded in Poland's external relations.

NOTES

1. I would like to acknowledge the valuable assistance of Dr. Marek Kozek in obtaining some of the material discussed in this chapter.

2. "No Place for Babies," *The Economist*, 4 February 1988, p. 50.

3. "Allarme AIDS a Mosca," *La Repubblica,* 22 February 1988, p. 10.

4. G. T. Ash, "The Empire in Decay," *New York Review of Books*, 29 September 1988, pp. 53–60.

5. Ibid.

6. "AIDS in the USSR," *Science* 240 (1988): 384.

7. By July 1989 approximately two million Bulgarians and resident foreigners had been tested: 77 Bulgarians and 72 foreigners were identified as HIV-positive, and 59 of the foreign seropositives (mainly African students) had been deported (*Nature* 341 (1989) 28 September, p. 275).

8. Following the publication of a decree on 29 August 1987, the Soviet authorities launched a large-scale screening program. In 1988 more than 18 million citizens (6 percent of the population) had been screened for HIV infection. Tests on 1,900 homosexuals revealed only 2 who were positive; none of the 120,000 intravenous drug users was found to be HIV-positive. A significant group of the infected (7 percent) were the children and heterosexual partners of HIV carriers. In all, 176 Soviet citizens and 378 foreigners living in the USSR have been diagnosed as HIV-infected. For the text of the decree, see, "Union of Soviet Socialist Republics: Subject Category IV A," *International Digest of Health Legislation* 38, no. 4 (1987): 770.

9. "Hungary: Legislation; Subject Category IV A," *International Digest of Health Legislation* 39, no. 4 (1988): 830.

10. J. Borneman, "AIDS in the Two Berlins," *October* 43 (August 1988): 223–237.

11. "Eastern Europe Faces a Western Epidemic," *New Scientist*, 8 April 1989, pp. 2–26.

12. Panos Dossier No. 1, *AIDS and the Third World* (London: Panos Institute 1987).

13. "Program walki z AIDS," *Zycie Warszawy*, 11 November 1988, p. 6.

14. Panos, *World AIDS*, no. 3 (May 1989), p. 4.

15. "Poland: Legislation: Subject Category IV A," *International Digest of Health Legislation,* 38, no. 4 (1987): 768.

16. The conference took place at Poznan University, in June 1988. The majority

of lawyers and medical experts attending the conference supported the move to liberalize existing legal arrangements. However, it is difficult to predict in which direction the propositions of the legal section of the AIDS Council will go because of newspaper articles pointing to the Soviet solution in this respect as being worthwhile.

17. "Bomba zegarowa," *Przeglad Tygodniowy*, 16 April 1987, p. 4.

18. "Poles Told to Bring Own Syringes," *New Scientist*, 7 July 1988, p. 32.

19. Ibid.

20. Teresa Bochwic, "Taniec ze smiercia," *Tygodnik Solidarność*, 6 October 1989, pp. 1, 6.

21. M. Sokolowska and B. Moskalewicz, "Health Sector Structures: The Case of Poland," *Social Science and Medicine* 24, no. 9 (1987): 763.

22. Ibid., p. 767.

23. V. Simko and B. Krompholz, "Aspects of Diseases," in H. Rotschild, ed., *Biocultural Aspects of Disease* (New York: Academic Press, 1981), p. 465.

24. Ibid., p. 470.

25. "Poles Told."

26. "AIDS to tylko jedno ogniwo," *Zycie Literackie*, 9 March 1988, p. 8.

27. "Poles Told."

28. "Mlodziez i seks," *Polityka*, 4 October 1986, p. 5.

29. "Poles Told."

30. The survey was carried out in September 1988 by Centrum Badan Opinii Spolecznej (Center for the Study of Public Opinion) on an all-national sample of 1,443 respondents. The preliminary results (unpublished) show the repressive attitudes of Polish society toward homosexuals. About 32 percent of respondents thought that homosexuality is a serious problem in Poland, mostly because of AIDS (32 percent), because it is abnormal (31.6 percent), and because it is a source of various pathologies (19 percent).

31. D. Altman, *The Homosexualization of America: The Americanization of the Homosexual* (New York: St.Martin's Press, 1982), p. 51.

32. "Sekcja specjalna," *Przeglad Tygodniowy*, 4 November 1987, p. 7.

33. Until the late 1970s, the Association for Family Development operated under the name Association for Family Planning. The change in name reflected a change in official ideology and of attitudes toward family planning, consistently under attack by the Catholic Church. The Church has just recently launched a legislative initiative to repeal Poland's relatively liberal abortion law and replace it with an absolute prohibition that would mean mandatory jail terms of three years for women who have abortions and up to five years for doctors who perform them.

34. More conservative statistics say that there are somewhere between 200,000–700,000 casual and 30,000–35,000 regular drug addicts. In 1986, 8,014 drug users sought medical treatment. In 1986, 1,025 cases of drug-related poisoning and 117 deaths were reported; the 1987 figures were 707 and 68, respectively. There are presently thirty-four rehabilitation wards and ten detoxification wards in hospitals, set up as a consequence of the Prevention of Drug Abuse Act (1985). The act also permitted voluntary organizations to establish advice and rehabilitation programs and allocated 1 percent of profits from alcohol sales to create a Drug Fund. For these and further details, see Margaret Watson, "Drug Use and Policy in Poland in the 1980s," *International Journal of Health Services* 19, no. 3 (1989): 443–456.

35. Panos, *World AIDS*, no. 3 (May 1989): 4.

36. Ibid.

37. P. Wojcik, *Problemy patologii i przestepcosci* (Warsaw: PAN, 1985).

38. According to media reports, all six prostitutes who tested seropositive were forced to change their occupations and submit to police control.

39. L. Czerchawski et al., "Human Immunodeficiency Virus Antibodies in Patients with Haemophilia and Other Inheritable Blood Clotting Disorders in Southwest Poland," *Archivum Immunologiae et Therapiae Experimentalis* 36, no. 1 (1988): 61–69.

40. "Poles Told.

41. "AIDS," *Jestem*, 3 March 1988, p. 8.

42. "Wirus strachu," *Polityka*, 23 January 1988, p. 7.

43. W. Narojek, "Perspektyw pluralizmu w upanstwowioinym spoleczwenstwie," unpublished paper, Warsaw, 1986.

44. M. Marody, "Antinomies of Collective Subconsciousness," *Social Research* 55, no. 1–2 (1988): 102.

45. *New Scientist*, 8 April 1989, pp. 25–26. Recent Soviet estimates (February 1989) put the number of seropositives at 600,000 by 1995 and the number of full AIDS cases at 200,000 by the year 2000.

46. "AIDS: Symulacja," *Konfrontacje*, 2 February 1988, p. 24.

47. J. Mann, "For a Global Challenge," *World Health* (March): 4–8.

48. F. Feher, "Crisis and Crisis-Solving in the Soviet Union," *Thesis Eleven*, no. 21 (1988): 12.

AIDS in Australia: Diffusion of Power and Making of Policy

While the earliest formation of AIDS policy in the United States was characterized by conflict and widespread disputes, initial impressions in Australia suggested national consensus and effective state action. In many respects Australia was a "lucky country" as far as AIDS is concerned. First, it had time to prepare itself for the epidemic before the disease actually reached its shores. Second, the Labour government, with a leading role played by an active and liberal Health Minister, created a favorable political climate for discussion of responses to AIDS and showed concern to consult very widely in forming policies. A national rhetoric reinforced the positive picture by proclaiming Australia as "world leader in fighting the disease, as the first country to introduce the universal screening of blood supplies."[1]

International recognition is generally valued highly in each nation, but in Australia, a "country without a region," it is especially important. The Australian public was told by the federal health authorities that there was international appreciation and admiration for the leadership and common sense the country had shown in its response to AIDS. The same official publication claims that "Australia has been one of the few countries in the world to establish effective nation-wide coordination of strategies in respect of AIDS." Australia has also tried to take a prominent international role, for example by sponsoring the United Nations' resolution on AIDS designed to promote international cooperation and coordination in the global fight against the disease and by assisting South Pacific and East Asian countries to develop prevention and educational programs.[2]

Differences between Australian and U.S. AIDS policies are also worth mentioning. While in the United States the intensity of disagreement about

AIDS policies illustrates how "the public rhetorical dramas of symbolic politics are a mechanism for coping with the fragmentation of political authority," Australian claims of unity and success seem to be an attempt to pacify and preempt the potential conflicts generated by diffusion of power.[3] A further contrast concerns the emphasis placed on research. Probably because of a belief that the country "can insulate itself from the rest of the world through rigid immigration and quarantine laws" and the inhibiting combination of egalitarian values and collectivist norms against risk-taking and innovation, Australia has supported efforts in the sphere of education and prevention rather than in searching for a cure.[4] Resources have been devoted to a dramatic public information campaign on the grounds that every Australian has a right to know about AIDS; but in contrast to the better-funded and more effectively planned research programs in the United States, research in Australia has been largely neglected.[5]

From 1988 onward, however, the policy of consensus in Australia has been under increasing challenge, both from medical professionals and, to a lesser extent, from the main opposition party, the Liberals. The emphasis of Australia's AIDS policy on consensus, compassion for AIDS victims, and social and community-based strategies may have been praised abroad; at home it has been confronted by increasingly "medicalizing" definitions of the disease and by demands for a return to more traditional models of public health measures. Since early 1988, in efforts to preserve the much-valued consensus on response, the federal government has tried in several ways to retain all of its symbolism and much of its substance. While in the United States, Britain, and Sweden the triumph of professionalism is now clearly revealed by the extent to which experts in clinical medicine, research, and public health are determining the response to AIDS, Australia is still enmeshed in debates about the priorities to govern decisions on testing, screening, and education. To what degree, therefore, have the well-publicized tensions between different groups influenced the actual course of AIDS policy? How far has the desired national AIDS strategy been achieved?

THE AIDS PROFILE

The first AIDS case in Australia was reported in 1982. By June 1989 a cumulative total of 1,350 cases had been reached, of whom almost half have died. Although in absolute numbers the incidence of the disease has not been large, the cumulative rate of 62 per million places Australia as the fourth most affected country in the world after the United States (286 per million), Switzerland (76.1), and France (75.7).[6] The most striking feature of the AIDS profile in Australia is still the overwhelming dominance of homosexual and bisexual men who, in constituting 87.7 percent of all cases, represent the highest proportion in any national profile. In consequence Australia shows a significantly higher male to female ratio of reported AIDS cases (24:1) than in the United States and Europe (9:1). Together these features suggest that the epidemic in Australia is some two or three years behind its counterpart in the United States. Moreover, the relatively low percentages of drug users (3.3 percent) and prostitutes (1.3 percent) among AIDS cases differentiates Australia from such countries as Italy, Spain, or even the United States.

As is characteristic of other advanced societies, the geographical concentration of AIDS cases in Australia—effectively in two urban areas—is marked. The epicenters of the epidemic are in New South Wales (mainly Sydney), which has reported 65 percent of all cases, and Victoria (mainly Melbourne), which has reported 21 percent. The remaining states are much less affected: Queensland (7 percent) and West and South Australia (3 percent each). A study of all diagnosed seropositive cases in West Australia between 1983 and 1987 indicated that HIV infection was associated with young men of low socioeconomic status living in metropolitan areas and belonging to two specific occupational groups: service, sport, and recreational workers, and professional and technical workers.[7]

As far as can presently be determined, the progress of the disease at an individual and collective level in Australia is also similar to that of other Western societies. The median period of survival after the diagnosis of full AIDS for patients who have been infected by homosexual partners is similar to that in other developed countries (11.4 months), although there was an early difference in the median length of survival of Australian patients whose initial symptom was Kaposi's sarcoma (12.4 months) as against 16 months in Italy, 17.3 months in San Francisco, and 21 months in the United Kingdom.[8] Now, however, the survival period has lengthened to 2.5 years and the fatality rate is declining, largely attributable to the effects of zidovudine. The annual number of deaths reached its highest hitherto recorded level at 199 in 1987 and dropped to 86 last year. Indeed, the latest figures show not only a fall in the number of deaths but also a fall in the rate of increase of new cases. In 1986 there was a 97 percent increase in the number of cases over 1985, but in 1987 the annual rate of increase fell to 60 percent and in 1988 to 24 percent.[9]

The projections encouraged by such figures are of course utterly fragile without some indications of the numbers of seropositives and the size of at least the primary high-risk groups. According to the most recent government estimation, seropositives in Australia number between 15,000 and 25,000, although the total number actually verified (November 1988) stood at 6,247. Current official predictions, which are much more conservative than those of two years ago, suggest that there will be cumulative totals of 3,000 AIDS cases and 1,500 deaths by 1991 (*Sydney Morning Herald*, 12 April 1989, p. 4).

New infections are still expected to occur mainly among the homosexual population, although the extent of gay activities and bisexuality is as uncertain in Australia as elsewhere. That said, data from recent surveys suggest that male homosexuality may be substantially less common than its estimated incidence in some other advanced industrial societies. As against the admittedly dated Kinsey finding that 37 percent of American males had had sexual contacts with other men, Ross (1988) reports that only 11 percent of his sample had had homosexual experiences in the past and a still smaller 6 percent in the previous twelve months. Among gay groups, however, education programs appear likely to reduce the incidence of infection.[10]

No such optimism is in order for intravenous drug users. The size of the ivdu community in Australia is very uncertain, lying somewhere between the 170,000 Australians who are reckoned to use illegal intravenous drugs casually and the estimated 50,000 hard-core users.[11] The encouragingly low early figures of between 1 percent and 3 percent seropositivity rates among ivdus have recently been revised sharply upwards to around 15 percent (*The Age*, 11 May 1989, p. 6), an increase that is hardly surprising when taken in conjunction with the reports that as recently as 1987, 90 percent of ivdus in Melbourne shared needles and—still more recently—that 12 percent of ivdus in Sydney continue to share needles with people known to be HIV-positive.[12] Moreover, in some states there are awkward legal restrictions on setting up effective prevention campaigns for drug users.[13]

Such evidence suggests that education campaigns, at least among the designated high-risk categories, have not been having the desired effects. Although a very significant part of the AIDS budgets has always been assigned for education campaigns (31 percent in 1986–1987), the federal government has still not managed to develop a uniform national education strategy. Precisely because of the great difficulty of making any direct connection between education and the rate of spread of the disease, the education-against-AIDS issue remains at the center of controversy. The view, which is quite common among Australian experts, that education campaigns have been ineffective is supported by various studies showing that only a minority of people have changed their sexual practices because of the AIDS scare. Research among 419 Sydney university students showed that while knowledge about AIDS was good, the impact of education campaigns on their sexual behavior was very limited.[14]

This observed discrepancy between belief and behavior is supported by other evidence: a Morgan Gallup Poll conducted in September 1987 found that only 5 percent of respondents claimed to have changed their behavior because of risk from AIDS and only 10 percent thought that the population at large was at risk.[15] The failure of the campaign to reach even the best-informed segments of the most significant age group, let alone the growing numbers of much less accessible homeless youth and drug addicts, seems plain. Indeed, even doctors themselves are not fully familiar with HIV infection and AIDS, as acknowledged in early 1989 by the president of the

Australian Medical Association, who remarked that "it is a fairly exotic and unusual disease for Australian doctors."[16]

To sum up, while the federal government was quick to introduce regulatory measures such as securing blood supplies and introducing mandatory reporting of full-blown AIDS cases, a national policy has yet to be formulated to supplement the hitherto mainly localized responses. Whereas other Western countries have defined AIDS primarily as a professional problem in the management of what is increasingly seen as a chronic condition,[17] Australia is still unable to develop a policy based on a consensus, both political and professional, that the epidemic is a disease like any other as far as research and treatment are concerned. This contributes to the government's inability to reconcile and coordinate the interests of various groups and to the growing separation between the official position and the demands of dissatisfied groups for a new understanding of the disease and what must be done to control its spread. The result has been "a stifling of speed, flexibility and creativity in developing preventive education and other AIDS policies and programs" (*The Australian*, 5 August 1988, p. 3). In what follows I shall therefore be considering the factors that may explain the particularity of the Australian response, examining them in relation to the specific features of the national political and health systems.

THE AUSTRALIAN CONTEXT I: THE POLITICAL SYSTEM

Australian society has always been marked by an activist, interventionist state. The convict origins of the country, the huge size of the continent, and its sparse population all called for centralized control of the polity. However, the principal form of centralized government in Australia lies not in Canberra, but "in the bureaucracies of the state governments."[18] Thus, under the federal structure of the Australian political system, the states have primary responsibility for the quantity and quality of welfare services, the development of economic resources, and the maintenance of law and order. Even while federal power has increased in recent decades, the states appear very resilient and their bargaining power remains strong. Moreover, with conservative parties holding office in some states and maintaining their traditional identification with anticentralist policies, and with the Labour Party in power at Commonwealth level, "anti-Canberra" feeling, reinforced by dislike of "socialists," makes cooperation between the federal government and some states very difficult.[19]

A further important characteristic of the Australian political context is the unqualified expectation by various organized groups that the state could and should respond to their demands.[20] Historically, in order to cope with these competing claims, the federal government has favored institutional solutions, setting up semijudicial procedures to distribute national resources

according to the guiding principle of equalization—a system that has necessarily also placed limits on public input into policy making. As Emy
indicates, the state is therefore regarded by many sectional interests as little
more than the sum of their administrative agencies. As a result of this
diffusion of power, the federal government finds it difficult to coordinate
policy and to achieve consensus on some reasonably objective criteria of
"public interest," especially at a time of crisis. These features of the Australian political system—its federal structure, the problems with coordinating policies and the diffusion of power, the difficulty of defining and
maintaining a sense of the public dimension of policy—have been important
in shaping AIDS policy.

The structural difficulties are aggravated by the role of the mass media,
which in Australia have become "more significant than politicians in setting
the agenda."[21] According to Altman (1986), the Australian media treatment
of AIDS has certainly been among the most irresponsible. In its battle with
AIDS, the federal government has been confronted by an uncooperative
mass media. Sensationalism, hysteria, exaggeration, false and superficial
stories have contributed to panic and have undermined the credibility of
the official line. In his first statement concerning AIDS the federal Health
Minister stated the case bluntly: "The most useful way of stopping panic
in the community would be for the media to get their facts right about the
issue.... We will be talking to the media and doing our best to get a realistic
appreciation of the AIDS problem...but there is a gross amount of exaggeration about it."[22]

THE AUSTRALIAN CONTEXT II: THE HEALTH SYSTEM

Although total Australian health expenditure continues to rise, it remains
low by comparison with the level of spending of major Western countries
such as Sweden, West Germany, and the United States. However, the system
of compulsory and universal health insurance (Australian Medicare) embod-
ies an ethic of distributive justice not so evident, for example, in the United
States. This creates a major difference for AIDS sufferers in Australia and the
United States. Moreover, the existing Medicare agreement meets the national
costs faced by public hospitals brought about by the increased number of
HIV-infected people seeking treatment with the drug AZT. People with HIV
infection are also eligible for financial assistance under existing government
social security schemes. Generally speaking, care for AIDS sufferers is very
good, especially in Sydney, where "you can get excellent care even if you
can't afford it and confidentiality provisions will ensure you'll be at no risk
[of] losing your health insurance or your job."[23]

Notwithstanding its positive dimensions, Australian health policy has also
been characterized by extreme controversy, by several brusque changes in
direction, and by the existence of political conflict about the insurance

system to an unusual degree. The conflict seems to have been more intense than in many other comparable countries and has generated substantial opposition by the medical profession to Labour government policies.[24]

At the time when AIDS struck Australia, the Labour government, which had been returned to office in 1983, was trying to reintroduce the national Medibank health insurance program, which had been abolished by the previous conservative coalition government during its 1975–1983 term. The program was intended to provide the Commonwealth with a mechanism to influence medical service costs through rebate determination; and it naturally led to a battle with the doctors' organizations, who opposed Labour's national health insurance proposal and waged a deeply antagonistic publicity campaign against it.

The political controversy between the federal government and medical practitioners in some way prepared the field for the future contact that took place in the new context of the AIDS crisis.[25] When the AIDS epidemic began, the political climate was therefore more favorable toward the gay lobby and toward a less medical model of approach to the disease. This is in clear contrast to the U.S. situation, where the epidemic of HIV infection began in a political climate characterized by "a fundamental shift in the locus of authority for health policy from the Federal government to state government and private sector and the willingness of public officials to let doctors and scientists continue to control spending with minimal oversight. Moreover, the strength of right-wing pressure groups seemed to preclude sympathetic policies for a disease that was most prevalent among homosexual men and intravenous drug users and that afflicted a disproportionate number of blacks and Hispanics."[26]

Under the federal arrangements set out in the Australian Constitution, the role of states in the delivery of most health services is more prominent than that of the Commonwealth, which can, however, impose conditions on grants given to the states and thus indirectly influence their specific policies. Although most of the constitutional power to control the spread of infectious diseases such as AIDS lies with the states, the Constitution contains a provision that Parliament may enact laws with respect to quarantine. In August 1984 the Governor-General proclaimed AIDS an infectious disease; since then AIDS has been a notifiable condition in all states, without, however, any further regulations having yet been made. Subsequently, the states themselves introduced new legislation or extended existing law to include AIDS. But because each state operates under a different health act, the legal status of HIV-infection, AIDS-related condition, and full AIDS varies from state to state. The three conditions may in fact be classified as "infectious," "notifiable," "proclaimed," "dangerous notifiable," or not mentioned at all, with varying legal consequences. Occasional absurdities become visible, such as the provision in West Australia, dating from its Health Act of 1911, which makes it an offense for an HIV-infected person to get on a bus without notifying the driver that he or she is infected. Given that the relationship between federal and individual state laws is confused or unclear, the federal government has expressed concern and opposition to any intemperate legislative action; and a recent working panel set up by the government has recommended that health legislation concerning AIDS should be reviewed.[27]

Among the states, Queensland was the first to pass an AIDS law (June 1983), making the disease notifiable on a compulsory basis, and, one year later, adding AIDS to the definition of venereal diseases under its Health Act of 1937. Draconian emergency legislation was introduced which made it a criminal offense for individuals to give false information about their eligibility to donate blood. In Western Australia, AIDS was proclaimed as both "infectious" and a "dangerous infectious disease," entailing extensive notification provisions that apply not only to doctors and hospital staff but also to anyone occupying the same premises as the AIDS victims. In June 1985 seropositivity was made notifiable on a compulsory basis; and in May 1989 new, exceptional, measures were introduced that proclaimed that anyone caught knowingly spreading AIDS would be quarantined, probably under a system of house arrest. In New South Wales the Venereal Disease Act was amended in August 1984 to provide for compulsory notification both of symptomatic seropositives and full-blown cases of AIDS. Victoria is currently preparing new legislation which, if carried, will give it the strongest laws of any state to detain AIDS patients whose behavior is believed to threaten the community. Although each state has already passed new laws imposing penalties for knowingly transmitting the virus, attempts to develop and clarify antidiscrimination legislation are proceeding slowly. For the time being, only Victoria has explicit provisions that allow anyone facing HIV-related discrimination to seek redress. In other states general antidiscrimination laws may provide limited protection.

Diversity of state and federal health acts, overlapping and unclear lines of responsibility, different systems of defining and reporting diseases—all contribute to the confusion involved in dealing with a health emergency. This fragmentation of the health system is exacerbated by the fact that Australia has no equivalent organization to the U.S. Centers for Disease Control. "We therefore muddle along, relying on hospital and university research workers and on hastily convened ad hoc committees, to cope with national medical and epidemiological emergencies such as the continuing spread of AIDS through our society."[28]

THE AUSTRALIAN CONTEXT III: THE GAY COMMUNITY

Generally, by the mid-1980s the overall legal situation for Australian homosexuals had improved, although the different states show substantial variations. Homosexual acts are still illegal in Queensland, Tasmania, and Western Australia, yet in New South Wales and South Australia it has become unlawful to discriminate on the grounds of homosexuality. The Australian gay movement that emerged at the beginning of the 1970s, to some degree influenced by the American gay movement, has remained "much more clearly anchored in the Left [than its U.S. counterpart] and hence more marginal to the commercial gay world."[29] Most of the political and legislative support for homosexuals in Australia has come, and continues to come, from the Labour Party and the socialist left. For the past two decades issues such as law reform and antidiscrimination have been the center of political activity of the gay community. However, the trend toward favoring homosexual law reforms "made it difficult for the movement to attract activists: the cause had lost its urgency."[30]

Although the gay movement in Australia grew out of the political left rather than a gay subculture, recognition of the movement was an offshoot of the Whitlam government's policy of multiculturalism, developed in the mid–1970s and emphasizing the diversity of communal existence in Australia. As Altman has pointed out, the discourse of multiculturalism, as much as of feminism, has played a major role in creating space for gays and has enabled the gay movement to capitalize on it in certain instances.[31]

Largely thanks to its strong links with its American counterpart, the Australian gay community was collecting information about AIDS as early as 1981; and a number of its leading figures, Altman himself being a representative example, acquired considerable expertise concerning the virus and its implications. Involvement in managing the AIDS crisis is important for gay activists not only because it has clearly been a matter of life or death for them but also because it has provided them with a unique opportunity to demand formal recognition of their legitimacy as a community. As Watson has argued, "AIDS has created the sense that the community at large, and politics at large, will never be able to talk about gay men and probably homosexuality in the way they have before."[32] Indeed, the urgency of the cause rallied many gays publicly in a way that had been harder to achieve in the years when the emphasis had been primarily on the legal restrictions on homosexuality.

The difficulties faced by governments in dealing with (sexual) practices that are presumed to be different from those of the majority did not really impede the early Australian health efforts. In contrast to the United States, where in the early years of AIDS a lack of familiarity with, and subsequent discomfort in discussing, the specific behaviors practiced by gays delayed sensible epidemiological responses,[33] cooperation between various research teams and the gay community resulted in a growing understanding of patterns of manifestations of the AIDS virus. Moreover, far more than in the United States, and due in part to the strong leadership provided by the federal Health Minister, the gay movement has had access to and support from government that can rival the most favorable position achieved in any other country.[34]

The success of gay-directed AIDS organizations, which were largely an extension of the existing political and communal gay movement, in getting financial support from federal and state governments can also be attributed to the political skills the gay movement developed in the protracted struggle for decriminalization. The first AIDS organization, the NSW AIDS Action Committee, was set up in Sydney in 1983, and parallel organizations were quickly established in other states. With subsequent support and funding from the federal government the Australian Federation of AIDS Organizations was established in 1985, to which all community AIDS organizations (AIDS Councils), operating through a network of volunteers and providing round-the-clock services to people with AIDS in each state, belong. The institutional position and direction of the AIDS Councils, however, varies from state to state. For example, in Tasmania and Queensland there are no official links between the AIDS Councils and the states' health departments, while in Victoria the AIDS Council is primarily concerned with gays with AIDS. In most states basic funding for voluntary organization has been provided on a share basis by the state and federal governments. Although it is officially recognized both that these organizations provide care and assistance at considerably lower cost than normal care services (the cost per day for a hospitalized AIDS patient is A$500 as against A$50 for funded care) and that the number of days a patient needs to spend in hospital is significantly reduced, state governments take the services for granted and use their (voluntary) provision to excuse their own lack of involvement. Speakers from AIDS Councils have regularly stressed that funding is inadequate and that the present system of annual funding for community groups is inappropriate, inflexible, and hinders the long-term planning of campaigns.[35] The adequate functioning of these organizations therefore is apt to depend upon local alliances with other nongovernment organizations such as churches. Involvement by the Catholic Archdiocese of Adelaide and the Anglican Church of Western Australia have been significant, as has the help given to the Queensland AIDS Council by the Sisters of Mercy. Without the initiatives and funding from the private sector, which covers up to 30 percent of all AIDS spending, governments would face greatly increased pressures for financial assistance. As the number of those needing care grows, there will be an increasing burden on community-based organizations. Moreover, the very demanding nature of full-time caring work is already producing "burn-out" among volunteers, most of whom have had little previous experience of managing so devastating a disease. The situation is of course especially difficult in areas outside the inner cities or in the country, where there is a lack of trained personnel.

Unlike the United States, where until recently there were no gay activists on AIDS government committees, representatives of the Australian gay community have been appointed to many federal and state AIDS bodies. However, that public presence does not mean that the paternalistic tradition of medicine in its failure to consult the affected group has not been visible in Australia. Indeed, the consequences of the conflict between the medical profession and gay-based AIDS organizations has affected government policy for the coming years.[36]

In sum, the gay movement's rapid and influential involvement in the battle against AIDS can be accounted for by its leaders' monopoly of knowledge about AIDS in the early stage of the epidemic, their opportunities and willingness to reach the risk group, the support and funding they received from the Labour government, and their skillfully organized political interventions. Furthermore, the high concentration of gays in the two major cities of Sydney and Melbourne largely compensated for the relative smallness of the Australian gay movement as a political constituency. The extent of organization and influence of the gay community on the AIDS issue adds one more element to the potentially high degree of conflict among the various actors—the federal government, the states, the medical profession, the mass media—involved in policy discussion or formulation. In determining the extent to which conflict has been actualized and has prevented consensual agreement on a "public interest" dimension of policy, the general framework of the AIDS policies themselves requires examination.

INSTITUTIONAL ARRANGEMENTS—DUAL ACCOUNTABILITY

Australia was preparing itself for AIDS even before the disease reached the country.[37] Particularly well informed and prepared were the gay community and medical researchers. From the outset both groups have played important roles in creating AIDS policy and have been incorporated into the "AIDS establishment." Representatives of the gay community played the role of watchdog in insisting that their constituency be consulted before any decisions that might affect it were taken. Their participation was important to the AIDS bureaucracy mainly as a source of information and contact with the highest risk group and in helping to plan and staff the relevant services. On the other hand, the AIDS Working Party, whose task was to monitor the AIDS situation and to advise the government on the best ways for preventing the spread of the epidemic, possessed only limited knowledge about the disease and gay lifestyle. Indeed, the medical experts who dominated the Working Party could appear resentful of the gay leaders' greater knowledge in both of these areas of substantial ignorance and uncertainty.

The turning point in the establishment of an institutional structure to manage AIDS came in November 1984 after the deaths from AIDS-related diseases of three Queensland babies who had received blood from a homosexual donor. The ensuing public panic triggered actions at both federal and state levels. Following an emergency meeting of state health ministers, a new agency (the National Advisory Committee on AIDS: NACAIDS) was set up to translate the medical recommendations of the AIDS Working Party (renamed the AIDS Task Force) into terms comprehensible to the general public. Appropriately for its task, NACAIDS was chaired by a prominent media personality and former magazine editor, Ita Buttrose. It was made accountable to the federal Health Minister and drew its diverse membership from the New South Wales and Victoria governments, AIDS community organizations, trade unions, organizations of hemophiliacs, and doctors. Its constituency was the AIDS Council, gays, prostitutes, and drug users. By contrast, the AIDS Task Force, composed of senior medical and scientific research staff, was accountable to the officials of the Australian Health Ministers Advisory Council and represented the constituency of the medical establishment.

By creating this double structure, the federal Health Minister was trying to reach a compromise between two commitments. One favored social and community-based strategies (strongly supported by senior advisers in his department); the other favored scientific and public health measures. However, the ambiguity in the responsibilities assumed by the two bodies imposed certain costs. General observations of systems of dual accountability cutting across levels of authority and institutions suggest that they hinder policy changes, with the result that policy tends toward "immobility, with a patchwork of incremental codas accumulating over time."[38] Every major issue connected with the AIDS epidemic has sparked controversy among participants in policy formation; and the ongoing disagreements have immobilized national policy. The AIDS Task Force has clashed publicly with the government and NACAIDS over strategies for dealing with the disease, leading to an (unsuccessful) attempt by the Health Minister to disband the Task Force itself in 1987 and later in the same year to the resignation of its chairman.[39] Simultaneously, poor relations were developing between the Commonwealth government and AIDS community groups. Consequently, at both state and federal level, the administrative structures established to manage AIDS were perceived as having become uncoordinated and increasingly directionless.[40]

In response to the difficulties the federal government decided in early 1988 to make organizational changes. As a result both the existing organizations, NACAIDS and the AIDS Task Force, were abolished and a new advisory body, the Australian National Council on AIDS (ANCA), was appointed.[41] ANCA's nineteen members were nominated for their expertise in medicine, science, law, and public policy. The selection indicates that the federal Health Minister wanted to provide his advisory bodies with a new image, which would be both less controversial and more closely aligned to the perspectives of the medical profession. The change necessarily led to disruptive discontinuities in the personnel responsible for devising and managing strategies, which were all the more significant in the light of the parallel lower-level changes in personnel concerned with AIDS in the Department of Community Health and Services.[42]

Subsequent developments in ANCA, notably the resignations and replacements of particular members, have rendered increasingly visible the impact of the medical lobby. For in the years 1988–1989 the medical profession, which had been a relative late-comer to the public AIDS scene, has come to engage in strong criticism of the government's management of AIDS, in particular for its failure to put sufficient emphasis on public health measures.

Despite the growing preference for medical expertise (ten of ANCA's members have a medical background, including a former president of the Australian Medical Association [AMA]), the Health Minister has found himself continuously under attack for "demedicalizing" the AIDS issue. Particularly hostile attacks have come from the conservative wing of the AMA, which is itself at odds with the present moderate leadership of the association. Even though only two ANCA members openly identify themselves with gay groups, the federal government is still attacked for displaying undue compassion and favoritism toward the gay community.[43] The recent appointment to the post of the government's chief scientific adviser, despite the opposition of some senior Health Department advisers who favored the kind of social and community-based strategies criticized by the new appointee, is an important indication of an AIDS bureaucracy more firmly committed to the priority of public health measures over civil rights concerns.

To sum up, the ambiguous pattern of responsibilities, changes in organizational structures, the high turnover of membership in the key committees, bureaucracies and voluntary organizations, an absence of a consensus about how the AIDS issue should be defined and managed—all these factors have produced an erratic and long-drawn-out set of debates that have still not seen any clear consensus. The two issues of education and testing provide obvious illustrations of the continuing controversies. In the first place, how should the public be educated, and which publics should be specific targets? In the second place, what kind of testing should be introduced, and who should be tested?

EDUCATION—OR POWER CONSTRAINED BY SALIENCE

In 1987, at a cost of A$3 million, the federal Health Department launched a national education program, coordinated by a steering committee from NACAIDS. The campaign was intended to shift the public perception of AIDS away from the media-fostered preoccupation with the high-profile risk categories and to focus attention on the longer-term risk that the disease presented to heterosexuals. That decision was justified by the market research commissioned by NACAIDS, which showed that up to 30 percent of young sexually active people are potentially at risk. In April 1987, therefore, a prime-time fear-inducing television advertisement, based on the striking (and now internationally notorious) figure of the Grim Reaper, began to frighten Australians to such a degree that it soon had to be withdrawn. The other components of the campaign—the provision via leaflets and radio messages of factual information on "safe sex" practices and grants to agencies and community organizations to assist them in handling requests for information—were in some cases no more successful. Indeed, the information brochure about AIDS was withdrawn after general condemnation of its vagueness and poor wording.

The promoters of the campaign used marketing professionals both to design the Grim Reaper clip and to evaluate its impact. The evaluating company, Australian Market Research (AMR), concluded that "less than two months after the campaign began, there is already evidence of behavioural change—22% of men and 14% of women said they had modified their sexual behaviour since AIDS became a concern."[44] That finding, in addition to AMR's prior estimate on the extent of risky practices, is not supported by the results of more detailed research.[45] Relying on "the boy wonders of the advertising agencies" rather than the several years' experience developed by gay leaders in selling unpopular messages about changing sexual behavior, NACAIDS and the government ran directly into criticism from gay leaders—the very group to which the public attributed the devising of the Grim Reaper message.[46] In the debate generated by the image it was pointed out that the campaign was misdirected, since the threat of heterosexual transmission was minimal. "The spectre of the Grim Reaper haunts the land but a credibility gap seems to be growing between the official line, that everyone from grannies to babies is at risk, and what appears to be reality—that AIDS still strikes primarily at homosexuals."[47] This claim was supported by members of the AIDS Task Force, who demanded the withdrawal of the Grim Reaper advertisement. They concluded that the real agenda behind the campaign was the diverting of attention away from the gay community by exaggerating the risk posed by AIDS to the general population. Ironically, NACAIDS and the federal health bureaucracy were faced both with public accusations of being dominated by the gay community and with criticism from the gay lobby.[48] Finally, the community-based organizations managing AIDS were unhappy with this educational strategy because it cost so much that minimal funds were left over for follow-up educational programs within the communities themselves.

All this criticism, however valid, does not address one underlying aim of the Grim Reaper campaign. A significant component appears to have been an attempt by the AIDS establishment to put AIDS on the political agenda, to make it a highly visible public issue in order to legitimate the allocation of urgently needed funds. Politicians and public opinion react on the "see-

and-touch" principle. Because of the long period of incubation of the disease, the real dimensions of the AIDS crisis were still invisible. The problem was therefore how to generate a response before the actual problem was publicly visible, by which time, of course, asymptomatic HIV infection would have spread far more widely. The task of shocking the public and politicians into action thus led to the symbol of the Grim Reaper.

The subsequent step in the campaign was an advertisement to be displayed on buses and trams from April 1988 onward. One of the posters proposed depicts a bus-length condom with the slogan "Cover yourself against AIDS," constituting the first attempt to address directly risky practices. It was, however, rejected by three states on the grounds that it was "distasteful." At the end of 1988 a new A$1.8 million campaign was launched, featuring two television advertisements and backed by youth magazine displays. This time the target groups were teenagers and drug addicts, but this campaign too ran into trouble. Because the clips featured men in bed, the privately owned television channels initially refused to screen them, relenting only when the "gay scene" was cut out. Moreover, the campaign has hitherto not been extended to country areas.

The federal government's educational effort was criticized not merely on the grounds of its content, chosen vehicles of communication, and target group, but principally because of the ineffectiveness of the dramatic and expensive commercials, especially on the behavior of at-risk groups. The basis of this criticism was that the use of television commercials and pamphlets to stop the spread of the disease was misconceived because, while possibly an effective means of conveying information, they cannot in themselves instigate long-term and secure changes in behavior. Although a comprehensive evaluation of the full impact of the education program is difficult, it seems that the absence of a uniform national strategy, an inability to address the AIDS issue in the necessary explicit language, and the lack of safe-sex literature allow doubts about its effectiveness. Why were A$11.24 million spent so inefficiently?

Since the boundary between sex education and discussion of "immoral acts" is relative to the beholders, an explicit "safe-sex" campaign leads almost inevitably to public protest by certain groups on behalf of what they perceive as moral concerns. Political leadership in support of educational programs potentially offensive to constituents has also been weak. A former senior member of the AIDS bureaucracy has concluded that "in terms of educating the populace the government has failed.... [Politicians are afraid of] an electoral backlash from the sector of the community strongly opposed to an explicit treatment of the subject in schools and on television."[49] The Liberal Opposition in Parliament, for example, insisted that programs "must not undermine the moral, ethical, family and social values on which our country is founded.... We are firmly of the view that any such program must be undertaken after full consultation and, hopefully, with the cooperation of the community and religious leaders."[50] In consequence the mass education campaign ultimately revolved around politicians' feelings of what the public would or would not tolerate rather than what the experts in areas of communications, marketing, medicine, and health education deemed necessary. Insofar as the education program was forced to respond to shared conventional meanings, therefore, power was limited by salience.[51] In such cases, when governmental power is constrained by salience and by the weight of public conservatism and when, consequently, the power to invent alternatives, which might meet salient problems, is diffused, the question can be asked whether the government should not acknowledge its limitations and delegate the responsibility for education to the community.

TESTING: TOWARD PLURALISTIC STAGNATION?

From the outset the controversial issue of testing was directly connected with the question of who should have the power to decide how Australia should deal with the AIDS crisis. Although at present only certain categories of people are subject to mandatory testing (including members of the army and persons in custody in South Australia, Queensland, and the Northern Territory), the debate over testing has reached a wide spectrum of the population.

The controversy has passed through two identifiable stages. At first it simply represented the prolongation of the disagreement between NA-CAIDS, acting in effect as the voice of the gay constituency, and the AIDS Task Force, expressing mainly the views of medical researchers, about the education programs. Members of the Task Force pointed to the fact that the numbers tested were falling, partly because, by avoiding singling out high-risk groups in its educational programs, NACAIDS did not actively encourage testing, and partly because gay rights activists directly discouraged participation in HIV testing. The further view was expressed by the gay community that testing should be an individual decision, on the grounds that in the absence of either a cure or a vaccine, the test was useless if behavioral change could be achieved in other ways. Moreover, its members remained concerned that the guarantee of confidentiality was by no means secure. During this first period neither the federal government nor its AIDS bureaucracy was directly criticized: in practice all sides recognized the need for testing as a source of the epidemiological data necessary to understand and combat the disease.

The second stage of the controversy over testing politicized the AIDS issue. It was triggered in August 1988 by the Liberal Opposition's health spokesperson, Wilson Tuckey, at the Third National Conference on AIDS. Although it was not the first time that the Opposition had raised the issue—on several occasions they had called in Parliament for the screening of immigrants, prisoners, and homosexuals entering Australia—Tuckey launched a sharp attack on federal government policy, claiming it had been captured by the gay lobby and labeling AIDS "a gay plague [stemming from] deliberate and possibly unnatural activity."[52] His statements resulted in a furious public debate. Tuckey's charges that AIDS organizations had become effectively the prisoners of gay groups who had hijacked the debate over policy and ensured that testing was carried out infrequently, were of course dismissed by the ANCA and by the federal Health Minister, with the assurance that the AIDS policies were governed by public health consideration and directed at protecting particular groups.

Characteristically, the sympathies of the largely conservative Australian press in reporting the debate lay with the Opposition, proposing that blood samples taken by medical doctors or in hospitals should routinely be tested—a suggestion that offered an open invitation for doctors to join the discussion. Hitherto doctors had been relatively less vocal than medical researchers in opposing the federal AIDS policy. But from that point on, the Australian Medical Association (which was already engaged in a policy of noncooperation with the Labour government after the reintroduction of Medicare), the Australian Doctors Fund (which seeks to reduce government intervention in medicine), and the Australian Association of Surgeons (which had a direct interest in the HIV status of patients undergoing operations) began a campaign for the compulsory testing of patients and for "medicalization" of AIDS policy. The case for testing is no longer argued on the basis of the need for epidemiological data but for the protection of health workers. They accused the government of ignoring the interests of the medical profession, failing to provide sufficient information, and attempting to conceal the risks faced by health workers—all for the purpose of protecting gays.

Interestingly, however, although protection and education of health workers had been indicated by the federal Health Minister as the third aim of the national strategy (after care for victims and prevention of the spread of infection), it had rarely been emphasized publicly, perhaps in order to avoid panic. Moreover, despite the fact that the government has issued AIDS infection guidelines, the medical profession has commonly acted publicly as if the instructions were unknown to them. The government soon learned the price of maintaining a low profile and strongly enforcing infection-control guidelines. In March 1989 a private Melbourne hospital refused to treat a man infected with HIV. As the ensuing furore grew, the collective voice of the medical profession became increasingly insistent on the need for wider testing and on the extent to which gay interests were controlling government policies. A decision to organize a conference of health workers on AIDS without inviting either politicians or representatives of the gay community was perceived as perfectly appropriate and as a clear statement of the medical profession's conviction that medical priorities in combatting AIDS have been undervalued relative to social implications. Such arguments, amply covered by the mass media, created further confusion in the public mind, increased the credibility gap, and left debates wide open to misinformation, manipulation, and unjustified fear.

Despite attempts by the Opposition parties to make AIDS a bipartisan issue, the involvement of the medical profession transformed policy debates into a battle over the definition of the problem. According to doctors AIDS is a technical medical matter that should be resolved by professionals on the basis of scientific knowledge. As such, it illustrates a more general truth about health systems: "the real battle in the health arena is precisely a definitional one: whether or not specific problems or issues should be labelled as being essentially "medical" in nature, and as taboo for nonexperts."[53] Furthermore, because the medical profession's capacity to dominate discussion is in "inverse relationship to the size of the stage on which a specific health care issue is fought out,"[54] its desire to diminish the role of "nonexperts" (in this instance, gay leaders and the state bureaucracy) is a necessary step toward getting its own way.

Lacking a clear political mandate and caught between two powerful pressure groups—the medical establishment and the gays—the federal government was immobilized. This situation can accurately be described as "pluralistic stagnation" in which the government's policy-forming and policy-executing capacities are inhibited by its inability to mobilize the necessary consent.[55] Accordingly, with the aim of overcoming fragmentation and perhaps of seeking a resolution of this impasse, the federal government has sought to involve further groups in policy formulation by issuing AIDS discussion papers for community consideration.

POLICY DISCUSSION PAPERS: DEMOCRACY AT WORK IN AN EMERGENCY?

Realizing the importance of building a consensus on the most effective responses to the AIDS virus, the federal government issued an extended Policy Discussion Paper in early 1988.[56] In its own words, its aim was to encourage and provoke informed debate on appropriate responses to the epidemic and to assist in the analysis of possible policy components.[57] The paper itself makes no recommendations but discusses a range of policy options and clarifies that an essential requirement is consensus and "the need to move towards accord at all levels of government and between government and community on a National AIDS Strategy."[58]

Calling for a national response can be seen as an attempt by the federal health system to take control of AIDS management and initiate new directions. In order to legitimize its eventual proposals, to have a weapon against dissenting politicians, the medical profession, gay groups, and state governments, and to fix the criteria on which a comprehensive and effective national strategy might be based, a new approach was adopted based on public forums. The federal Health Minister established six panels to provide a site for private submissions and public consultation on AIDS in relation to the Policy Discussion Paper. Over a period of five weeks in early 1989 politicians, health officials, medical experts, academics, and community activists traveled to the major cities in Australia to receive written and oral submissions on the problems associated with AIDS and to stimulate local debates among specialized and lay participants. Their task was to gather a range of reactions from which a common position could be constructed. The panels were also intended as a route for the transmission of grievances and complaints connected with discrimination against people with AIDS and to analyze the impact of differences in the legal frameworks existing in various states and relevant to the management of AIDS. Between them six panels conducted 38 public meetings, held 210 private hearings, and received 1,800 submissions from individuals and organizations as well as responses from all state governments.[59]

Observations of public debates in Queensland suggest that it was a rather useful exercise not only in exchanging information between panel members and the public but in compelling each participating group to notice and respect the different definitions of the situation presented by others in a public forum. The significance, indeed the achievement, of the meetings has been in this confrontation between various points of view and the mutual realization of how much cooperation and flexibility is required from everyone involved in formulating and implementing AIDS policy.

By reinstating AIDS policy making as a clearly public process—moving it from a closed technical arena into the public spotlight in open discussion, entailing reference to equality and fairness—the panels could be perceived not only as mechanisms to arrive at a program but also as a means of improving the quality of the final decision and endowing it with considerable legitimacy. Given these possibilities, it seems that the panels were designed to bypass the politicians' fear of conservative voters and to create consensus and cooperation between the various groups involved in AIDS policy making without seriously compromising the government's objectives.

AIDS is, however, not only a social problem. Discussions of the disease that do not recognize its biomedical aspect or the urgency of the situation do not seriously confront the issue of its successful control. While an admirably democratic attempt to solve the AIDS problem—or rather to dissolve the constraints faced by the government in its AIDS policy—a public consultative process does not imply an enormous sense of urgency. The question indeed arises: how far can democratic processes go in a situation defined as an emergency? In practical terms the answer has been partly preempted. One of the most powerfully organized groups, the medical profession, has refused to abide by the rules of the game implicit in the establishment of the panel discussions and has begun an independent campaign, having caught the ear of the mass media.[60] Even the government's chief medical and scientific adviser, by supporting testing in some situations where health workers are exposed to HIV, has expressed a view in contrast with the panel recommendation that testing should only be conducted with counseling, consent and confidentiality.

In such circumstances both the discussion paper and the panels can appear more like a public relations exercise in democracy, an impression reinforced by the reactions of the mass media to the recommendations of the panels. The proposals that heroin be legalized and prostitution and homosexual acts be decriminalized were immediately described as "unrealistic" and their adoption by the government as "unlikely."[61] The *Sydney Morning Herald* concluded that "it would not be surprising if both the White Paper and the Government's final decision were different from the panel's recommendations."[62] Moreover, opinion polls suggest that few Australians agree with many of the panels' recommendations. On one hand, 65 percent were opposed to the decriminalization of small quantities of heroin for personal use; but on the other, people appear willing to go much further than the panel proposed on the issue of testing.[63]

Publication of the recommendations may have exhausted one means of generating public support, but it has not closed the controversies surrounding AIDS policy, as was hoped. The government's attempt to create more space for its actions, to rid itself of the kind of paralyzing constraints made visible by the proposed changes to broadcasting and censorship laws, will soon be challenged again. Not only are more groups (nurses, civil rights activists, and drug users) actively joining the debate and proposing new alternatives,[64] but new scientific developments (such as the invention of home-testing kits for AIDS or the news from California that HIV can apparently live in the body for more than three years before causing changes in the blood that allow easy detection) will soon demand that the health authorities grapple with new problems. Given the volatile and conflict-ridden environment for the organization of responses, discontent among the groups directly responsible for combatting the disease is likely to deepen and public skepticism and confusion to grow.

CONCLUSION

Studies of Australia's experiences in managing other disasters show that its politico-administrative system does not provide a framework conducive to rapid and coordinated response.[65] The fragmentation of power, overlapping responsibilities, and conflicts between different levels of power—these dimensions of the Australian political system are ruthlessly exposed by the study of the formulation and implementation of policies on AIDS. The same studies also point to the importance of political intervention as a means of overcoming organizational rigidities. In the case of AIDS, however, the activist and liberal policies pursued by the government have not reduced—

indeed, they have paradoxically encouraged—the disputes among interested parties and have made the necessary consensus harder to achieve. The insistence on encouraging active participation has resulted in the fragmentation of policy and a continuing delay in formulating a national strategy more than six years after the first AIDS case in Australia.

The complexity of AIDS as a medical, individual, and social phenomenon demands a multiplicity of responses at different levels from different institutions. In Australia the responses that have taken place at the level of public policy have given a very significant role to social considerations. Apart from tending to downplay the importance of the biological dimensions of the disease, such an approach is also poorly adapted to digesting new knowledge about HIV, confronting its implications in new sets of choices, and embodying their outcomes in policy. The federal government acted from the start in accordance with the optimistic traditions of progressive preventive social medicine, on the assumption that its definition of the disease could not be challenged.

However, as this chapter has shown, the space given to social considerations in Australia has been coming under increasing attack by the medical profession. Thanks to the growing scientific knowledge about HIV and the ambivalence in the gay community on whether to emphasize members' role as primary sufferers or to insist that heterosexuals are equally at risk, the influence of nonmedical groups on public policy has been waning and the traditionally powerful health professionals have been reasserting their authority. In this trend Australia appears to be following the process of renewed professional control visible elsewhere in the West. Yet because of the space conceded to the representatives of the most-affected group by the federal political authorities and the health officials in the two states where AIDS cases have been concentrated, Australia still has a unique chance to devise and implement new programs in which "human rights and public health will march hand in hand."[66]

NOTES

1. Commonwealth Department of Health, *Australia's Response to AIDS* (Canberra: Canberra Publishing Co., 1986), p. 1.

2. Australia has been involved in the WHO's Global Program on AIDS (GPA) in its closest region by supporting the South Pacific countries financially and providing expertise. The Australian government has announced a contribution of A$2 million to the GPA by 1990–1991. In July 1987 Australia hosted a conference of ministers from the Pacific region and the West Asia region to work out ways of encouraging cooperation in dealing with AIDS in this region of the world (Policy Discussion Paper, 1988, pp. 224–229).

3. D. Fox et al., "The Power of Professionalism: Policies for AIDS in Britain, Sweden, and the United States," *Daedalus* 112, no. 2 (1989): 106.

4. D. Altman, *AIDS in the Mind of America* (New York: Doubleday, 1986), p. 186.

5. The neglect of research is visible in the structure of the AIDS budget. The first Commonwealth funding on AIDS was announced in November 1984. Over A$5 million was provided in direct grants to the seven states and territories, $2.7 million of which was to establish AIDS screening programs. In the first four years of the epidemic, until December 1988, some A$50 million had been spent on grants for community projects (15 percent), blood screening (16.6 percent), education (15.1 percent), advertising (14.5 percent), counseling and testing (8.8 percent), and AIDS research (9.2 percent). The Commonwealth matching grants to the states are based on a requirement that half of the amount is to be spent on prevention, education, and counseling, and half on treatment and support outside hospitals (Policy Discussion Paper, 1988, pp. 73–80). The AIDS budget for 1989 consists of A$3.34 million on general community education, A$3.5 million on biomedical AIDS research, and A$7.5 million on education programs directed at high-risk groups. AIDS educators have requested a budget of A$14.8 million for 1990, representing an increase of A$6 million over 1989. The same claim was advanced by medical researchers to double research funds (*The Age*, 15 April 1989, p. 20). Funding has been a controversial issue from the beginnings of the AIDS crisis. The question of funding AIDS research has brought major disagreement between the federal government and the medical profession. Medical researchers, in arguing that funding for AIDS research would have to increase in order to keep pace with other developed nations, were able to point out that Australia spends only a fraction of what major industrial nations spend on AIDS research. They have warned the government that the lack of commitment to a realistic level of research funding could have serious consequences in the future and have emphasized the necessity of establishing an antiviral drug industry to produce the drugs that Australia presently has to import. Frustration at the lack of financial support for AIDS research programs has triggered resignations of such AIDS experts as Professor Tony Basten.

6. The figures on the incidence of AIDS cases are taken from WHO, *Weekly Epidemiological Record* 42 (14 October 1988): 319. A rather higher figure of 1,300 cases in Australia by June 1989 is given by *The Australian*, 3 July 1989, p. 3.

7. C. D'Arcy et al., "Population-Based Epidemiology of Human Immunodeficiency Virus Infection in Western Australia," *Medical Journal of Australia* 150, no. 7 (1989).

8. B. Whyte et al., "Survival of Patients with the Acquired Immunodeficiency Syndrome," *Medical Journal of Australia* 150, no. 7 (1989).

9. *The Age*, 12 April 1989, p. 3. Although a recent downturn in the numbers of new notifications of HIV infection is quite evident, it is too early to draw a firm conclusion as to whether or not the epidemic in Australia has peaked. However, it is worth noticing that these statistics are quite similar to data from other Western countries: in 1987 the rate of increase in France, Italy, and the United States was a little above 50 percent.

10. A survey of 1,000 Sydney homosexual men shows that the education program has lowered new infection rates from 4 percent in 1985 to 1 percent in 1988 (*The Australian*, 15–16 April 1989, p. 9). Similar results were provided by researchers from Melbourne (Policy Discussion Paper, 1988, p. 49).

11. These figures are taken from a NACAIDS study, cited in *The Australian*, 3

July 1989, p. 3. Other figures are given by the Department of Community Services and Health, *Intravenous Drug Use and AIDS*, Consultation Paper No. 4, 1989, p. 2, which claims that up to 500,000 Australians have used illicit drugs intravenously, and *Time*, 23 January 1989, p. 13, which suggests a figure of 50,000–70,000 casual users of heroin, amphetamines, and cocaine.

12. See L. Edgoose and J. Baillie, "AIDS and Intravenous Drug Abuse: Risk Behaviour," *Medical Journal of Australia* 146, no. 5 (1987): 279–280; *The Australian*, 3 January 1989, p. 1. The use of condoms among ivdus also appears to be infrequent.

13. In all states possession, use, and trafficking of drugs is illegal. Although some existing legislation stands in the way of prevention of HIV infection (e.g., supplying of equipment for injection is illegal in Tasmania), a needle-exchange program in the most affected state, New South Wales (NSW), is recognized as important and has succeeded in distributing 1.5 million syringes each year (*Sydney Morning Herald*, 13 May 1989, p. 13). However, the legislation designed to protect needle and syringe exchange has not been entirely clear and effective. People returning dirty syringes to the needle exchange agency may be charged with self-administration of the drug (or in Queensland with prior possession of the drug based on possession of trace elements found in the dirty syringe, Department of Community Services and Health [DCSH] 1989, Consultation Paper No. 2, p. 7). Besides the attempts to educate drug users on AIDS prevention, methadone programs are operating in Victoria, South Australia, Western Australia, Queensland, and NSW (where about 5,000 addicts and prisoners are on the program). However, studies show that only 15 percent of all addicts have any contact with a treatment agency and that most addicts see methadone very much as a second-choice drug (*Time*, 23 January 1989, p. 12). The Health Department has established two organizations designed to involve users and former users in the prevention of AIDS among drug users and to provide support for those already infected. Groups such as Users Advocacy Association and Injector Services have been established in all states, and a federal peak group called the IV League was set up at the end of 1988 (*Sydney Morning Herald*, 13 May 1989, p. 13). Characteristically, the major reason for the emergence of these groups lay in the opinion of many users and former users that such organizations as the AIDS Councils are principally for middle-class gay men and unsympathetic to addicts.

14. Alison M. Turtle, "AIDS-Related Beliefs and Behaviours of Australian University Students," *Medical Journal of Australia*, 150, no. 7 (1989): 371–376.

15. G. Bell and P. Cornford, "AIDS: The Worst is Still to Come," *The Bulletin*, 6 October 1987, pp. 59–63.

16. *The Age*, 11 March 1989, p. 1.

17. See Fox et al., "Power of Professionalism," pp. 93–111.

18. D. Horne, "Who Rules Australia?"in *Australia: The Daedalus Symposium* (North Ride: Angus and Robertson, 1985), p. 175.

19. Federalism provides the opportunity for state governments to make an issue of resistance and obstruction when some electoral advantages can be won. This was visible in the sphere of AIDS policy, where states have a tendency to give priority to services and the Commonwealth has a tendency to give priority to preventive education. This conflict was particularly clear during the negotiation of the allocation of funds from the Commonwealth to the Queensland Health Department. "It seems that all Canberra wants to do is to provide funds for education programs and not

have primary medical programs which Queensland believes are urgently required," commented the Queensland Health Minister. As a reaction to the social and moral evils in Canberra (which "promotes promiscuity rather than discouraging it"), Queensland opposed the federal policy and was much slower than other states in planning and organizing education and counseling services. Fortunately, the fall of the arch-conservative premier Joh Bjelke-Petersen in late 1988 enabled Queensland to bring its AIDS program into line with the rest of the country.

20. For this attitude see the chapters by H. Emy, "The Diffusion of Power," and S. Encel, "The Bureaucratic Ascendancy," in A. Parkin, J. Summers, and D. Woodward, eds., *Government, Politics and Power in Australia* (Melbourne: Longman, 1982). This paragraph draws heavily on Emy's conclusions.

21. Horne, "Who Rules Australia?" p. 182.

22. Neal Blewett, quoted in A. Brass and J. Gold, *AIDS in Australia: What Everyone Should Know* (Sydney: Bay Books, 1985), p. 133.

23. *Sydney Morning Herald,* 10 June 1989, p. 6.

24. Valuable accounts of the Australian health system and its conflicts can be found in M. C. Brown, *National Health Insurance in Canada and Australia* (Canberra: Australian National University Publishing Services, 1983); Gwen Gray, "The Termination of Medibank," *Politics* 19, no. 2 (1984): 1–17; and G. Palmer, "Politics, Power and Health: From Medibank to Medicare," *Social Alternatives,* 23 October 1983, pp. 19–22.

25. As one newspaper put it, "The battle with doctor's groups softened [the federal Health Minister's] attitude toward any underdog doing battle with medical ogres." *Courier Mail,* 22 August 1988, p. 8.

26. Fox et al., "Power of Professionalism," p. 105.

27. See M. C. McGuirl and R. N. Gee, "AIDS: An Overview of the British, Australian and American Responses," *Hofstra Law Review* 14, no. 1 (1985): 107–133.

28. Brass and Gold, *AIDS in Australia,* p. 134.

29. Dennis Altman, "The Gay Movement: Homosexual Politics in the United States and Australia," *Social Alternatives* 6, no. 2 (1987): 17–22. For the gay movement's political affiliations see A. Landsdown, *Blatant and Proud: Homosexuals on the Offensive* (Cloverdale: Perceptive Publications, 1984).

30. T. Matthews, "Australian Pressure Groups," in H. Mayer and H. Nelson, eds., *Australian Politics: A Fourth Reader* (Melbourne: Cheshire, 1981), p. 229.

31. Altman, "Gay Movement," pp. 17–22.

32. Watson, "Life after AIDS," *Australian Left Review* 107 (1988): 12–15.

33. Lewis H. Kuller and Lawrence A. Kingsley, "The Epidemic of AIDS: A Failure of Public Health Policy," *Milbank Quarterly* 64, no. 1 (1986): 56–78.

34. Altman, "Gay Movement," p. 21.

35. See DCSH, *Education and Prevention—HIV/AIDS,* Consultation Paper No. 3, Canberra, 1989.

36. Gay leaders were informed by the medical experts on AIDS that the medical profession "does not normally deal directly with patients." *Courier-Mail,* 22 August 1988.

37. "There were high-tech research teams waiting, epidemiologists eager to hunt down every contact of every case, and federal grant monies earmarked 'AIDS' ready to send." Brass and Gold, *AIDS in Australia,* p. 1.

38. Douglas D. Ross, "Power, Salience and Public Policy," in R. Byestone, ed., *Public Policy Formation* (Greenwich, Conn.: JAI Press, 1984), p. 55.

39. The Task Force chairman is generally reckoned to have outmaneuvered the Health Minister. His own account of the incident is to be found in *The Australian*, 27 December 1987.

40. See, for example, the comments in *The Australian*, 5 August 1988, p. 3.

41. In addition to ANCA the following bodies had also been created at federal level to manage AIDS by 1988:

- the National AIDS Forum, consisting of all members of ANCA and twenty-two members directly involved in work with people with AIDS. The Forum's role is to provide input and support to ANCA, and its public image and visibility remain very low;

- the Parliamentary Liaison Committee on AIDS, an all-party body from the Senate and House of Representatives established by the Health Minister at the request of the Opposition. Its function is to inform politicians about AIDS so that they in turn can inform their electorates;

- the Intergovernmental Committee on AIDS, staffed by public servants from the Commonwealth and from each state or territory (two from each). Its role is to coordinate the efforts of Commonwealth departments in the control of AIDS and to advise the federal Health Minister on the interaction of federal, state, and territory responsibilities for developing AIDS policy;

- People Living with AIDS, an organization with both federal and state-level branches, comprised of seropositives and concerned with the organization of support, treatment, and care for AIDS sufferers. Recently it has been involved in a controversial treatment program—against medical advice—in which people treat themselves and are examined by private doctors.

All state governments have established advisory bodies similar to ANCA.

42. This turnover was noted—and considered an important factor in preventing the emergence of a national AIDS policy—by a government-established panel in 1989. DCSH, *Education and Prevention—HIV/AIDS*.

43. See, for a recent example, *The Age*, 29 April 1989, p. 1.

44. NACAIDS, Survey on Effects of Grim Reaper Campaign, Press release, Canberra, 29 May 1987.

45. See the studies cited in notes 14 and 15 above.

46. The phrase on the ad boys is taken from Adam Carr, "The Grim Reaper: Bowling-Ball or Boomerang?," *Australian Society*, July 1987, p. 30, who provides further details on the abortive campaign.

47. Bell and Cornford, "Worst Is Still to Come," p. 59.

48. *The Australian* of 15 April 1989 claimed that "the gay community has persuaded Dr. Blewett and Co to blur the truth, to deny the obvious nexus" (p. 2).

49. J. Dwyer, "AIDS in Australia," in V.Cosstick, ed., *AIDS: Meeting the Community Challenge* (Homebush: St Paul Publications, 1987), p. 199.

50. Hansard, *Commonwealth of Australia: Parliamentary Debates—House of Representatives*, 1987, vol. 154, p. 1936.

51. As Ross argues, "the broad conventions provide a stable, boundary-setting context for specific adjustment of power to salience" ("Power," p. 41).

52. In June 1989 the Liberal Party released its detailed AIDS policy, proposing that any patient refusing a request to take the test would be referred to a specialized AIDS unit or could be treated as if infected. In both cases health workers would be

given indemnity against legal action for discrimination. The policy does not support compulsory AIDS testing for all hospital patients. It does, however, support compulsory testing for prisoners entering and leaving jail, all refugees, and intending migrants. If returned to power the Opposition will endeavor to "streamline AIDS organisations and advisory bodies to overcome the present problem of having too many committees wanting to have an input on every decision" (*The Australian*, 16 June 1989, p. 5).

53. R. Klein, *The Politics of the National Health Service* (New York: Longman, 1983), p. 57.

54. Ibid., p. 105.

55. See Ian Marsh, "Politics, Policy Making and Pressure Groups: Some Suggestions for Reform of the Australian Political System," *Australian Journal of Public Administration* XLII, no. 4 (1983): 434.

56. *AIDS: A Time to Care, a Time to Act. Towards a Strategy for Australians* (Canberra: AGPS, 1988).

57. Ibid., p. 3.

58. Ibid., p. 88.

59. C. Ward, "Towards a National AIDS Policy," *Bulletin of the Legal Service* 14, no. 2 (1989): 63–65.

60. In March 1989 an array of medical associations decided to sponsor an AIDS summit to assert doctors' rights in the treatment of HIV infection. Because "so called AIDS-experts and others with no background in medical science [are trying to] downplay the risk to health workers [we need] a forum, one that's not dominated by the Government, homosexuals, or AIDS experts," said an AMA spokesman (*The Australian*, 9 March 1989, p. 1). The conference was attended by more than 100 surgeons and other health care workers. It was planned by doctors as a test of the federal government's management of the AIDS epidemic. A key speaker at the meeting, the surgeon Lorraine Day from San Francisco, caught the mass media's attention with a strong, alarmist call for the testing of all patients in surgery, regardless of their wishes. The conference was dominated by claims that the government had placed too much emphasis on the civil rights of AIDS patients and high-risk groups and not enough on traditional public health measures, especially routine testing. However, the fact that the constituent groups of the AMA are embroiled in a more general power struggle entails that the association's stance on AIDS is not either monolithic or unequivocal. So, while the conservative faction headed by Bruce Shepherd called for compulsory testing, it was out-maneuvered by the moderates and the call was rejected. A further point of division among doctors is on making heroin legally available, an issue with obvious implications for the management of AIDS among ivdus and one which is expected to be considered at the next AMA summit. The coming conference will be sponsored and financed by Shepherd's organization, the Australian Doctors Fund.

61. The Government Working Party on AIDS will formulate the White Paper on AIDS policy on the basis of the six consultation papers released by the individual panels in May 1989. The panels recommended that:

• homosexuality, prostitution, and possession of drugs for personal use be decriminalized.

• information on HIV infection be covered by privacy laws.

• discrimination on the basis of HIV infection be outlawed except to protect public health.

- testing be available to everyone at high risk.
- mass compulsory screening for HIV of the general population not be carried out.
- funding be provided to all community AIDS organizations in each state, with uniform funding guidelines for people affected by HIV disease.
- a national conference for Aboriginal AIDS workers be held.
- a needle and syringe exchange program be set up in all states.
- methadone programs be set up in all states.
- the federal government review laws relating to censorship and broadcasting standards to remove any "unreasonable impediments to education and prevention programs and to ensure the promotion of such programs in a non-discriminatory manner."
- the Commonwealth exercise the option of amending the Broadcasting Act (1942) to require the licensees of television and radio stations to broadcast HIV advertisements at no cost during periods determined by the Australian Broadcasting Tribunal.

62. *Sydney Morning Herald,* 9 May 1989, p. 10.

63. *The Age,* 11 May 1989, p. 2.

64. These new proposals have been stimulated by the panel's recommendations or derive from the individual states launching their own solutions to the AIDS issue. The NSW Council of Churches, for example, has criticized the AIDS campaign as "promoting homosexuality, promiscuity and intravenous drug use by not adopting a moral stance" (*Sydney Morning Herald,* 24 April 1989, p. 5); the leading agency in the field of drug rehabilitation, the James McGrath Foundation, is opposed to any legalization of heroin; and health workers such as nurses are providing an increasingly audible and independent voice in debate. The states too appear to be acting on their own initiative more frequently. A new law has been introduced in Western Australia to provide for the quarantining by house arrest of anyone caught knowingly spreading AIDS; and the Queensland state government has recommended premarital testing as well as the testing of all patients from high-risk groups without their consent and of all prisoners at their release.

65. For two case studies of disaster management see Neil Britton, "An Appraisal of Australia's Disaster Management System Following the Ash Wednesday Bushfires in Victoria, 1983," *Australian Journal of Public Administration* 45, no. 2 (1986): 112–127; Lynne Chatterton and Brian Chatterton, "Drought: The Problems of Policy Implementation in a Crisis," in S. Encel, P. Wilenski, and B. Schaffer, eds., *Case Studies in Australian Public Policy* (Melbourne: Longman, 1981).

66. Brett Tindall, "Fourth International Conference on AIDS," *Medical Journal of Australia* 150, no. 2 (1989): 87–92.

AIDS, Development, and the Limitations of the African State

Constructing an adequate understanding of the AIDS epidemic in Africa depends on whether one is prone to taking the short or long view regarding the course of infectious diseases and their relationship to human society. The short view, and the one most discussed in the literature on AIDS, begins with the formal recognition of the disease by medicine, then moves forward to document its specific clinical manifestations and direct effects, and backwards to trace the natural history of the pathogen.

The longer view begins at the same point but tries to situate the present disease within the broad historical, social, ecological, cultural, and political relationships that mediate humanity, sickness, and the environment.[1] Both views are necessary if we are to understand how the epidemic will project itself into the complex web of social interdependencies and potentialities that characterize specific nations, and more generally, how the presence of the disease will mark the future direction of human society.[2] Consequently, both views are also essential to the question I now wish to raise, namely, under what constraints do African states labor in their attempts to halt the spread of this epidemic? Addressing this question is critical if we are to develop a realistic assessment of the present and future effectiveness of AIDS prevention and treatment strategies and policies of these nations.

The building of a deeper analysis of AIDS and its amenability to the efforts of African states requires the pursuit of a number of issues. This chapter will focus on the relations between AIDS and patterns of development and underdevelopment in Africa, and the related limitations both impose upon African states, and, conversely, those imposed by these states on AIDS prevention and treatment efforts. It is my intent to inquire into the extent to which AIDS conspires with local conditions and the modern African state to place obstacles to its eradication.

The emphasis on development necessitates excluding the consideration of a number of other important issues such as the effect on state action of civil war and rebellion (Uganda, Sudan, Angola, South Africa, for example), the large number of refugees in many of these nations, and the cross-cultural problems associated with prevention, surveillance, diagnosis, and treatment efforts in multitribal societies. Yet these issues must be examined as well, and it is hoped that research into the social consequences of the epidemic will continue to expand in these areas.

DIMENSIONS OF THE EPIDEMIC IN AFRICA

The biological history of AIDS in Africa has only recently started to emerge. Serologic studies of stored blood now locate the earliest known entry of the human immunodeficiency virus type 1 (HIV–1) into the African population as occurring in Zaire in 1959.[3] Retrospective AIDS diagnoses of Africans in Europe, and increases in AIDS indicator diseases (cryptococcal meningitis, chronic diarrhea, generalized Kaposi's sarcoma) in Central Africa, have dated the growth of HIV–1 infection since the mid- to late 1970s.[4] Yet despite this early entry of the AIDS virus into the continent, the possibility that HIV was infecting Africans was not recognized until 1983 when European doctors reported AIDS-like illnesses in their African patients.[5] Further research initiated by Western scientists on individuals with similar symptoms and immunologic problems in Rwanda and Zaire, along with the subsequent isolation of the AIDS virus by Montagnier and Gallo and availability of antibody screening procedures, made it finally possible to confirm that Africans were indeed infected with the same or a similar virus affecting those in the West.[6]

According to the World Health Organization (WHO), of the fifty-one countries on the African continent providing data on persons diagnosed with AIDS, forty-five have reported at least one or more persons, resulting in a cumulative total of 14,939 persons with AIDS.[7] (See Table 10.1.) Although they are important, these numbers reflect little of the whole story. They are severely compromised by problems of appropriate diagnosis, inadequate laboratory facilities (quality control, trained personnel), inaccurate record keeping, political manipulation, and government recalcitrance. They also do not reflect those suffering from AIDS who have never been in contact with official medicine.[8] Even Jonathan Mann, director of WHO's Global Program on AIDS, suspects that the underreporting of AIDS is "huge."[9] Others have estimated that as many as 50,000 to several hundred thousand lives may have already been lost to AIDS in Central Africa, and that 1 million Africans may die of AIDS in the next decade.[10]

The question of the prevalence of HIV–1 infection is even more difficult

Table 10.1
Africa: Nations Reporting over 100 Cumulative AIDS Cases 1988

Country	Cumulative Aids Cases
Burundi	1408
Central African Republic	432
Congo	1250
Cote D'Ivoire	250
Ghana	145
Kenya	2097
Malawi	583
Rwanda	987
Senegal	131
South Africa	120
Tanzania	1608
Uganda	4006
Zaire	335
Zambia	993
Zimbabwe	119
	14,464

Source: World Health Organization, August 1988.

to assess, with figures varying widely from two, to five, to "several million" persons possibly already carrying the virus in Central Africa. These figures are variously interpreted based upon the results of a host of small sample studies of HIV–1 infection in specific African countries and in specific target populations.[11]

With such wide-ranging figures, a vocal skepticism surrounding the production of these numbers can be heard. There are those who contest these rather startling estimates and the methods by which they are calculated. They argue that for a number of reasons—from erroneous blood tests to political manipulation—these statistics are at worst highly exaggerated or, at best, misleading.[12] In addition to these criticisms, future projections of

AIDS in Africa, it is contended, must be tempered by recent research from the respected SIDA Project in Zaire, which has produced some evidence suggesting that the rate of infection may be leveling off in certain areas of Zaire and Zambia.[13]

The issue of numbers is further complicated by the discovery of HIV–2 in West Africa, and its subsequent isolation in Africans with AIDS and ARC.[14] The clinical expression of this related virus and its prevalence have yet to be determined, but the ramifications of this discovery for disease surveillance, diagnosis, blood screening, and vaccine development should not be underestimated.

While all the major infection patterns associated with AIDS can be found on the continent of Africa, it is by now well known that patterns of HIV–1 transmission, as well as the population affected, differ in Central and Eastern Africa (those areas most affected) from those patterns associated with the epidemic in the West.[15] AIDS in this part of the world is a predominantly heterosexually transmitted disease equally distributed among men and women. But, as in the West, over 90 percent of those who are dying from AIDS are between the ages of 20 and 49, with the highest number of infected persons in Africa being between the ages of 16 and 29.[16]

Susceptibility to infection through sexual transmission seems to be facilitated by the presence of genital ulcers, other sexually transmitted diseases, and chronically activated immune systems made so by constant subjection to other infections.[17] Infection has also occurred, although how much is still debatable, through the transfusion of contaminated blood and through the use of nonsterile needles and syringes. This form of transmission is not based on illegal IV drug use as in the West, but occurs both in legitimate medical facilities that lack supplies and trained personnel and through the proliferation of injections offered by local healers outside the official medicine.[18]

Fear has also been expressed that traditional communal practices and rituals associated with scarification, circumcision, and removal of the clitoris may also lead to HIV infection. None of these practices as of this date, however, has been indicated by field research to have actually increased transmission of the virus.[19]

The rising numbers of children being infected through perinatal transmission of HIV is also of much concern. In some parts of Central and East Africa between 2 and 15 percent of pregnant woman are seropositive for HIV. Up to half of the children born to these women will be infected.[20] In Zambia, for example, there may have been as many as 6,000 children infected with HIV during 1987.[21] In addition, there is some evidence of the possibility of children being exposed to the virus through the use of unsterile instruments in critical child immunization programs, and through the transfusing of contaminated blood to children with malaria-related anemia.[22]

Among African nations the incidence of HIV–1 infection is mostly centered in urban areas, with high prevalence in cities such as Kinshasa and Kigali. For example, research indicates a tenfold increase in HIV infection among pregnant women in Kinshasa from 1970 to 1980. However, HIV infection is seemingly rare, or of low prevalence, in rural Zaire, Rwanda, and Kenya.[23] The exception to this generalization is, of course, in the rural regions of western Tanzania and southwestern Uganda surrounding Lake Victoria, where AIDS has been repeatedly documented. The predominance of AIDS in the cities may change. As some have argued, the risk of wide-spread diffusion of HIV infection to those rural towns and villages located near truck routes, railways, lakes, and rivers is very real.[24]

DEVELOPMENT, DISEASE, AND AIDS

The relationship between social and economic development and the health and illness of a population is a complex one. What are the connections between the real and potential effects of the AIDS epidemic on the course of development within African nations, and, turning the question around, what are the effects of development and underdevelopment on the course of the AIDS epidemic in Africa? The former question requires an under-standing of the interdependence of health and important forms of social and economic activity, while the latter forces a historical analysis of how social, political, and economic activity has contributed to the current con-struction of health and illness.

As noted, the numbers tell little of the real story. Most of the concern over AIDS and development in Africa surrounds the social and economic consequences of the losses associated with those segments of the population being infected with HIV. Some worry that the rising incidence of pediatric AIDS threatens to seed future generations of Africans with the AIDS virus in addition to diminishing recent gains made in child survival.[25] Others are fearful of the more immediate effect that AIDS is having on the urban educated elite and those who constitute Africa's skilled labor.[26]

In many African cities, physicians are seeing persons with HIV infection who represent a wide spectrum of the bureaucratic, professional, and tech-nical workers who go to make up Africa's middle classes.[27] Premature deaths in these groups due to AIDS are having, and will have, enormous ramifi-cations for all members of those societies. By 1990 the collective loss from these deaths in Tanzania, Uganda, Central African Republic, Rwanda, Bu-rundi, Zambia, and Zaire could rise to almost a billion dollars. By 1995 these deaths in Zaire may account for an annual loss of 8 percent ($350 million) of that country's GNP.[28]

Depending on the future course of the epidemic in Africa, the loss of productive power portends only to become greater. Besides the impact on skilled labor, the ongoing health and other costs associated with AIDS will loom as an ever increasing threat to the livelihood of those still in the job market. Compared to the low annual per capita amount spent on health in African nations ($5 average), the costs of treating persons with AIDS are overwhelming. In Zaire the direct cost of treatment for persons with symptoms of AIDS ranges from a minimum of $132 to more than $1,500. The cost of just one hospitalization episode in Zaire for AIDS is more than three times the average monthly income.[29]

Despite what one may think about the low financial priority given to health programs in African countries, it is clear that these costs, and those that are projected, will have some serious effects. First, it must be remembered that much of the cost of health care in these African nations is underwritten by employers. In Zambia mining industry employers are already "alarmed" at the impact of the rising cost of sick pay and its effect on profits and competitiveness. This industry alone accounts for 20 percent of that nation's GNP, and mining employers are already considering screening their workers and future hires for HIV.[30]

Second, these increased costs associated with AIDS must be seen within an environment of mounting national debt—the African international debt is some $200 billion—declining national incomes, and a general retreat in foreign assistance programs.[31] For those countries dependent on tourism for their critical supply of foreign exchange, the epidemic has made the volatile and fragile nature of this business even more apparent in view of its negative impact on tourist revenues.[32] Given these circumstances, the AIDS epidemic in Africa provides one more reason for those with capital, foreign or domestic, to look elsewhere when investing their resources, when traveling, or when contemplating starting up new industries.[33]

Besides the impact the AIDS epidemic may have on industrial development, there are potential consequences for agricultural development as well. If the epidemic does continue to follow market routes into the rural areas, and does so to the extent that many fear, then it may pose a serious threat to food production. The economies of many African countries are tied to the capacity of local farming to feed the population. In both Zimbabwe and Kenya, 80 percent of the gross domestic product comes from the agricultural sector.[34] The loss of large numbers of the young adults upon which these nations depend for farming labor could mean even more disastrous food shortages in the future.

From this brief description it is clear that the AIDS epidemic confronts African states with a challenge that they are ill equipped to take on, and with potential social and economic consequences of devastating proportions. But as important to our understanding of AIDS as these effects are, there is still the question of how the process of development or, depending on one's point of view, the underdevelopment of African states has affected the course of the epidemic.

Any discussion of this question must begin by addressing how the pattern of Western colonial development in Africa has carved its legacy into the bodies of Africans. By this we mean that the health and sickness of Africans is still mediated in very powerful ways by the effects of Western colonization. These effects have taken three historical forms: the introduction of new pathogens by Westerners into African populations with little or no previous immunological experience of their effects; the creation of sickness-producing social formations in Africa as a product of colonialist development and expropriation of African resources; and the disruption of the fragile evolutionary balance among culture, environment, pathogenic organisms, and the human immune system through land use policies and displacement of indigenous populations.

As Westerners began to colonize Eastern and Southern Africa during the eighteenth and nineteenth centuries, many African communities were decimated from the repeated and combined effects of diseases brought in by foreigners that were either unknown to Africans or that had previously been kept in check through limited contact between Africans and the West. Sicknesses such as measles, smallpox, cholera, influenza, tuberculosis, whooping cough, and polio took a heavy toll on populations that had little prior immunity. Western history of the colonization of Africa, in contrast, emphasizes the impact of diseases, such as malaria, that resulted in the deaths of many European settlers and soldiers. Within the European experience, Africa became known as the "white man's grave" and a "dark" and "disease ridden" continent.[35]

The politics and struggle that emerged out of Western colonialist development, and that surround these two very different ways of experiencing disease in Africa, have been infused into the AIDS epidemic. The controversial "African origin" theory of AIDS, which became popular in the West in late 1985 (and which continues to be taken as fact in the face of significant challenges, and whose believers dismiss African notions that it is the West that has seeded AIDS in Africa), reflects a one-sided version of AIDS history. The adverse reactions in Africa over this theory are not so much over any controversy about the inherent benefit of establishing the scientific location or place of origin of the epidemic, but are a consequence of the battle between African sensitivities over the historic injuries sustained at the hands of the West, and the continuing self-serving and myopic image that the West has of its own role in the eradication of disease on that continent. The hostility of Africans over this issue and others related to AIDS is a mark of this deep and ongoing struggle against the effects of colonial and neocolonial subjugation.

Charles Hunt argues that the demographic and clinical picture of AIDS in Africa varies from that in the West precisely because of the different social, political, cultural, and historical environments within which the AIDS virus (and the epidemic) in Africa must find its expression.[36] Hunt writes that the dominant reality of that environment is determined by the historic relations of dependency between Africa and the West, the effects of that dependency on the health of Africans, and, in particular, how the West has forced upon Africans catastrophic changes in social, cultural, and economic life that have upset the fragile evolutionary balance between disease and African society.

For example, it should be recognized that the forms of labor market organization and rural agricultural development historically imposed upon Africans by colonialists have largely dictated the course of this disease.[37] The emergence of centers of colonialist production such as plantations, mines, and railroads, required the drafting of large numbers of laborers from rural areas. The conditions under which these Africans worked, the low wages they were paid, the crowded and unsanitary towns and cities in which they lived and that were spawned by these enterprises, and the predominantly male migrant workforce far from family and cultural life—all had disastrous effects on the health of African society. As more of the land was expropriated by Westerners, or abandoned by Africans for lack of sufficient labor power, many Africans were forced to emigrate to those towns and cities where conditions affecting their health were even more threatening. This reconstitution of African social life as a result of the imposition of Western economic demands, and its negative effects on families and cultural bonds, produced dramatic rises both in prostitution and in the spread of sexually transmitted diseases now typical of African cities.[38] This is the African environment into which the AIDS virus has been introduced. Thus it is critical for our understanding of AIDS in Africa that we appreciate the effects that this historical production of persons highly vulnerable to disease has, and will continue to have, on the course of this virus.

It is also from this historical long view that we must frame our understanding of the relation of African poverty to AIDS, as well as the chronic underdevelopment of health resources (and its effects on the epidemic), and most important, the particular historical role of the African states in the development and perpetuation of these conditions.

As the epidemic moves more directly into the African underclass, among those who are illiterate, far from the reach of media campaigns and health agencies, chronically malnourished, ill, and too poor to purchase condoms, the ability of AIDS prevention efforts to make a difference is even more radically constrained. Moreover, as African states continue to underfund health services, even basic blood screening is highly limited; therefore the most effective technical response to the epidemic, that of ensuring uncontaminated blood, is denied to Africans. And to the extent that the state participates in the widening of class divisions and has a vested interest in current economic, political, and social conditions that support the dominant classes—the formation of which are rooted in colonial history—the more obstacles there are that block the efforts of those who want to address the more fundamental social "causes" and ramifications of the AIDS epidemic.

Finally, there is one more sense in which this history of development has had an effect on the epidemic. If we look at the history of malaria in Africa, we find that Western-imposed development disturbed long-standing patterns of both inherited and acquired biological immune responses to malaria, responses that emerged over years of repeated exposure and eventual adaptation to the disease. Just as important to the rise of malaria was the destruction of cultural traditions that in one way or another reduced exposure to the mosquito vector.[39] The major population shifts resulting from the colonial policies previously mentioned often had the effect of reducing individual adaptation to this disease by radically interrupting the repeated infection necessary to maintain immune resistance. This process thus set the stage for a more severe episode with malaria when the individual was reexposed, but, more important, this immune deficit was passed on to descendants who are now unable to share in the benefits of collective immunity developed by previous generations.

In addition, through the expansion of agricultural production, as well as the consequent forcing of African herding activities into those geographic areas traditionally avoided because of their association with disease and its vector, many African communities and tribes experienced dramatic increases in malaria transmission.[40] Similarly, when Africans died from the smallpox brought by the Europeans, some communities were so hard hit that agricultural practices associated with keeping tsetse fly exposure and infection at a tolerable rate could not be maintained.[41]

With regard to the AIDS epidemic, there is some evidence to suggest that the social dislocation already discussed has exacerbated the epidemic by upsetting naturally occurring adaptation to HIV. In relatively isolated rural areas in Zaire research indicates that low HIV prevalence has been stable for at least the last ten years.[42] This is in high contrast to the tenfold increase of HIV infection in Kinshasa over that same period.[43] Those who were seropositive in this research were likely to have previously lived outside the area, usually in Kinshasa or local trading centers. It may be, as these researchers speculate, that "AIDS could have existed and remained stable in rural areas of Africa for a long period," and that the "disruption of traditional life styles and the social and behavioral changes that accompany urbanization may be important factors in the spread of AIDS in central Africa."[44] We would only add that "urbanization," far from being some sort of naturally occurring and essentially neutral or progressive phenomenon, as implied by these researchers, is a specific political/historical process shaped by Western colonial and postcolonial policies, which continue to influence negatively the health and welfare of many Africans.

THE LIMITATIONS OF THE STATE

Current AIDS programs in Africa, and here we are mostly concerned with Central and Eastern Africa, are predominantly the product of international urging and intervention. For example, through the work of the WHO, $19 million has been pledged by donor countries to a five-year AIDS control program for the nations of Rwanda, Ethiopia, Kenya, Tanzania, and Uganda.[45] Efforts to expand this program to other countries in the area are also under way. Within the WHO's agenda these programs are designed to help these governments develop national plans, help develop programs that teach people how to prevent the spread of further infection, and support the research necessary to expand the knowledge base about the epidemic. The WHO has been quite successful in these preliminary strategies, but the real success of these programs depends on the will and ability of African states to act.

As suggested by the discussion on AIDS and development, the forces acting upon the spread of this disease may be larger or more intractable than is suggested by the short view of the epidemic. In the context of mass poverty, chronic disease, and limited health services, AIDS acts in a way that magnifies, and is itself magnified by, these conditions. While similar to other diseases, AIDS differs from many in terms of its fatal consequences, in its particular targets, and in its consequences for the exacerbation of other diseases. In terms of whom it targets—at present the African middle class—AIDS destroys the forces that would lead the fight against its spread: those teachers, community opinion leaders, and members of the educated elites who would be the most effective vanguard in the prevention process. In addition, because HIV infection destroys human immune capabilities, those who are infected have less resistance to other illnesses. For example, the growth of incidence of tuberculosis as a result of HIV infection is remarkable within these African states.[46]

With the care of these persons limited to diagnosis and minimal palliative treatment, and the cure nowhere in sight, options for state action are restricted. While some of the needs in prevention are ones that are determinable, technical, or fixed (albeit costly) by nature—such as the screening of blood—and thus in theory at least doable, many of those tasks charged to the state have to do with the very difficult and open-ended problem of preventing AIDS through changing sexual behavior. This is a task, one should add, that often lacks a clear focus and concrete modes of delivery and evaluation, especially within the African context.

Thus the nature of the epidemic, even outside its mediation by underdevelopment, poses for the state the kind of dilemma it may be least suited to undertake. It is forced to pursue the modification of behavior at highly individuated and intimate levels, levels at which it has least authority, legitimacy, and capacity to influence, and which have traditionally, in the case of sexual behavior, been the most difficult areas of human life to script en masse. One can argue that this state scripting of sexuality is more likely to be successful in the West, where more and more areas of human life are being bureaucratized and subjected to the homogenizing impact of the mass media and the detailed surveillance apparatus of modern disciplinary structures. In many of the countries in Africa that we are discussing, these panoptic structures of modernity are either only in embryonic form or nonexistent.[47]

There are also areas of prevention dictated by the course of the disease which may, if pursued, conflict with major legitimation strategies and policies of these new African states. For example, almost all of the African state boundaries established during the colonial era cross tribal constellations, and include within those boundaries numerous tribal, linguistically diverse, and sometimes hostile groups. Within this context, the process of state formation demands the internalization of the new "civic" order as opposed to the tribal order as a way of building loyalty to the state and its emerging elites. For these new states in particular this process of shifting identifications has been described as the "indigenization of the state through the promotion of a generic culture."[48] The politics of this antitribalist indoctrination includes the appropriation, commodification, or destruction of the symbols and practices representative of the tribal cosmology and authority. It has also meant the active suppression of those who articulate or support tribal solidarity.[49]

This state legitimation strategy has the potential to undermine AIDS prevention efforts that stress involvement with the authority structures of tribal communities. Those programs that attempt to use locally preferred leadership as an entry point into the understanding and changing of sexual behavior run the risk of challenging state authority. All of this depends upon the particulars of specific countries, of course. Kenya has an active antitribalist policy and appears to be focusing its AIDS messages within the two official state languages of English and Swahili.[50] Thus its AIDS programs reinforce state power as it is acted out in its cultural policy, which mitigates against indigenous tribal identifications. The closer prevention programs move to more local ways of speaking about sexuality, as well as to grassroots understandings of health and illness that are affiliated with tribal traditions and leadership authority, the closer those programs come to direct conflict with broader state objectives.

In Uganda, the situation is so desperate, the government so in need of assistance as a result of both the extent of the epidemic and the long history of bloodshed from civil war, that tribal identifications are still part of official state discourse. This is shown in the AIDS campaign where posters present the message "Love Carefully" in the twenty-two languages that make up the linguistic and tribal mix of that country.[51]

The ability of African states to act on AIDS is shaped not only by the different patterns of the disease itself but also because of the specific local conditions with which both the epidemic and the machinery of the state are situated. By this we mean that the current and future spread of the epidemic is mediated by the degree of urbanization and industrialization of the nation; the particular patterns of market exchange that integrate core and peripheral trading centers; the quality and density of transportation networks; the priority of health objectives within state resource allocations; the proliferation of the health service structures; the level of class and tribal conflict; the nature of the constituencies affected and politicized by the epidemic; the political particularities of how AIDS came to be known in the country; and specific local events that have contributed to any and all of these dimensions. All of these factors, as they are influenced by patterns of development and the conditions of underdevelopment, either restrict or empower African state actions to deal with the epidemic.

But the possibilities for African states to act competently and compassionately in dealing with the AIDS epidemic are in the end compromised by the diminished roles Third World states can assume in the pursuit of their own interests. While it is not our intention to review contending theories of what constitutes the nature of the developing state, or the parameters of its possible actions in the modern world, it is important to be aware that the ability of African states effectively to address the domestic consequences of the epidemic is inextricably tied to their position in the international world capitalist economy. The binding of these states to this world economy in general has the impact of reducing the resources they have to bring to bear on the epidemic. The commitments of these states to the payment of international debt, including that administered by the International Monetary Fund, are viewed as a priority over AIDS, given the consequences of nonpayment for the overall viability of African states to attract needed credit and capital. Yet that commitment has historically restricted the capacity of these states to inject needed monies into meeting their own broad domestic needs, especially those related to health. The repayment and servicing of these debts can take as much as 50 percent of the capital sorely needed for welfare and health of local populations.[52] Unfortunately AIDS has hit those countries in Central Africa that are most in debt to the West.

In a twist to this theme, the Congress of the United States in the recently passed Foreign Assistance Act is denying new assistance to countries that are late in paying on loans from the U.S. government. This includes monies from the U.S. Agency for International Development, which is the agency handling U.S. AIDS assistance to Africa. Defaults on U.S. loans by countries such as Tanzania could result in the severance of critical supplies and funds for AIDS.[53]

Further, in the very complex and dense network of connections of these states and their elites to large multinational corporations, we often find these states responding more to the needs of corporations for markets than to the deprivations of their populations. As we have argued elsewhere, the historical expansion of Western medical markets in Africa has often led to inappropriate allocation of scarce resources by these states to the health care sectors with limited impact on the health of the vast majority of citizens. The development of urban hospitals and the purchasing of expensive management services, drugs, and medical supplies have often tended to favor the capital accumulation desires of corporations at the expense of real strategies against disease and the effects of injury.[54]

The AIDS epidemic, with its expensive testing routines, high-cost medications like AZT, and wide-ranging treatment requirements, has set the stage for the corporate battle over the AIDS dollars coming from donor countries. Some have already expressed fears on how the importing of AIDS-related supplies, equipment, and drugs will affect the deteriorating balance of trade in African countries.[55]

AIDS IN KENYA

In several respects the AIDS epidemic in Kenya reflects many of the political dynamics discussed above. Kenya's 22 million people have experienced the damaging effects of British colonialism as well as the problems associated with independence. But Kenya's reputation is that of an African success story, a nation now on the road to modernization with assistance from the West. Or so it would seem.

The first case of AIDS in Kenya was reported in 1983. Kenya's National AIDS Committee was formed in the autumn of 1985, and in November of that year Kenya became the first African nation to report its AIDS cases to WHO. The accuracy of those reports, however, resulting from both the practical problems of diagnosing HIV and probable government tampering with the numbers, continues to be called into question.[56] Guidelines on the disease were issued to senior doctors in Nairobi by the Ministry of Health in late January 1986.[57]

In February 1987, the Ministry announced that by March Kenya would become the first African nation to screen all of its blood supply for the AIDS virus.[58] Later press reports argued that Kenya had only eight labs to perform this testing and thus no real capacity or "adequate facilities to screen blood for HIV."[59] In January 1988, Kenya made AIDS a reportable disease and began an effort to require doctors and nurses to send the names and addresses of their patients with AIDS to the Ministry of Health.[60]

Most of the activities over AIDS in Kenya are the result of both the WHO AIDS prevention and control program in that area, and the efforts of major nongovernmental organizations (NGOs). As indicated earlier, Kenya was one of the first African countries to be enlisted into the WHO's five-year program along with Rwanda, Ethiopia, Tanzania, and Uganda. As a result of several meetings of donor agencies held under WHO auspices in 1987, Kenya launched its anti-AIDS campaign with U.S. $2.94 million in pledges as well as a request for U.S. $11.32 million over the next four years.[61] Over half of its first-year budget is reported to be allocated to testing kits and the training of laboratory technicians.[62] Under this program, Kenya has completed a medium-term plan for AIDS control and prevention and has signed technical services agreements.[63]

AIDS activities under the program and in cooperation with NGOs such as the Kenyan Red Cross Society have primarily focused on mass education. This includes brief radio programs, the production of a thirty-minute film, and the distribution of 700,000 leaflets, 9,000 booklets, and 20,000 posters (in both Swahili and English).[64] AIDS education is also incorporated into government-sponsored family planning and maternal/child health programs.

One of the most publicized efforts in Kenya has to do with the education of prostitutes on AIDS and condom use. This well-documented and well-researched program to reduce risk behaviors in Nairobi prostitutes, sponsored by the Kenya Medical Research Institute, the University of Nairobi, and others, has shown demonstrable increases in condom use when education is provided through culturally relevant modalities (one-to-one counseling, *barazas*, skits, singing) and the distribution of free condoms.[65]

All of these efforts in AIDS prevention and control are commendable, especially in the light of Kenya's own colonial legacy, which is still heavily inscribed in the country's political and social life and its health care structure. Colonial Kenya experienced the same major shifts of population described earlier with the development of its agricultural and industrial sectors. Nairobi, for example, grew "from a few Europeans living in tents and corrugated iron buildings in 1899, to a multiracial city of 20,000 by 1920."[66] Other cities in Kenya have also experienced rapid growth, especially after the 1940s.

As early as 1911, males in Nairobi outnumbered females by six to one. With the subsequent emergence of prostitution in this new environment, venereal syphilis began to spread rapidly. Furthermore, the intervention of colonial health authorities in the 1920s and 1930s often led not to the prevention of this disease but to its rapid spread.[67]

While post-independence Kenya is less subjected to mass migration and its effects, the enormous prostitution trade, the heavy travel of workers between rural and urban areas, and the high levels of unemployment speak to Kenya's colonial inheritance, its impact on access to health care, and the particular form of the epidemic it is experiencing. Government investment in health is generally low in Kenya, and although health officials are still not convinced that AIDS is a high priority, foreign money attached to AIDS assistance programs has stirred some official interest.

One must remember, however, that church-based services still form a large part of the health care sector. Thirty percent of all hospital beds are church-supported, as are hundreds of health facilities that serve the rural areas.[68] These organizations are often rooted in colonial traditions and bring their Western morality baggage with them. So while these organizations offer much potential for fighting AIDS, they also present formidable barriers to AIDS prevention efforts.[69]

Finally, the hostility of Kenya's own leadership to reports or criticisms on its problems with AIDS reflects the subtext of historical struggle with the West alluded to earlier.[70] Yet, we can also see in these reactions the use of the epidemic as a device to consolidate the power of local elites through the invoking of this long-standing animosity between Africa and the West. It must also be said that Kenya's poor human rights record testifies to the willingness of this elite to sacrifice the well-being of its people for political gain.[71] Thus, while the forcing of AIDS prevention efforts through this historical gauntlet does little to halt the disease, to ignore the effects of these power relations on the course of the epidemic may undermine the value of even the most well-designed prevention program.

OBSERVATIONS

As I have indicated, the limitations of the African state in dealing with the AIDS epidemic have to do with the nature of the disease, the particular social, political, and economic conditions of the states involved, and the modern situation of Third World states as they exist within the world economy. The seriousness of these limitations is relative to the strategies and goals sought after and the means by which they are to be achieved. For example, tasks the state is better placed to accomplish may be those that require centralized and standardized operations and that are compatible with Western technology that is already available (such as in the screening of blood). Other work, as in the education of individuals in safer sexual behavior, may be better accomplished by diverse, private, and more local constellations of groups, organizations, and those in the ranks of tribal leadership.

One difficulty with this approach, of course, is that the absence of a vocal and politically active AIDS constituency that incorporates within it the voice of persons with AIDS—an absence that is characteristic of these states—deprives the state of the kind of political incentive to move on AIDS that local pressure groups can provide. Further, these states are also in desperate need of the leadership and energy those groups frequently offer. Without this resource the state must then become all things to all people, which in practical terms is an impossible responsibility. Yet, if the state perceives these private initiatives as a threat to its own legitimacy for reasons we have already mentioned, the success of these efforts, and consequently the success of the entire AIDS prevention and control effort, is in jeopardy.

In sum, the combination of state formation in Africa, the international context of state development, and the legacy of colonialism conspire on a number of levels both to exacerbate the epidemic and to restrict the ability of the state to respond. Further, the nature of the disease itself, its magnifying effect on other illnesses, its particular contribution to the deterioration of social and economic relations, and the difficult strategies it requires for prevention, situate the African state in an arena of action in which it is least competent. The crisis that this situation presents should not discourage those involved in AIDS control and treatment efforts. It does demand, however, that serious consideration be given to the broad political dimensions that the epidemic draws out, and that have historically compromised the health of all Africans.

NOTES

1. One example of a text taking the long view is A. Brandt's *No Magic Bullet* (New York: Oxford University Press, 1985).

2. AIDS has become an object of concern for futurists as well as historians. See for example J. Platt, "AIDS and the Year 2000," *The Futurist*, Fall 1987, pp. 9–17.

3. See discussion in P. Piot et al., "AIDS: An International Perspective," *Science* 239 (1988): 574.

4. Ibid.

5. N. Clumeck et al., "Acquired Immune Deficiency Syndrome in Black Africans," *The Lancet* I (19 March 1983): 642; N. Clumeck et al., "Acquired Immune Deficiency Syndrome in African Patients," *New England Journal of Medicine* 310 (23 February 1984): 492–497.

6. See P. Van de Perre et al., "Acquired Immune Deficiency Syndrome in Rwanda," *The Lancet* 2 (14 July 1984): 62–65; P. Piot et al., "Acquired Immunodeficiency Syndrome in a Heterosexual Population in Zaire," *The Lancet* 2 (14 July 1984): 65–69; R. J. Biggar, "The AIDS Problem in Africa," *The Lancet* 1 (11 January 1986): 79–83.

7. World Health Organization, August 1988.

8. See, for example, A. Fortin, "The Politics of AIDS in Kenya," *Third World Quarterly*, July 1987, pp. 906–919.

9. United Press International, 15 February 1987.

10. See *Newsweek*, 11 November 1986; *Time*, 16 February 1987; Panos Dossier No. 1, *AIDS and the Third World* (London: Panos Institute, March 1987), p. 35; J. Mann et al., "The International Epidemiology of AIDS," *Scientific American*, October 1988, p. 85.

11. Ibid.

12. See F. Konotey-Ahulu, "AIDS in Africa: Misinformation and Disinformation," *The Lancet* 2 (1987): 206–207; Wanume Kibedi, "AIDS and African Viewpoint," *Development Forum*, March 1987, p. 6. See also Biggar, "AIDS Problem in Africa," on early overestimation of HIV prevalence in Africa, p. 80.

13. *Washington Post*, 21 March 1988.

14. Piot et al., "AIDS: International Perspective," p. 577.

15. Ibid., p. 576.

16. Panos, *AIDS and Third World*, p. 40.

17. Piot et al., "AIDS: International Perspective," p. 574.

18. Ibid.; also Fortin, "Politics of AIDS in Kenya," pp. 914–919.

19. Mann et al., "International Epidemiology of AIDS," p. 85.

20. Piot et al., "AIDS: International Perspective," p. 575.

21. L. Heise, "AIDS: New Threat to the Third World," *World Watch*, January/February 1988, p. 24.

22. Ibid.; *New York Times*, 22 January 1988.

23. See discussion in N. Nzilambi et al., "The Prevalence of Infection with Human Immunodeficiency Virus over a Ten-Year Period in Rural Zaire," *New England Journal of Medicine* 318 (1988): 276; Piot et al., "AIDS: International Perspective," p. 574.

24. W. Wood, "AIDS North and South: Diffusion Patterns of a Global Epidemic and a Research Agenda for Geographers," *Professional Geographer* 40, no. 3 (1988): 268.

25. Heise, "AIDS: New Threat," pp. 23–24; Mann, ". . . for a global challenge," *World Health*, March 1988, p. 6.

26. Panos, *AIDS and Third World*, p. 40.

27. *International Herald Tribune*, 23/24 January 1988.

28. Heise, "AIDS: New Threat," p. 25; Piot et al., "AIDS: International Perspective," p. 578.

29. *New Scientist*, 17 March 1988, p. 31.

30. Panos, *AIDS and Third World*, p. 41; *New Scientist*, 17 March 1988.

31. Panos, *AIDS and Third World*, p. 35. See also *New York Times*, 19 October 1987.

32. Panos, *AIDS and Third World*, p. 35. See also the report in the *Daily Nation* (Nairobi), 14 January 1987, on one Nairobi firm losing over $3 million in contracts with British travel agencies after the first news of AIDS in that country was first published in the international press.

33. See J. Tinker, "AIDS in Developing Countries," *Issues in Science and Technology*, Winter 1988, p. 45.

34. P. Epstein and R. Packard, "Ecology and Immunology," *Science for the People*, January/February 1987, p. 10.

35. Ibid.

36. C. Hunt, "Africa and AIDS: Dependent Development, Sexism and Racism," *Monthly Review*, February 1988, p. 12.

37. Ibid.

38. Ibid., p. 13.

39. Epstein and Packard, "Ecology and Immunology," p. 12.

40. Ibid.

41. *New Scientist*, 14 January 1988.

42. Nzilambi et al., "Prevalence of Infection."

43. Ibid., p. 278.

44. Ibid., pp. 278–279.

45. *UN Chronicle*, March 1988, p. 33.

46. Panos, *AIDS and Third World*, p. 9.

47. For a discussion of surveillance and modern disciplinary structures see Michel Foucault, *Discipline and Punish* (New York: Vintage, 1979).

48. J. Philibert, "The Politics of Tradition: Towards a Generic Culture in Vanuatu," *Mankind* 16, no. 1 (April 1986).

49. See Ngugi wa Thiong'o, *Detained: A Writer's Prison Diary* (London: Heinemann, 1981).

50. See Fortin, "Politics of AIDS in Kenya," p. 914.

51. Heise, "AIDS: New Threat," p. 22.

52. *New York Times,* 10 October 1987.

53. Section 518 of the Foreign Assistance Act (H.R. 4637) passed by the U.S. Congress in July 1988 reads: "No part of any appropriation contained in this act shall be used to furnish assistance to any country which is in default during a period in excess of one calendar year in payment to the United States of principal or interest on any loan made to such countries by the United States pursuant to program for which funds are appropriated under this Act."

54. A. Fortin, "AIDS and the Third World: The Politics of International Discourse," paper presented at the Fourteenth World Congress of the International Political Science Association, Washington, D.C., September 1988; see also L. Doyal, *The Political Economy of Health* (London: Pluto Press, 1979), pp. 270–271.

55. Heise, "AIDS: New Threat," p. 25.

56. Fortin, "Politics of AIDS in Kenya," pp. 911–912.

57. Ibid., p. 914.

58. *New York Times,* 24 February 1987.

59. *New Scientist,* 7 January 1988, p. 36.

60. Ibid., p. 37.

61. Ibid., p. 36.

62. Ibid.

63. Panos Institute, *AIDS and the Third World* (Philadelphia: New Society Publishers, 1989), p. 162.

64. *New Scientist,* 7 January 1988, p. 36; *New York Times,* 24 February 1987.

65. E. N. Ngugi et al., "Prevention of Transmission of Human Immunodeficiency Virus in Africa: Effectiveness of Condom Promotion and Health Education among Prostitutes," *Lancet* 2 (1988): 887–890.

66. Marc H. Dawson, "AIDS in Africa: Historical Roots," in Norman Miller and Richard C. Rockwell, eds., *AIDS in Africa: The Social and Policy Impact* (Lewiston, N.Y.: Edwin Mellen Press, 1988), pp. 58–59.

67. Ibid., pp. 59–60.

68. Edward H. Greeley, "The Role of Non-governmental Organizations in AIDS Prevention: Parallels to African Family Planning Activities," in Miller and Rockwell, *AIDS in Africa,* pp. 132–134.

69. Ibid., pp. 136–137.

70. For a summary of these reactions see generally Fortin, "Politics of AIDS in Kenya."

71. See, for example, *Kenya: Torture, Political Detention and Unfair Trials* (London: Amnesty International Publications, July 1987).

Barbara A. Misztal and David Moss

Conclusion

The preceding chapters compose an interim report on the ways in which the appearance and spread of HIV infection have been managed in its first decade. They range across societies with populations of between 9 million (Belgium) and 227 million (the United States), governed under authoritarian or liberal democratic political systems, offering different mixes of public and private responsibility in their systems of health care, and displaying wide contrasts in the social and cultural organization of sexual identity, drug use, and sudden death. Perhaps unsurprisingly, the various national accounts do not yield the materials for a rigorous comparison, not only because different dimensions and determinants of responses to AIDS have seemed important to their authors but also because much of the primary research that would license more refined conclusions has yet to be carried out or reported. Nevertheless, the very diversity of factors examined in the individual country discussions might be considered less a failure of editorial control than a vindication of the relativistic approach to AIDS that provided the initial impulse for this volume. Mere juxtaposition is certainly no substitute for controlled comparison; but at this stage of the epidemic the reverberations from the establishment of significant relationships linking knowledge, interests, and policy formation may be a more valuable sensitizing device for future analyses.

FACTORS SHAPING RESPONSES

By 1988 all countries covered in this book had created new institutions to advise on the problems presented by AIDS and had aimed education programs at the population at large. However, it is clear that at the national level, the formulation of overall strategies to manage AIDS has everywhere been cautious and generally slow. In France—at the forefront of scientific research on the virus—AIDS was not declared a "national cause" until 1987; the first direct government educational campaigns directed at individual households began in the United States and Italy only in 1988; and Australia was still in the throes of devising a national strategy. At the subnational levels of region, state, and municipality, of course, many proposals had been made and often implemented by public authorities. But the symbolic power and practical range offered by national political initiatives had been used sparingly as governments grappled with public discussion and justification of strategies dealing with hitherto largely taboo issues.

Governmental inaction has largely been judged either as justified caution in the face of scientific uncertainty over an entirely unexpected infectious epidemic or as the deliberate refusal to address a health problem initially affecting mainly marginal and widely stigmatized social groups. Those assessments, usually reached by differently positioned participants with contrasting personal and public interests, are beyond reconciliation. Two points should, however, be made. First, research success in identifying the cause and transmission patterns of HIV has certainly been unprecedentedly rapid;[1] and precisely the range of choices made possible by its success (most crucially, the availability of testing) has generated the very policy dilemmas that have ensured the impossibility of any uncontroversial formation of government policy. Second, while scientific and epidemiological uncertainties have characterized all societies attempting to control the spread of infection, the factors that appear to have shaped policies in our sample countries are very diverse. The internalist chronicle of the translation of scientific advances into public health measures therefore needs to be accompanied by an externalist account of agenda-setting and interest-group conflicts.

The nine country studies suggest that, besides the occasional refusal to take measures that were known to be unenforceable, seven sets of factors—separately or in combination—ought to be considered in analyses of the management of AIDS. Not all have been equally present or salient in each society, but they cover the most significant relationships between the key social actors in policy formation.

The International Context

Fortin's description of the weight of Africa's colonial past in not only provoking contemporary patterns of disease but also in ensuring that the postcolonial governments of multiethnic and war-torn societies have a restricted range of health protection strategies available to them indicates the leading role of foreign influences, although some can now only be regretted, not revised. It is clear that for developing countries the patterns of economic and financial dependency in restricting practical policy options for their governments have repercussions not only insofar as the government's general array of policy options may be limited but also in the specific determinations of policy imposed from abroad, directly by foreign powers or indirectly through the bilateral arrangements sponsored by WHO. In the specialized field of research Parker indicates that in Brazil the national research agenda on AIDS is funded by outside agencies, notably from the United States, which are therefore enabled to determine the nature of the research to be conducted. In a more positive vein, it should be noted that the active concern expressed by WHO, coupled with offers of very substantial funds to establish education and prevention programs, was an important factor in stimulating African countries to acknowledge the growing local incidence of AIDS and to overcome their initial, often justified, hostility to foreign interest.[2]

In developed societies the international context is noted by several contributors as a factor in national policy formulation insofar as the impressions likely to be created beyond national frontiers by policy decisions appear to influence response strategies. In several instances the meanings attributed to AIDS are enmeshed in a national feeling of pride. Thus Pollak draws attention to the deliberate de-dramatization policy in France, which was designed to recover a primacy threatened by the Montagnier-Gallo dispute by leading the way in the display of rational and humane management responses. In Belgium the compulsory screening of all African students imposed in 1987 was mitigated after opposition by universities and human rights organizations. Moreover, Hubert argues that the primary target for Belgian AIDS education was chosen in part because of the political difficulties in addressing directly the Central African origins of early HIV infection in the country. In Poland, too, as Misztal suggests, the desire to match other countries in tolerance and civility led to the very gradual and undramatic divulgence of information in order not to arouse what was evidently feared as likely to be a profoundly intolerant social reaction. The rhetoric employed by Australia's health officials has also insisted on its world leadership role in the management of infection. More pragmatically, the volume of people circulating between West Germany and the German Democratic Republic has forced both governments into discussion of policy coordination; and, remarkably, the first point in the communiqué issued by the leaders of the two Germanies after the first official postwar meeting affirmed the agreement to conduct joint research on AIDS.[3] That the scientific controversy between Montagnier and Gallo could be settled by an agreement reached at the presidential level between Mitterrand and Reagan shows how far the global incidence of AIDS has ensured a national competitiveness in all aspects of disease control.

The Changing Social Profile of Disease

In each society HIV infection has been portrayed as linked firmly, if never exclusively, with a particular social group or category: gays in the United

States, ivdus in Italy, prostitutes in Central Africa, foreign students in Belgium and Eastern Europe. The accumulating knowledge of the relative riskiness of particular *practices* has not so far weakened the role of those *social categories* as the primary orienting grid either for statistical compilation or in prevention campaigns. An obvious factor relevant to responses is the particular national profile of HIV infection and AIDS cases, which may not only vary considerably among countries grouped together in global statistics but is liable to progressive or discontinuous changes along several dimensions. In some countries (the United States) the change is gradual, with ivdus occupying an increasingly large share of new cases. In other countries (Italy between 1985 and 1986) the shift may be quite rapid, leading to a dramatic shift in the position of a hitherto subordinate risk category. Where these changes are accompanied by a shift in the social location of the disease (as in Brazil and France, where the increased role played by lower-middle-class and lower-class groups, to be found at increasing distances from the original centers of infection and intervention, is clear), then the problems for adequate responses are especially severe. Indeed, shifts in the social and geographical locations of infection are likely to require new strategies of prevention and education. Ivdus are less accessible than gays in all societies; but a drift of HIV infection downwards in the social hierarchy of gays may also weaken the impact of gay organizations' work since the newly infected come from strata that do not provide members for, nor are easily reached by, the initial largely middle-class gay groups.

The Social Identity of Transmission Categories

The attachment of high risk to particular categories has been double-edged in its effects. Most obviously it has generated the possibility of further daily stigmatization of already "deviant" and socially powerless groups—although it is remarkable and encouraging how few instances of open discrimination are actually reported in the preceding pages. But the same identification has necessarily marked out a (not very clearly bounded) set of individuals as a potential action-set, bearing equal risks but potentially empowered to act publicly on behalf of their own and others' well-being. It is therefore an empirical question how far the individuals marked out by the name of a particular transmission category do indeed regard a significant dimension of their social identity as embodied in that name.

Because so little is presently known about sexual cultures in any society, Parker's account of homosexuality in Brazil is especially valuable. By describing the conflict between official sexual categories and the everyday understandings of participants, he shows the problem of identifying a "gay community," especially among the lower middle and lower classes now increasingly infected by HIV in Brazil, and the consequent difficulty in the effective organization of men who do not ground their social identity in same-sex encounters. The nonexclusivity of gay and heterosexual practices is not discussed in the other chapters, although reports from Italy suggest an analogous importance for the active/passive distinction in the formation of sexual identity.[4] Bisexuality is an alternative, if rarely discussed, passage route for HIV between gay and heterosexual communities, but estimates of its actual significance for the spread of the virus depend heavily on the meaning to be attached to the term "partner" in the self-reports and ethnographies of sexual relationships.

The Extent of Organization in "High-Risk" Communities

Even where being gay or using drugs is acknowledged as a basis for identity and claims to solidarity, societies vary in the extent to which those "deviant" communities possess enduring institutions accessible to outsiders and able to carry out the tasks associated with education, prevention, and caring. The most stable gay communities, which predate the recognition of AIDS, are undoubtedly to be found in the United States where, as Pollak notes for France, gays may constitute separate representative sections among their professional organizations. The least secure, among the societies we consider, appear in Poland, where a combination of religiously inspired disapproval, party puritanism, police harassment, and the refusal of legal registration for gay organizations leaves their members dispersed and largely invisible to one another.

By comparison with the other "high-risk" groups, gays have nonetheless occupied a relatively privileged position. Intravenous drug users are more often bound into exploitative or competitive relations by their addiction, which combines with their outlaw status to destroy most of the capacity to act as a pressure group. Prostitutes represent an equally disadvantaged category, but in any case their infection rate outside Africa seems to have been surprisingly low. Many of the initiatives related to those categories appear to have been brought by outsiders, often in collaboration with ex-members, and to be local temporary measures, likely to last—in the absence of institutional support—no longer than the personal enthusiasms of their initiators. The remaining categories—hemophiliacs, children with AIDS, foreign students, heterosexuals—are too dispersed or too broadly categorized or too powerless to generate an organized group in their own right prior to infection itself. The extent to which these risk groups can build on their self-organization to achieve a hearing and support from nonmembers is a further question to be examined below.

The Participatory Traditions of Civil Society

The cases reported in this volume show wide variation in the traditions and extent of voluntary organization in civil society. At one extreme stands the United States, where not only are voluntary organizations part of the American way of life, as Quam and Ford stress, but also, in the area of health in particular, individual recourse to the law and collective organization through mutual support groups of sufferers have been increasingly popular. Strategies of both individual self-help and collective solidarity characterize the U.S. experience with AIDS and represent a major channel for the energies (although somewhat less of a channel for financial resources) devoted to education and management.

At the other extreme can be found societies in which, for historical or contingent reasons, citizens' associations, where they exist at all, have been unable to exercise pressure on political elites or to contribute very effectively to managing the problems posed by the disease. African postcolonial societies have seen few enduring mobilizations around health issues; and in any case the years immediately preceding the appearance of AIDS were often more devoted to the destruction of solidarities and local resources through civil wars and communal violence. A different picture is offered by the cases of Brazil and Poland, in which the appearance of the first AIDS cases in the early 1980s coincided with widespread alienation of civil society from the political process. The generalized disenchantment in the wake, respectively, of the failure of Diretas Jà in Brazil and of the proscription of Solidarity in Poland was largely responsible for inhibiting any popular pressure to place a difficult and novel issue like HIV infection on the political agenda and to compel politicians to take up unequivocal public positions on the methods for its control. In Poland some space was found for individual initiatives only in the interstices of, or camouflaged within, existing state institutions. Continental European societies lie somewhere between these extremes, providing space for volunteer efforts and pressure on public decision making but also strongly influenced by the historically central role of the state in social protection and welfare. Sufficient variation exists, however, to enable Pollak to contrast the limited role played by voluntary organizations in France (and, we would add, Italy) with the much greater reliance placed on their efforts in Germany, the Netherlands, and Switzerland.

The Extent of Political Consensus

One remarkably constant theme to emerge from all country studies is the extent to which AIDS has been kept out of party political conflict. Both in countries where the parliamentary political spectrum is narrow (the United States, West Germany, Belgium) and where it stretches from extreme left to extreme right (France, Italy), few of the contentious issues of HIV management divide supporters and opponents along party lines. Parliamentary reports are usually jointly authored by members of different parties, and the relevant committees have been determinedly bipartisan. When extreme proposals have been formulated, as by the Front National's leader Le Pen in France in 1987, their impact has been to underline publicly the consensus among other parties rather than to succeed in rupturing it. Other instances, such as the Liberal Party's growing criticism of the Labour government's policy in Australia in 1988–1989, confirm that the attacks derive from the right and usually are less concerned with specific policy differences than with their opponents' willingness to grant space to the views of the gay community and civil rights organizations. In any case it seems likely that the only conditions under which political disagreements can be provoked is where both contestants become aligned with more directly involved participants (notably the gay and medical communities) and when conflict over AIDS policies represents simply the prolongation of broader and long-entrenched politico-professional disputes.

Political consensus has also been maintained by the creation of advisory bodies on AIDS to which all controversial questions can be referred. Such bodies have been dominated by professional scientists and doctors, who constitute their sole membership (as in the case of Belgium between 1983 and 1988) or are assisted by social scientists and state officials (as, for example, in West Germany). Such bodies enable governments to distance themselves from direct involvement by providing nonpolitical fora for conflicts over the issues of testing, screening, funding levels, and so on, with the added advantage that the disputes—if not entirely disguised—take place in a much less accessible and accountable arena than a parliamentary chamber or committee room. As the Australian case indicates, the creation of separate expert bodies for specific tasks may lead to conflict between the two agencies or with the government itself. But in most Western and Eastern societies the distance established between such organizations and the ordinary political process also insulates their debates and decisions from calamitously conflictual intersection with existing sources of party or factional controversy.

The Resources and Structure of the Medical System

As a disease, HIV/AIDS is the immediate responsibility of the health services whose direct impact on responses depends on their resources and structure. Notwithstanding the several transmission routes for HIV, many countries classify AIDS as a sexually transmitted disease—a determination that automatically places sufferers in a network of existing health institutions, legal obligations, and treatment practices. That classification is therefore likely to be much more than an uncontroversial administrative convenience; in the French case, indeed, it has evoked powerful associations with the war years and foreign conquest. In any case the treatment centers for STDs, at least in Europe and the United States, have been both chronically underfunded and overstretched, not least because of the rising incidence of syphilis and gonorrhea in the years immediately preceding the appearance of AIDS itself; Italy, for example, saw syphilis cases more than double between 1977 and 1986. Whether or not AIDS is classified as an STD, the burden of care falls much more widely on the hospital services.

Under pressure, governments have increased their budgets for AIDS, first gradually, then substantially, in order to fund growth in the numbers of hospital beds, trained personnel, and specialized centers for HIV testing. In some cases the local health services have constituted part of the problem rather than a means towards its solution. In Poland and the USSR hospitals have been a major site for the transmission of infection because of the need to reuse syringes and the lack of effective cleaning materials; and the Polish government has had to grant health workers a considerable rise in salary in order to obtain cooperation in confronting the risks of AIDS. Contaminated blood remains a major source of infection outside the affluent West: in Brazil efforts to ensure HIV-free blood have included a ban on the commercialization of all blood and blood products.

As Quam and Ford indicate for probably the most decentralized health system in our sample, the flexibility provided by local autonomy in health care delivery may not be economical or effective in an emergency. Not only may there be no central body able to give authoritative guidance—or ensure that guidance, once given, is followed—but the tasks of predicting impacts and evaluating services become very hard to carry out. Decentralized health responsibilities, coupled with central funding and a very uneven regional distribution of the disease, also ensure the fragmentation of a potentially powerful pressure group and a greater difficulty in persuading central governments to take action. Both in scope and quality, therefore, health services vary widely, calling for very different kinds of involvements from sufferers themselves and volunteers. Where health care depends greatly on private insurance, the refusal of insurance companies to enroll HIV-positive applicants generates higher hospital costs or much more elaborate home-care arrangements based on volunteers.

COMPARING TRAJECTORIES OF RESPONSE

At the risk of violence to the more nuanced and discriminating accounts of national cases reported here, it seems possible to identify two distinct periods of response in Western countries, the more recent being characterized by two partly contrasting tendencies shaping demands for intervention. In Eastern Europe, Kenya, and Brazil the two-stage periodization appropriate to the West can be identified, although in each case the type of interventions being periodized in that way are rather different.

As far as Western societies are concerned, the two periods run from 1981 to 1986 and from 1987 to the present. The break, in late 1986-early 1987, marks a transformation not only in the perceived nature of the disease each society had come to confront but also in the relations between the major actors involved in making and implementing policy. In the phase that began in 1987 two tendencies have become visible, although the force that each carries in any particular society is not uniform. On one hand, the growing body of knowledge about at least some aspects of the virus and its manifestations has led to an increasingly technical approach to AIDS management; on the other hand, the tasks that governments are increasingly being called upon to assume demand a more interventionist stance. The first process tends to drive AIDS issues out of the political arena still more firmly, while the second—by multiplying the number of actors and issues to be regulated—tends to produce more conflicts requiring central resolution.[5] It is far from clear how the balance will be struck in the coming years.

The Early Years: 1981–1986

Along the medico-scientific axis the first phase can be conveniently demarcated by the descriptions of the first patients with AIDS in 1981 and the recommendation that the virus causing the disease be named the human immunodeficiency virus in 1986. Thereafter, with only muted and minority dissent, the relation between HIV and AIDS has been assumed to be direct.[6] Between those dates the uncertainties over the duration, transmission, and consequences of infection were especially intense and allowed particular space for lay claims and interventions. It has been suggested that, in the United States at least, additional room was provided by the decentralization and increasing privatization of responsibilities for health care in the early 1980s, accompanied by a decline in the traditional loci of medical authority.[7] An analogous shift is noted for Italy over the same period, ensuring that mobilization to put pressure on the central government over health issues is more difficult but, given the dominance of the public provision of health services, without providing significantly greater opportunities for lay intervention.

As Quam and Ford note for the United States—and as every Pattern 1 country report confirms—the roles played by the gay community in the early years of the epidemic have been multiple and essential. Most work has been carried out at the local level; nowhere do the governmental advisory bodies or commissions on AIDS appear to have formally incorporated representatives of gays. Access to the central authorities by the primary community affected in the early years (outside Africa) was therefore indirect, through connections with a governing political party (as in Australia) or alliances with medical experts (as in France) or in negotiations on the spending of state subsidies (as in West Germany). In the primary centers of disease gays not only took on the tasks of education, practical prevention campaigns, and care for the sick but also participated in epidemiological research, seropositivity-rate ascertainment, and the testing of new drugs. The scale of gay response, and the visible public commitment to protect health, was probably as significant a factor in ensuring the authority of the community's representatives as the more general questioning of medical and scientific expertise.

Government responses displayed the caution noted above. After the availability of the ELISA test in 1985 steps were everywhere taken to ensure that supplies of blood and blood products were free of HIV contamination, although—as the cases of Brazil and Kenya, and to a lesser degree Poland, demonstrate—it has not always been possible for governments to ensure that their regulations were made effective in the face of inadequate funding, unavailability of test equipment, and the continuing donor demand, driven by poverty, for clandestine blood banks not subject to restrictive quality controls. All the societies surveyed here have established, where usable mechanisms were not already in place, centralized surveillance systems for the epidemic, although the requirements on disease notification continue to vary. In the United States, Italy, and France, but not in West Germany (or the UK), AIDS is a notifiable disease. ARC and HIV infection are required to be reported only in some states in the United States, although suggestions that the reporting of HIV infection be made mandatory have been heard elsewhere.

The possibility of testing/screening to establish infection and the subsequent treatment of the infected has been the key locus of the conflict between individual liberty and public health protection. On the evidence presented in this book governments have so far shown a considerable reluctance to advertise concern for the general population by dramatic and coercive measures to test and to quarantine—an encouraging sign needing only to be qualified by the reminder that in many instances considerable, if long neglected, coercive powers were already on the statute books. At the national level the United States has introduced compulsory testing for immigrants and military recruits; but while individual states have introduced tests for various categories, the more idiosyncratic decisions (for example, the testing of marriage license applicants in Louisiana) have already been repealed. In West European countries, mandatory testing of general categories has not been introduced anywhere except in the German state of Bavaria, where support for retention of the measure appears to be falling in the wake of federal government opposition. Illustrative of West European stances is the fact that no country except Greece has imposed mandatory testing on one of the socially weakest, and in some cases most obviously exposed, categories: the prison population. In the East governmental power has been used to impose testing on foreign students, prostitutes, identified gays, and ivdus, as well as on prisoners and hospital patients. In Europe generally the different balance struck between civil rights and public health distinguishes liberal from popular democracies.

Since 1987: The Second Phase

The inauguration of the second phase was signalled by national governments embarking on more active and directed strategies of containment. In the less developed world the change was powerfully reinforced by the establishment of the World Health Organization's Special Program on AIDS, encouraging donor agencies to support initiatives such as Kenya's five-year program to control AIDS, which was launched in January 1988. In the West new directions or new commitments have been everywhere apparent. A set of political bodies in Belgium took up their first public positions on AIDS, an extensive education campaign was begun, and the membership of the major advisory body was extended to the representatives of new groups (Hubert, p. 103); the Council of (regional) Health Ministers in West Germany issued its first report, closely followed by the widespread diffusion of information (Pollak, p. 124); Poland initiated the systematic checking of all donated blood (Misztal, p. 173); in France AIDS was now declared a "national cause" (Pollak, p. 98); the Italian and Brazilian governments established their advisory committees and surveillance units (Moss, p. 144; Parker, p. 66); the first substantial increases in budget allowances were negotiated from the U.S. Congress in the wake of the Institute of Medicine's 1986 report *Confronting AIDS* (Quam and Ford, p. 30); and Australia launched its first national "Grim Reaper" educational campaign (Misztal, p. 202). Whatever regional or municipal authorities had been doing for perhaps several years, national governments began to translate into much broader schemes.

The flurry of activity now increasingly visible is sometimes polemically attributed to the spread of infection into the heterosexual population, which spurred homophobic governments, less concerned with the fate of gays and ivdus, into their first committed strategies of response. On a count of AIDS cases alone, the spread was anticipated rather than actual; for even where the ivdu transmission category was most significant, the actual numbers of heterosexuals infected, calculated as a cumulative total or as new cases, remains small.[8] In assessing the determinants of the new scale of response, other factors need to be taken into account.

In the first place, the diffusion of infection from center to periphery in almost all societies by the late 1980s gave the epidemic an obvious national dimension demanding appropriately national-level responses and guidance. As the smaller centers began to develop expertise and support structures, too, the migration of the infected to the larger centers—which in France ensured that one in six AIDS cases in Paris in 1986 was from the provinces— was certain to diminish. Second, the revelation of the length of time between HIV infection and the appearance of the symptoms of ARC and AIDS demanded educational campaigns for increasingly younger groups, to be provided through the school system, which in many societies is the direct responsibility of the state. Third, the immense efforts made by gay groups in the first phase were encountering barriers to further development. The appearance of HIV infection in gay groups outside the social and geographical catchment areas of the organizations of the gay movement, the psychological burden of long-term care provided by mostly untrained volunteers, and the prolonging of the duration of illness by the deployment of new drugs, notably AZT, and better self-management imposed new tasks which it was difficult to expect that the gay community could fulfill without institutionalized assistance. In Australia a high turnover even among health officials has been noted as a significant hindrance to effective disease management. Fourth, the spread of HIV among ivdus, which by 1989 accounts for roughly half of all new AIDS cases reported in Europe, has required human and financial resources and organizational structures to be generated from outside that community of sufferers. Additional pressure is applied by the concomitant growth in cases of pediatric AIDS, as a direct consequence of wider infection among ivdus. Fifth, the simple acceleration in the numbers of cases has combined with the preceding four factors to ensure financial obligations at a level that can only be met by governments.

The expansion of the epidemic confronted national politicians and health authorities not merely with vastly increased costs but also with a range of new claimants for attention. New communities of sufferers with their spokespersons, new categories of local health personnel and municipal administrators, new defenders of public health at the workplace, new business interests, new experts in the interpretation of the accumulating scientific knowledge of HIV infection—all these additional categories of potential participants in decision making have encouraged a revision of the earlier interactional patterns of policy formation.

The pressures experienced by the earlier allies are visible in the conflicts reported from many countries from 1987 onwards. One point of tension appears in the relations between central and local authorities. In West Germany, Bavaria institutionalized its dissent from the policies of the federal government by imposing its own testing laws, and disputes over the nature of the individual responsibilities of the infected reached the legal system. In France the Southeast region, where a growing proportion of new AIDS cases are located, entered into direct conflict with the central health authorities in Paris over the acceptability of registration of seropositives. In Italy the Lombardy regional government openly criticized the dilatoriness of the national Health Minister and rejected his attempt to set aside the hitherto anonymous reporting of AIDS cases. Disputes could indeed be expected to appear both where local authorities saw themselves as directly responsible for meeting a new threat and where they had already established a working strategy of containment now threatened with disruption by the initiatives of a remote central government.

A second shift appears, perhaps less clearly, in the relations between the government and the gay community. In West Germany, indeed, both the federal government and some regional authorities came into conflict with the AIDS *Hilfen* and began actively to seek new partners in the work of education and prevention. To the extent that HIV has become an increasing threat to ivdus and the heterosexual population, too, the centrality of gays as sufferers and educators in the first phase of the epidemic must necessarily be diminished. New interest groups and different perspectives on the key policy dilemmas occupy more public space. As the Australian case shows, one of the most significant bearers of positive initiatives has been the medical profession itself; and the replacement of the two units of the AIDS Task Force and NACAIDS (in which medical and community expertise enjoyed substantial parity) by ANCA, dominated by scientific advisers, exemplifies a more general trend.

The absence of secure knowledge in the early years of AIDS, coupled with the articulate lay competition represented by the well-informed leaders of the gay community, prevented the medical profession from occupying its traditionally authoritative role in disease management. Indeed, generalized claims to authority based on an allegedly uncontentious expertise were probably weakened by the Three Mile Island episode and the Chernobyl disaster and by the more public scrutiny of professional power in a financially cold climate. Only in France did the rather special circumstances of the prestige enjoyed by Montagnier and the close links established between researchers and gay organizations such as AIDES allow the medical professionals clearly to dominate the public approach to AIDS from the outset.

However, in the later part of the decade, the balance between lay and professional influence shifted in favor of professional groups. First, the extremely rapid accumulation of scientific data provided the basis for a restoration of their definitional power and uncontested input into policy. As Barrilleaux and Miller note in general, highly organized professional groups with knowledge and experience of the workings of the health bureaucracy always prosper at the expense even of the most attentive segments of the public as the specific problem becomes more abstract and complex.[9] Second, the emergence of ivdus as the major risk group in developed countries entailed that, because illegal drug users had few representative groups, the public voice of the directly affected became much weaker than when gay groups were able to speak for the primary category of sufferers. Third, the simple increase in the numbers of medical and paramedical staff coming into direct, even routine, contact with seropositive and AIDS patients for the first time created an increasingly vocal constituency with its own (not necessarily homogeneous) views on how the disease should best be managed in the interests of both patients and carers. Moreover, while the figures for the number of health workers contracting AIDS in the course of their professional work remain very small (twenty-five in the United States by the end of 1988), the increasing risk to surgeons has led to the public mobilization of a more prestigious and powerful group than the lower-level occupational categories hitherto regarded as principally at risk.[10]

The achievement of dominance by the medico-scientific community does not imply its continuing unity. As the case of France indicates, the increases both in the resources available and in the prestige of contributing to the control of the epidemic are so considerable as to have generated sharp, and public, conflicts to command the new field. Among doctors the splits visible in the Australian Medical Association have led to quasi-rival scientific conferences, as well as providing material for the growing policy divergences between the Labour government and the Liberal opposition.

Because many medical professionals—and other professionals, notably employers, whose continuing success in their own careers depends on knowledge of the likely longevity or infectiousness of their associates, clients, and workforce—support the gathering of such knowledge through mandatory testing, it is likely that the reluctance to impose the test that characterized policy in the first phase will come under increasing pressure. If indeed modifications are achieved, it remains open whether opinion will favor the screening of entire categories or the delegation of decisions on whether to use the test to individual institutions. In either case more coercive policies are likely to be facilitated by the generalized illegality and social disapproval of the increasingly significant category of the infected—intravenous drug users. To the extent that AIDS ceases to be an emergency and becomes routinized by the very institutions that were created to organize the early responses or by incorporation into the ordinary health services, testing itself may cease to be so controversial an issue. But before HIV/AIDS can be managed as one more chronic disease, the effects of the first, dramatically rapid and entirely silent, spread of infection in the late 1970s will have to be seen and contained, especially in the less developed world.

POLICY COMPARISONS: TOWARD A RECIPE FOR SUCCESS?

Reception of AIDS as an emergency has made visible some forgotten or hidden aspects of health policies and structures. It has variously underlined the inequalities in national health protection, the inadequate provision of resources and the substantial ignorance about the shape of sexual lives in all cultures. Prospectively, HIV has also revived interest in general strategies of prevention and education and has forced consideration of alternative approaches to long-standing, AIDS-related problems. For example, the need to halt the spread of infection among ivdus has suggested that the aim of rendering drug dependence safer might be more appropriate than the attempt to eliminate it altogether, especially when the rate of drug supply is effectively outside any one government's control.

Whatever the disease has so far revealed, the evidence that would enable us to compare strategies of response and derive clear lessons from their successes and failures is not yet in. The reluctance in the early period of management to impose generalized testing itself prevents the reconstruction of any clear picture of the epidemiological profile of infection and therefore any convincing comparison between policy initiatives and subsequent changes in seropositive rates and progression to AIDS. Moreover, the evidence of these chapters emphasizes the influence of historical factors on policies: the refusal of the French government to classify AIDS as a sexually transmitted disease because of the associations of the relevant legislation with the Vichy period; the impact of political disillusion on the politics of response to AIDS in Brazil; and the significance of the colonial past on the distribution of ill health in postcolonial African societies. Rational health policies on AIDS are constructed within the spaces offered by local history, social organization, and culture, and they differ accordingly. How the real and perceived consequences of both infection and response will influence national policy discussions and decisions remains presently as uncertain as the transformation of the virus itself and the outcome of the search for a cure. What seems more secure is the forecast that our nine countries' experiences in managing AIDS, viewed from a decade hence, will require very different accounts.

NOTES

1. Considerable controversy has occurred over the desirable levels of funding to be granted to research on HIV/AIDS. One attempt to evaluate the allocation to AIDS-related research in the United States argues that work on AIDS does not appear to be overfunded in relation to other causes of death and disability. E. Hatziandreu, J. Graham, and M. Stoto, "AIDS and Biomedical Research Funding: Comparative Analysis," *Reviews of Infectious Diseases* 10, no. 1 (1988): 159–167.

2. See the comments by Jonathan Mann and James Chin in *New Scientist* 1665 (20 May 1989): 23.

3. John Borneman, "AIDS in the Two Berlins," *October* 43 (1988): 223.

4. The alleged rigidity of the distinction in Southern Europe, in contrast to the United States, has been suggested as a barrier to the spread of infection among gays in Italy, Spain, and Greece and therefore as an explanation of the greater salience of ivdus in those countries; see S. Franceschi et al., "Homosexual Role Separation and Spread of AIDS," *The Lancet*, 7 January 1989, p. 2.

5. For a comparison between the United States, Sweden, and the UK that indicates the growing technical pressures exerted by professionals, see D. Fox, P. Day, and R. Klein, "The Power of Professionalism: Policies for AIDS in Britain, Sweden and the United States," *Daedalus* 112, no. 2 (1989): 93–112.

6. For a recent, heavily criticized, rejection of the direct connection, see Jad Adams, *AIDS: The HIV Myth* (New York: St. Martin's Press, 1989). Some of the criticisms are summarized in *New Scientist*, 29 April 1989, pp. 6–7.

7. Fox et al., "Power of Professionalism," p. 105.

8. Considerable uncertainty remains as to whether the spread of HIV among the heterosexual population is likely; R. May, R. Anderson, and S. Blower, "The

Epidemiology and Transmission Dynamics of HIV-AIDS," *Daedalus* 12, no. 2 (1989): 163–201.

9. C. J. Barrilleaux and M. E. Miller, "The Political Economy of State Medicaid Policy," *American Political Science Review* 82, no. 4 (1988): 1089–1107.

10. For some U.S. surgeons' appraisals of the risk, and the suggestion that HIV may be transmitted in the vapors produced from body fluids by surgical instruments, see *New Scientist*, 13 May 1989, p. 9.

Bibliographic Essay

Materials on HIV/AIDS increase as rapidly as the venues (journals, workshops, conferences) where they are hosted. The January 1989 issue of the monthly bulletin *AIDS Information* contained details of 209 original papers published within the previous month: the July issue counted 277, an increase of one-third in six months. Indeed *AIDS Information*'s first six issues for 1989 covered 1,265 contributions to scientific, medical, and public policy research on HIV/AIDS, so that by the end of the year as many papers were published in 1989 alone as were indexed on Medline for the entire four-year period 1983–1986. At least three new English-language AIDS-dedicated journals appeared in 1989, bringing the total to ten, with the number of publications disseminating updated bibliographic information monthly or bi-monthly standing at seven. Twelve major conferences on specific aspects of AIDS were announced for the second half of 1989 alone. Clearly the volume of material now being produced is as sure a guarantee of the limited life span of most single contributions and bibliographies as it is an encouraging manifestation of scientific and public attention.

Apart from its inevitable datedness (covering only materials in print at mid-1989), this bibliographic essay has two other limitations. First it only covers materials in English. The lists of references at the end of each chapter contain details of relevant journals and other sources in the various national languages. It would have been too unwieldy to try to produce an adequate composite bibliography for nine countries, covering publications in at least seven languages. The second limitation is an indirect effect of the first: most substantial publications in English (i.e., beyond the level of letters to the editors of journals) deal with the experience of English-speaking societies, for the most part the United States, the United Kingdom, and Anglophone Africa. The essay therefore regrettably does not help readers who wish for guidance through materials on Latin America or specific European countries.

JOURNALS AND BIBLIOGRAPHIC SOURCES

Databases

Material relevant to the social and epidemiological aspects of AIDS can be found in very many places and is most conveniently identified through electronic databases such as Medline. A useful guide to relevant databases, search procedures, and the growth of knowledge on AIDS up to 1987 is: S. Roberts, L. Shepherd, and J. Wade, "The scientific and clinical literature of AIDS: development, bibliographic control and retrieval," *Health Libraries Review*, 4 (1987), 197–218. Medline covers the general medico-scientific publications (e.g., *JAMA*, *BMJ*, *The Lancet*, *American Journal of Public Health*), which report and comment on the most recent findings as well as hosting original and review articles.

Bibliographic Sources

Bibliographic sources concerned strictly with HIV/AIDS continue to increase. The most useful, with the date of first appearance, are: *AIDS Information* (1985), *AIDS Newsletter* (1986), *AIDS Record* (1986), *ATIN: AIDS Targeted Information Newsletter* (1987), *AIDS Research Today* (1987), *Current AIDS Literature* (1988: formerly *AIDS and Retroviruses Update* [1986]) and *WHO AIDS Technical Bulletin* (1988). *AIDS Information*, for example, has a section on "public policy, social and legal": abstracts of articles may be provided.

HIV/AIDS-Dedicated Journals

The journals and newsletters specifically concerned with HIV/AIDS contain material relevant to sociological and public policy analysis: *AIDS* (1986), *AIDS Forschung* (1986), *AIDS Patient Care* (1987), *AIDS Research and Human Retroviruses* (1987: formerly *AIDS Research* [1984]), *The AIDS Letter* (1987), *Journal of Acquired Immunodeficiency Syndromes* (1988), *AIDS Education and Prevention* (1989), and *AIDS Care* (1989). The newsletter *WorldAIDS* (1989), published by the Panos Institute, is principally devoted to non-Western societies, as is the Institute's regularly revised *AIDS and the Third World*. The U.N. journal, *Development Forum*, has carried detailed local reports of AIDS in Africa.

Special Issues

A number of journals have published special issues on AIDS that address a wide range of medical, social and policy concerns in a single forum and are usually accompanied by substantial bibliographies. An inclusive collection is *Science* 239(5 February 1988), 4840: greater emphasis is given to medico-scientific details in *Scientific American*, 259, no. 4 (October 1988). In the field of public policy responses *The Milbank Memorial Quarterly* 64, suppl. 1 (1986), entitled "AIDS: The Public Context of an Epidemic," contains valuable essays by historians and social scientists, as does "In Time of Plague," *Social Research* 55, no. 3 (1988). More recent contributions, which include papers by some of the authors in the preceding two collections, can be found in the successive issues of *Daedalus* 118, nos. 2 and 3 (1989), entitled "Living with AIDS"; and health policy issues are pursued in the *American Journal of Public Health* 78, no. 4 (1988). Two issues of *Law, Medicine and Health Care,* 14, nos. 5–6 (1986) and 15, nos. 1–2 (1987), both edited by L. Gostin and W. J. Curran and entitled, respectively, "AIDS: Science and Epidemiology" and "AIDS: Law and Policy," range widely over scientific and social issues.

Legal concerns, particularly in the United States, mark the *Hofstra Law Review* 14, no. 1 (1985), while the *Journal of Medical Ethics* 15, no. 2 (1989) brings together legal, philosophical, and psychosocial considerations. Anthropological accounts of the representation, management, and prevention of AIDS, drawing primarily on research in the United States, comprise *Medical Anthropology* 10, nos. 2–3 (1989), reprinted as Ralph Bolton, ed., *The AIDS Pandemic: A Global Emergency* (New York: Gordon and Breach, 1989). A more activist perspective characterizes *October* 43 (1988), subsequently published as D. Crimp, ed., *AIDS: Cultural Analysis/Cultural Activism* (Cambridge, Mass.: MIT Press, 1988). Modeling the future course of HIV/AIDS is the central focus of the *Journal of the Royal Statistical Society,* Series A, 151, Part 1 (1988): specifically actuarial approaches to the same topic can be found in papers by working parties set up by the professional bodies in different countries, a consolidated report by the Institute of Actuaries in England taking up most of the *Journal of the Institute of Actuaries* 115(1989), 727–837.

BOOKS AND ARTICLES

Epidemiology

Basic statistics that track the changing global, national, and social distribution of HIV/AIDS are published regularly by the World Health Organization in the *Weekly Epidemiological Record* and by the Centers for Disease Control in its *Morbidity and Mortality Weekly Report.* Global analysis is provided by Peter Piot et al., "AIDS: An International Perspective," *Science* 239(5 February 1988), 573–579, and by J. M. Mann et al., "The International Epidemiology of AIDS," *Scientific American* 259, no. 4 (1988), 82–89. For the United States a convenient summary, noting the statistical impact of changes in disease definition, is "Update: Acquired Immunodeficiency Syndrome—United States 1981–1988," *JAMA* 261, no. 18 (12 May 1989), 2609–2617. The results of ninety-two studies of HIV infection among intravenous drug users (ivdus) in the United States are surveyed in Robert Hahn et al., "Prevalence of HIV Infection Among Intravenous Drug Users in the United States," *JAMA* 261, no. 18 (12 May 1989), 2677–2684. An intensive local study of the worst-affected New York borough is Ernest Drucker and Sten H. Vermund, "Estimating Population Prevalence of Human Immuno-deficiency Virus Infection in Urban Areas with High Rates of Intravenous Drug Use: A Model of the Bronx in 1988," *American Journal of Epidemiology,* 130, no. 1 (1989), 133–142.

Figures for HIV/AIDS in African societies, and details of selected seroprevalence studies, are given in Barbara O. de Zalduondo, Gernard I. Msamanga, and Lincoln C. Chen, "AIDS in Africa: Diversity in the Global Pandemic," *Daedalus* 118, no. 3

(1989), 165–204. The future demographic impact of AIDS in the Third World is discussed by R. M. Anderson, R. M. May, and A. R. Maclean, "Possible Demographic Consequences of AIDS in Developing Countries," *Nature* 332 (17 March 1988), 228–234: the authors broaden the analysis in Robert H. May, Roy M. Anderson, and Sally M. Blower, "The Epidemiology and Transmission Dynamics of HIV-AIDS," *Daedalus* 112, no. 2 (1989), 163–201.

Social Science Research on HIV/AIDS

The recency of AIDS, and the urgency of getting potentially policy-orienting results into public circulation, means that, to date, most research projects designed by social scientists have been restricted in scope: the more ambitious projects, launched in the late 1980s, have yet to be completed. An annual register of AIDS-related sociological research, largely confined to the United Kingdom, has been compiled by COBRA (Coordinating Organization for Behavioural Resarch on AIDS, University of Wales, U.K.), *Register of Current Research.* An account of the novel research method employed in the most extensive longitudinal study in the United Kingdom is A.P.M. Coxon, "Something sensational . . . the sexual diary as a research method in the study of the sexual behavior of gay males," *Sociological Review* 36, no. 2 (1988), 353–367. The difficulties of designing feasible, valid, and useful social research projects on AIDS are explored by Karolynn Siegel and Laurie J. Bauman, "Methodological Issues in AIDS-Related Research," and Jane Zich and Lydia Temoshok, "Applied Methodology: A Primer of Pitfalls and Opportunities in AIDS Research," both in the collection by Douglas A. Feldman and Thomas M. Johnson, eds., *The Social Dimensions of AIDS: Method and Theory* (New York: Praeger, 1986). More recent explorations are included in C. Turner, H. Miller and L. Moses, eds., *AIDS, Sexual Behavior and Intravenous Drug Use* (Washington, D.C.: National Academy Press, 1989). Similar issues in developing countries are examined by E. Maxine Ankrah, "AIDS: Methodological Problems in Studying its Prevention and Spread," *Social Science and Medicine* 29, no. 3 (1989), 265–276. For Africa, N. Miller and R. C. Rockwell, eds. *AIDS in Africa: The Social and Policy Impact* (Lewiston, N.Y.: Edwin Mellen Press, 1988) contains programmatic research agendas alongside accounts of the spread, and reception, of HIV infection across the continent.

How sociological research on HIV/AIDS in Western societies can build on what is known about sexual conduct and communities, and the extent to which what is known is unreliable, out-of-date, or inadequate, is the focus of John H. Gagnon, "Disease and Desire," *Daedalus* 118(1989), 47–77: pre-AIDS studies of gay, lesbian, and drug-using communities are noted there. Despite recent efforts to use survey data (Robert E. Fay et al., "Prevalence and Patterns of Same-Gender Sexual Contact Among Men," *Science* 243[20 January 1989], 338–348), our widely acknowledged substantial ignorance of the range, intensity, and volatility of sexual activity and drug use has the consequence that micro-data of sociological interest are largely confined to small-scale studies of changes in behavior since AIDS (considered in "Responses Among 'High-Risk Communities' " section below).

One prominent dimension of HIV/AIDS examined by social scientists and others is the manner in which the disease has been publicly discussed and represented. Susan Sontag's *AIDS and its Metaphors* (New York: Farrar, Straus and Giroux,

1989) is the best known: its lack of persuasiveness is clearly revealed by Andrew Scull, "Mortal Meanings," *Times Literary Supplement* (10–16 March 1989), 239–240, who metes out equally severe treatment to another work in the same genre, Sander L. Gilman, *Disease and Representation: Images of Illness from Madness to AIDS* (Ithaca, N.Y.: Cornell University Press, 1988). More circumscribed analyses, concerned principally with the United Kingdom, are contained in Peter Aggleton and Hilary Homans, eds., *Social Aspects of AIDS* (London and Philadelphia: Falmer Press, 1988), and Peter Aggleton, Graham Hart, and Peter Davies, eds., *AIDS: Social Representations and Social Practices* (Basingstoke, U.K.: Falmer Press, 1989). Talk about AIDS in seven religious groups is analyzed in Susan Palmer, "AIDS as Metaphor," *Society* (January–February 1989), 44–50.

A second obvious field for sociological research is the nature, distribution, and behavioral significance of beliefs about AIDS among the general public or specific groups. Leon Eisenberg, "Health Education and AIDS," *British Journal of Psychiatry* 154 (1988), 754–767, includes a section on levels of public knowledge about HIV/AIDS mainly in the United States; J. P. Moiatti, L. Manesse, and C. Legales, "Social perception of AIDS in the general population: A French Study," *Health Policy* 9, no. 1 (1988), 1–8, deal with France; M. W. Ross et al., "Knowledge of AIDS in Australia: A National Study," *Health Education Research* 3 (1988), 367–373, show how negative attitudes to AIDS are correlated with ignorance about it; and Ian Warwick, Peter Aggleton, and Hilary Homans, "Constructing commonsense—young people's attitudes about AIDS," *Sociology of Health and Illness* 10, no. 3 (1988), 213–233, compare beliefs among lesbian, gay, and heterosexual youth in the United Kingdom. Acquiring knowledge about HIV/AIDS is of course a necessary but not sufficient step toward changing sexual or drug behaviors: some reasons for the gap are offered by Harvey V. Fineberg, "Education to Prevent AIDS: Prospects and Obstacles," *Science* 239(5 February 1988), 592–596.

Institutional Responses

The most general account is of course R. Shilts, *And The Band Played On* (New York: St. Martin's Press, 1987): among its many reviewers Sandra Panem, "A Drama and Questions," *Science*, 239(1988), 1039–1040, provides constructive grounds for her judgment that the book is "flawed but important." More narrowly focused, on the Public Health Service, is Sandra Panem, *The AIDS Bureaucracy* (Cambridge, Mass.: Harvard University Press, 1988) and, on political and bureaucratic responses, D.Guston, *Institutional Tensions in the Federal Government's Response to AIDS* (Cambridge, Mass.: MIT Press, 1989). An interesting insider's view of the Presidential Commission's *Report on the Human Immunodeficiency Virus Epidemic* (Washington, D.C.: U.S. Government Printing Office, 1988) is Kristine M. Gebbie, "The President's Commission on AIDS: What Did it Do?," *American Journal of Public Health* 79, no. 7 (1989), 868–870.

For countries other than the United States much less is available. Details of programs in place in several countries are described by national officials in World Health Organization, *AIDS: Prevention and Control* (Oxford: Pergamon Press, 1988): the Australian authorities' early responses are set out in Margaret Duckett, *Australia's Response to AIDS* (Canberra: Australian Government Publishing Service, 1986); and responses to, and local research on, AIDS in Southeast Asia are described in the contributions to the ASAIHL Conference on AIDS held in Hong Kong, June 28–30, 1989. A comparative survey of the first legal responses in three English-speaking countries is provided by Marlene C. McGuirl and Robert N. Gee, "AIDS: An Overview of the British, Australian and American Responses," *Hofstra Law Review* 14, no. 1 (1985), 107–135; a more recent comparison, similarly concerned with legal and administrative responses, is sketched by Daniel M. Fox, Patricia Day, and Rudolf Klein, "The Power of Professionalism: Policies for AIDS in Britain, Sweden and the USA," *Daedalus* 118, no. 2 (1989), 93–111. The necessity for international collaboration is emphasized by Lincoln C. Chen, "The AIDS Pandemic: An Internationalist Approach to Disease Control," *Daedalus* 116, no. 2 (1987), 181–195, while the factors that hamper it are suggested by Nicholas Christakis, "Responding to a Pandemic: International Interests in AIDS Control," *Daedalus* 118, no. 2 (1989), 113–134. Criticisms of WHO's response, in particular its funding policies, are examined by Sharon Kingman, "AIDS Brings Health into Focus," *New Scientist* 122, no. 1665 (20 May 1989), 19–24.

Law and Ethics

Overviews of legal issues associated with HIV/AIDS can be found in Bernard M. Dickens, "Legal Rights and Duties in the AIDS Epidemic," *Science* 239(1988), 579–586; Michael Kirby, "AIDS—Legal Issues," *AIDS* 2, suppl. 1 (1988), S209–S215; and Michael Kirby, "AIDS and Law," *Daedalus* 112, no. 3, (1989), 101–122. The effects of different legal systems on striking a balance between public health and individual rights are examined by Alistair Orr, "Legal AIDS: Implications of AIDS and HIV for British and American Law," *Journal of Medical Ethics* 15, no. 2 (1989), 61–67. Most discussions of the conflict, potential or actual, between public and private interests have been American, reflecting its tradition of concern with the defence of individual freedoms. Ethical issues are addressed in a series of essays by Ronald Bayer: see in particular his *Private Acts, Social Consequences: AIDS and the Politics of Public Health* (New York: Free Press, 1988). The *Hastings Center Report* (December 1986) brings together six historically informed examinations of the ethical considerations to guide public health policy. Discussions of specific issues reflect the extent to which advances in the scientific understanding of modes of transmission, periods of maximum infectivity, and the effects of drugs administered at different stages of infection have been digested. Recent contributions include: Ronald Bayer, "Ethical and Social Policy Issues Raised by HIV Screening: The Epidemic Evolves and So Do the Challenges," *AIDS* 3, no. 3 (1989), 119–124; John J. Potterat et al., "Partner Notification in the Control of the Human Immunodeficiency Virus," *American Journal of Public Health* 79, no. 7 (1989), 874–876; and N. A. Christakis, "The Ethical Design of an AIDS Vaccine Trial in Africa," *Hastings Center Report* 18, no. 3 (1988), 3–37.

An indispensable review of AIDS legislation across every U.S. state has been compiled by Larry O. Gostin, "Public Health Strategies for Confronting AIDS: Legislative and Regulatory Policy in the United States," *JAMA* 261, no. 11 (17 March 1989), 1621–1630. Accounts that set AIDS in relation to earlier public health emergencies and the legal-administrative responses to them are available in Daniel Fox and Elizabeth Fee, eds., *AIDS: The Burdens of History* (Berkeley and Los Angeles: University of California Press, 1988), and Allan M. Brandt, "AIDS in Historical Perspective: Four Lessons from the History of Sexually Transmitted Diseases," *American Journal of Public Health* 78, no. 4 (1988). On quarantine see the historical essay by David Musto, "Quarantine and the Problem of AIDS," *Milbank Quarterly* 64, suppl. 1 (1986) 97–117, and Michael Quam and Nancy Ford, "AIDS Quarantine: The Legal and Practical Implications," *Journal of Legal Medicine* 8, no. 3 (1987), 353–396. H. L. Dalton, S. Burris, and the Yale AIDS Law Project, eds., *AIDS and the Law: A Guide for the Public* (New Haven: Yale University Press, 1987) provides a thorough survey of the legal and administrative responses by government, public institutions, and the private sector to HIV/AIDS in the United States.

Information on legal initiatives in countries other than the United States has been published by WHO, *Tabular Information on Legal Instruments Dealing with AIDS and HIV Infection* (WHO/GPA/HLE 88.1, June 1988). Details of national legislation on HIV/AIDS can also be found in the section "communicable diseases" of the quarterly *International Digest of Health Legislation*, although coverage is neither full nor always up to date. The *IDHL* also carries valuable reviews of books in English and other languages on legal aspects of HIV/AIDS, primarily dealing with Europe and the United States.

Funding

Whether sufficient resources have been committed to AIDS research, education, treatment, and care is a vital, but often loosely formulated, question. Two attempts to make it more rigorous are Evridiki Hatziandreu, John D. Graham, and Michael A. Stoto, "AIDS and Biomedical Research Funding: A Comparative Analysis," *Reviews of Infectious Diseases* 10, no. 1 (1988), 159–167, and William Winkenwerder, Austin R. Kessler, and Rhonda M. Stolec, "Federal Spending for Illness Caused by the Human Immunodeficiency Virus," *New England Journal of Medicine* 320, no. 24 (1989), 1598–1603, which elicited a response by David E. Rogers, "Federal Spending on AIDS—How Much is Enough?" *New England Journal of Medicine* 320, no. 24 (1989), 1623–1624. A detailed disaggregation of direct and indirect government expenditure related to HIV/AIDS in Australia between 1984 and 1988 is contained in the Policy Discussion Paper, *AIDS: A Time to Care, a Time to Act* (Canberra: Australian Government Publishing Service, 1988).

Effects of Specific Initiatives

Sufficient time has passed for the impact of some responses, official or officially sponsored, to have been evaluated. The costly and unanticipated consequences of the imposition of premarital testing in Illinois are reported in Bernard J. Turnock and Chester J. Kelly, "Mandatory Premarital Testing for Human Immunodeficiency Virus: The Illinois Experience," *JAMA* 261, no. 23 (16 June 1989), 3415–3428. The impact of other kinds of testing choices are more difficult to assess: Laura J. Fehrs et al., "Trial of Anonymous Versus Confidential Human Immunodeficiency Virus Testing," *The Lancet* (13 August 1988), 379–381, are nonetheless able to show that in Oregon anonymity provides an increased incentive to test. Needle-exchange schemes have represented a controversial initiative especially in the United States, not least because, as Pascal Imperato has pointed out in the *Journal of Community Health* 14, no. 2 (1989), 61–62, it is extremely hard for supporters to show that the schemes do not in practice encourage the unwanted consequences that their critics predict. Details of the workings of exchange schemes in Amsterdam and the United Kingdom are provided in the *National Institute of Drug Abuse Research Monograph Series* no. 80 (1988), and in Gerry V. Stimson et al., "Syringe Exchange Schemes for Drug Users in England and Scotland," *British Medical Journal* 296 (18 June 1988), 1717–1719.

Responses Among "High-Risk Communities"

The Gay Community

As a general account of the gay community in the time of AIDS Dennis Altman, *AIDS in the Mind of America* (New York: Anchor, 1986) is a useful supplement to Shilts' book. The extent of individual changes in sexual behavior has been the topic of many micro-studies: their findings, covering the period 1981–1988, are summarized in Marshall H. Becker and Jill G. Joseph, "AIDS and Behavioral Change to Reduce Risk: a Review," *American Journal of Public Health* 78, no. 4 (1988), 394–409, and Anne M. Johnson, "Social and Behavioural Aspects of the HIV Epidemic—A Review," *Journal of the Royal Statistical Society* A 151, Part 1 (1988), 99–114. Subsequent analyses include, for England and The Netherlands, respectively: Brian A. Evans et al., "Trends in Sexual Behavior and Risk Factors for HIV Infection Among Homosexual Men," *British Medical Journal* 298, no. 28 (28 January 1989), 215–218, and J. P. Godfried et al., "Changes in Sexual Behavior and the Fall in Incidence of HIV Infection Among Homosexual Men," *British Medical Journal* 298 (28 January 1989), 218–221. A discussion of lesbians and AIDS is included in the more general analysis by Diane Richardson, *Women and the AIDS Crisis* (London: Pandora, 1987).

Intravenous Drug Users

Accurate descriptions of the social context and relations of intravenous drug use are necessarily much harder to come by. The U.S. evidence is summarized in Don C. Des Jarlais, Samuel R. Friedman, and David Strug, "AIDS and Needle-Sharing within the IV-Drug Use Subculture," in Douglas A. Feldman and Thomas M. Johnson, eds., *The Social Dimensions of AIDS: Method and Theory* (New York: Praeger, 1986) 111–126, and the need to distinguish between old and new ivdus is stressed by Samuel R. Friedman et al., "AIDS and the New Drug Injector," *Nature* 399 (1 June 1989), 333–334. Roy Robertson's *Heroin, AIDS and Society* (London: Hodder and Stoughton, 1987) deals with the British experience. Most accounts are concerned with heroin users, so that the world of cocaine injection—which appears to be more closely linked to HIV infection than heroin injection—remains unexplored.

As Don C. Des Jarlais and Samuel Friedman observe in "AIDS and IV Drug Use," *Science* 245 (11 August 1989), 578, it is remarkable that, notwithstanding the absence of drug users' organizations to provide education and peer-group support, behavioral change has taken place at all: the details, and the barriers to definitive risk reduction, are examined in Samuel R. Friedman et al., "AIDS and Self-Organisation among Intravenous Drug Users," *International Journal of the Addictions* 22, no. 3 (1987), 210–219. Other evidence is contained in the general surveys by Becker and Joseph and by Johnson mentioned in "The Gay Community," section above. However, while changes in drug-use practices are significant, evidence from Italy (Giovanni Rezza et al., "Needle Sharing and Other Behaviours Related to HIV Spread Among Intravenous Drug Users," *AIDS* 3, no. 4 [1989], 247–248) emphasizes that sexual relations among ivdus may be an equally important path of transmission. The classificatory preference for "risk groups," based on a single feature, rather than "risk practices" has, however, helped to render that fact invisible.

Prostitutes

Although prostitutes can be women, men, or men presenting themselves as women, most of the meager scientific literature is concerned with women and the risks that they pose for male clients. In her summary of findings on the scale of infection in various societies Sophie Day ("Prostitute Women and AIDS: Anthropology," *AIDS* 2, no. 6 [1988], 421–428) underlines the differences in the meanings and practices of "prostitution" in the West, sub-Saharan Africa, and Asia. A similar cross-cultural perspective is taken by Beth E. Schneider, "Women and AIDS," *Futures* 21, no. 1 (1989), 72–90, who discusses the more general issue of the place of women in the changing patterns of HIV infection. Focused studies of the effects of health education among prostitutes in African societies include John O. Chikwem et al., "Impact of Health Education on Prostitutes' Awareness and Attitudes to Acquired Immune Deficiency Syndrome (AIDS)," *Public Health* 102 (1988), 439–445, which deals with Kenya, and E. N. Ngugi et al., "Prevention of Transmission of Human Immunodeficiency Virus in Africa: Effectiveness of Condom Promotion and Health Education Among Prostitutes," *The Lancet* (15 October 1988), 887–890, which covers Nigeria.

Accounts by Seropositives and People with AIDS

Views of HIV/AIDS by people living with infection have so far been mostly expressed *viva voce* in such fora as the International Conferences on AIDS. Some extracts from the Washington Conference of 1987 have been reproduced by Paul Farmer and Arthur Kleinman, "AIDS as Human Suffering," *Daedalus* 112, no. 2 (1989), 135–160, and are transcribed in *New England Journal of Public Policy* 4, no. 1 (1988). An exception to the absence of accounts in print is Emmanuel Dreuilhe, *Mortal Embrace: Living with AIDS* (New York: Hill and Wang, 1988). It is not only likely that with the development of life-prolonging drug therapies accounts by the infected will appear increasingly frequently, it is also, as Farmer and Kleinman argue, highly desirable that they should do so, since their voices will be an essential element in discussions of all aspects of the future management of HIV/AIDS.

Index

Contributors

NANCY FORD is Associate Professor of Legal Studies and Director of the Center for Legal Studies at Sangamon State University, Springfield, Illinois.

ALFRED J. FORTIN is Assistant Professor in the Department of Psychiatry, John A. Burns School of Medicine at the University of Hawaii, Honolulu.

MICHEL HUBERT teaches at the Facultés Universitaires Saint-Louis in Brussels.

BARBARA A. MISZTAL is Lecturer in the Division of Humanities at Griffith University, Brisbane.

DAVID MOSS is Senior Lecturer in the Division of Humanities at Griffith University, Brisbane.

RICHARD G. PARKER is a visiting professor and researcher in the Instituto de Medicina at the Universidade do Estado do Rio de Janeiro.

MICHAEL POLLAK is a researcher at the Conseil National de Recherche Scientifique in Paris.

MICHAEL QUAM is Professor of Anthropology and Health Services Administration at Sangamon State University, Springfield, Illinois.

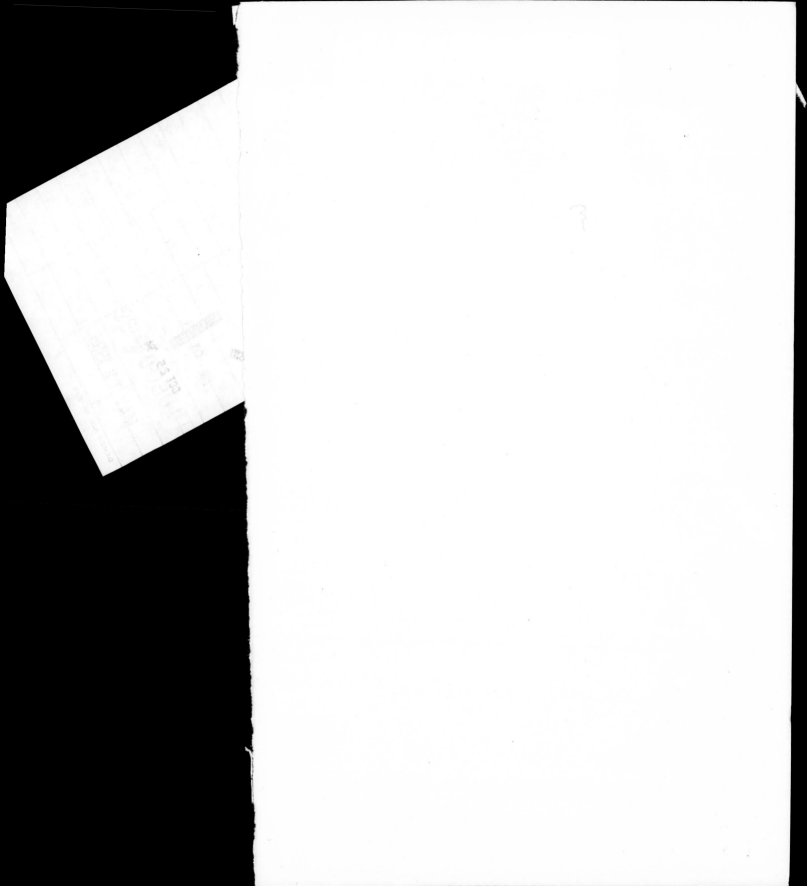

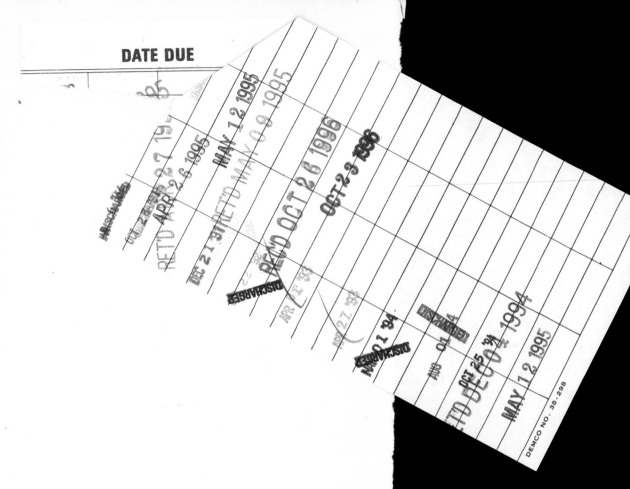
RE